Self-Controlled Case Series Studies

A Modelling Guide with R

Chapman & Hall/CRC Biostatistics Series

Shein-Chung Chow, Duke University of Medicine
Byron Jones, Novartis Pharma AG
Jen-pei Liu, National Taiwan University
Karl E. Peace, Georgia Southern University
Bruce W. Turnbull, Cornell University

Recently Published Titles

Repeated Measures Design with Generalized Linear Mixed Models for Randomized Controlled Trials
Toshiro Tango

Clinical Trial Data Analysis Using R and SAS, Second Edition
Ding-Geng (Din) Chen, Karl E. Peace, Pinggao Zhang

Clinical Trial Optimization Using R
Alex Dmitrienko, Erik Pulkstenis

Cluster Randomised Trials, Second Edition
Richard J. Hayes, Lawrence H. Moulton

Quantitative Methods for HIV/AIDS Research
Cliburn Chan, Michael G. Hudgens, Shein-Chung Chow

Sample Size Calculations in Clinical Research, Third Edition
Shein-Chung Chow, Jun Shao, Hansheng Wang, Yuliya Lokhnygina

Randomization, Masking, and Allocation Concealment
Vance Berger

Statistical Topics in Health Economics and Outcomes Research
Demissie Alemayehu, Joseph C. Cappelleri, Birol Emir, Kelly H. Zou

Medical Biostatistics, Fourth Edition
Abhaya Indrayan, Rajeev Kumar Malhotra

Applied Surrogate Endpoint Evaluation Methods with SAS and R
Ariel Alonso, Theophile Bigirumurame, Tomasz Burzykowski, Marc Buyse, Geert Molenberghs, Leacky Muchene, Nolen Joy Perualila, Ziv Shkedy, Wim Van der Elst

For more information about this series, please visit:
https://www.crcpress.com/go/biostats

Self-Controlled Case Series Studies

A Modelling Guide with R

By

Paddy Farrington

School of Mathematics and Statistics, The Open University, UK

Heather Whitaker

School of Mathematics and Statistics, The Open University, UK

Yonas Ghebremichael Weldeselassie

University of Warwick Medical School, UK

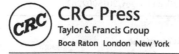

CRC Press

Taylor & Francis Group

Boca Raton London New York

CRC Press is an imprint of the
Taylor & Francis Group, an **informa** business

CRC Press
Taylor & Francis Group
6000 Broken Sound Parkway NW, Suite 300
Boca Raton, FL 33487-2742

First issued in paperback 2021

© 2018 by Taylor & Francis Group, LLC
CRC Press is an imprint of Taylor & Francis Group, an Informa business

No claim to original U.S. Government works

Version Date: 20180406

ISBN-13: 978-1-03-209553-0 (pbk)
ISBN-13: 978-1-4987-8159-6 (hbk)

Library of Congress Cataloging-in-Publication Data

Names: Farrington, Paddy, author. | Whitaker, Heather, author. |
Ghebremichael Weldeselassie, Yonas, author.
Title: Self-controlled case series studies : a modelling guide with R / Paddy
Farrington, Heather Whitaker, Yonas Ghebremichael Weldeselassie.
Description: Boca Raton, Florida : CRC Press, 2018. | Includes
bibliographical references and index.
Identifiers: LCCN 2018002262| ISBN 9781498781596 (hardback : alk. paper) |
ISBN 9780429491313 (e-book)
Subjects: LCSH: Medicine--Research--Methodology. | Clinical
trials--Methodology.
Classification: LCC R850 .F37 2018 | DDC 610.72/4--dc23
LC record available at https://lccn.loc.gov/2018002262

Visit the Taylor & Francis Web site at
http://www.taylorandfrancis.com

and the CRC Press Web site at
http://www.crcpress.com

To Beckie, Dylan, Finlay,
Isla, Benhur, HiabEl and Lulya

Contents

Note: Starred (*) sections may be skipped.

Preface   **xiii**

1 Introduction   **1**
   1.1 Control and self-control in epidemiology   1
   1.2 Self-controlled methods   2
   1.3 Guide to contents   4
   1.4 Computer package and data   4

2 Epidemiological overview   **7**
   2.1 Genesis of the SCCS method   7
   2.2 Rationale for the SCCS method   9
       2.2.1 Case series   9
       2.2.2 Self-control 10
       2.2.3 Data requirements 11
   2.3 Some illustrations 13
       2.3.1 Using only cases 13
       2.3.2 Controlling confounding 16
   2.4 Assumptions and alternatives 18
       2.4.1 Assumptions of the SCCS method 18
       2.4.2 What if the assumptions are not satisfied? 19
   2.5 Bibliographical notes and further material 20

3 The SCCS likelihood   **21**
   3.1 Why start with the likelihood? 21
   3.2 Likelihood for the standard SCCS model 22
   3.3 Properties of the SCCS likelihood 26
   3.4 Example: MMR vaccine and aseptic meningitis 27
   3.5 The general SCCS likelihood 32
   3.6 MMR vaccine and aseptic meningitis: derivation of the
       SCCS likelihood 33
   3.7 Assumptions of the SCCS method 36
       3.7.1 Assumption 1: Poisson or rare events 36
       3.7.2 A counter-example: negative binomial events* 37
       3.7.3 Assumptions 2 and 3: validity of conditioning 37
       3.7.4 A more formal demonstration* 39

      3.7.5   Assumption 4: independent ascertainment   40
  3.8   Derivation of the SCCS likelihood*   41
  3.9   Bibliographical notes and further material   45

4   The standard SCCS model   47
  4.1   Proportional incidence models   47
  4.2   Fitting the standard SCCS model   49
  4.3   The R package SCCS: standard SCCS model   51
      4.3.1   A single point exposure: MMR vaccine and ITP . . .   51
      4.3.2   Reshaping the MMR vaccine and ITP data   55
      4.3.3   Extended exposures: antidepressants and
               hip fracture   57
  4.4   Data formats for repeated exposures   59
      4.4.1   Intermittent treatments: NSAIDs and GI bleeds . . .   60
      4.4.2   Multiple vaccine doses: convulsions and
               DTP vaccine   62
  4.5   Multiple exposure types   65
      4.5.1   Exposures of several types: convulsions, Hib
               and MMR vaccines   66
      4.5.2   Multiple exposures of several types: NSAIDs,
               antidepressants and GI bleeds   68
      4.5.3   Multiple doses of different vaccines: convulsions,
               DTP and Hib vaccines   70
      4.5.4   Overlapping risk periods: convulsions and DTP   73
  4.6   Comparing models: likelihood ratio tests   74
      4.6.1   Comparing models: ITP and MMR vaccine   75
      4.6.2   Combining multinomial categories*   76
  4.7   Interactions: effect modification and stratification   77
      4.7.1   Interactions: sex, ITP and MMR vaccine   78
      4.7.2   Interactions between exposures: GI bleeds, NSAIDs
               and antidepressants   81
  4.8   Indefinite and extremal risk periods   83
      4.8.1   Curtailed observation: antidiabetics and fractures . . .   84
      4.8.2   Indefinite risk periods: MMR vaccine and autism . . .   87
      4.8.3   Initial risk periods: NRT and MI   90
  4.9   SCCS analyses with temporal effects   92
      4.9.1   Calendar time: GBS and influenza vaccine   93
      4.9.2   Seasonal SCCS model: OPV and intussusception . . .   95
  4.10   Parameterisation of the standard SCCS model*   100
  4.11   Bibliographical notes and further material   101

5   Checking model assumptions   103
  5.1   Rare disease assumption for non-recurrent events   104
      5.1.1   Evaluation of absolute risks: convulsions
               and stroke   105

      5.1.2   Quantifying the bias for non-recurrent events*   106

  5.2 Poisson assumption for potentially recurrent events   107

      5.2.1   Investigating recurrences   107

      5.2.2   Recurrences for MMR and ITP data   109

      5.2.3   Recurrent convulsions and MMR vaccine   111

  5.3 Event-dependent observation periods   114

      5.3.1   Investigating event-dependent observation periods . .   115

      5.3.2   Planned and actual observation periods:

               NRT and MI   117

      5.3.3   Heavy censoring: antipsychotics and stroke   119

      5.3.4   Censoring of observation periods*   125

  5.4 Event-dependent exposures   127

      5.4.1   Investigating event-dependent exposures   128

      5.4.2   Event-dependence of exposures: ITP and MMR   130

      5.4.3   Event-dependence with multiple exposures:

               NSAIDs, antidepressants and GI bleeds   134

      5.4.4   Long-term dependence: influenza vaccine and GBS . .   137

      5.4.5   Interpretation of pre-exposure risk period*   140

  5.5 Modelling assumptions   143

      5.5.1   Checking the model   143

      5.5.2   Risk periods and age groups: MMR and convulsions .   144

      5.5.3   Homogeneity of effect: MMR and convulsions   147

  5.6 Asymptotic assumptions   149

      5.6.1   Permutation test for the aseptic meningitis data . . .   150

      5.6.2   Permutation test for the ITP data   151

  5.7 Bibliographical notes and further material   154

6 Further SCCS models 157

  6.1 Semiparametric SCCS model   157

      6.1.1   Formulation of the semiparametric model   158

      6.1.2   Semiparametric model for the MMR and ITP data . .   160

      6.1.3   Semiparametric model for the MMR and

               autism data   162

      6.1.4   Further details of the semiparametric model*   163

  6.2 SCCS model with spline-based age effect   166

      6.2.1   Splines for the relative age effect   167

      6.2.2   Spline model for age: MMR vaccine and ITP   170

      6.2.3   Spline model for age: antidepressants and

               hip fracture   173

      6.2.4   Precision of estimators: MMR and autism   176

      6.2.5   Modelling with M-splines*   179

  6.3 SCCS models with spline-based exposure effect   181

      6.3.1   Splines for exposure effects   182

      6.3.2   Spline model for exposure: MMR and autism   185

6.3.3   Spline model for exposure: antidiabetics
and fracture 187
6.3.4   Nonparametric model: MMR and convulsions 189
6.3.5   Nonparametric model: acute risk of hip fracture 191
6.3.6   Further material on spline-based models* 193
6.4   SCCS model for multi-type events 195
6.4.1   Modelling multi-type events 195
6.4.2   Febrile and non-febrile convulsions 197
6.4.3   Antidiabetic drugs and fracture site 201
6.4.4   SCCS likelihoods for multi-type events* 203
6.5   SCCS models for quantitative individual exposures   207
6.5.1   Modelling quantitative exposures 207
6.5.2   Headaches and blood pressure 209
6.6   SCCS models for environmental exposures 211
6.6.1   SCCS likelihood for environmental exposure data . . . 212
6.6.2   Air pollution and asthma 215
6.6.3   Ambient temperature and RSV 218
6.7   Bibliographical notes and further material   222

7   **Extensions of the SCCS model**   **225**
7.1   SCCS for event-dependent exposures   225
7.1.1   Estimating equations and counterfactual exposures . . 226
7.1.2   Unique exposures: influenza vaccine and GBS 232
7.1.3   Multiple doses: rotavirus vaccine and intussusception . 233
7.1.4   Model comparisons: OPV and intussusception 236
7.1.5   Multiple exposures: respiratory infections and MI . . . 240
7.1.6   SCCS for event-dependent exposures:
a special case* 243
7.1.7   General method for event-dependent exposures* . . . 248
7.2   SCCS for event-dependent observation periods 253
7.2.1   A two-stage modelling approach 254
7.2.2   Nicotine replacement therapy and MI 257
7.2.3   Respiratory tract infections and MI 259
7.2.4   Antipsychotics and stroke 262
7.2.5   Experimenting with initial values 266
7.2.6   Adjustment for event-dependent observation
periods* 269
7.2.7   Estimating the weights* 272
7.3   Deaths in SCCS studies 275
7.3.1   Death as the outcome event 276
7.3.2   Bupropion and sudden death 277
7.3.3   Hexavalent vaccines and sudden infant deaths 280
7.3.4   Partner bereavement and death 282
7.4   Bibliographical notes and further material   283

8 Design and presentation of SCCS studies **285**

  8.1 Choice of design 285

      8.1.1 The primary time line 286

      8.1.2 Risk periods 287

      8.1.3 Case ascertainment and observation periods 289

      8.1.4 Age groups 292

      8.1.5 Some examples of design choices 292

      8.1.6 Self-controlled risk interval designs 295

  8.2 Sample size and power 298

      8.2.1 Estimating the sample size: no age effects 299

      8.2.2 Power assessment by simulation 301

      8.2.3 Estimating the sample size: with age effects 304

      8.2.4 Simulated power with age effects present 306

      8.2.5 A formula for the sample size* 311

  8.3 Efficiency and identifiability 313

      8.3.1 Relative efficiency of the SCCS method 314

      8.3.2 Impact of design on parameter estimates 318

      8.3.3 Estimability and identifiability in SCCS models 322

      8.3.4 More on identifiability and relative efficiency* 325

  8.4 Presentation of SCCS studies 329

      8.4.1 Results tables for SCCS studies 329

      8.4.2 MMR vaccine and ITP: relative incidence table 329

      8.4.3 Multiple exposures: NSAIDs and antidepressants . . . 331

      8.4.4 Graphical displays for SCCS studies 333

  8.5 Measures of attribution in SCCS studies 335

      8.5.1 Attributable fraction and attributable risk 336

      8.5.2 Attributable risk: MMR and ITP 337

      8.5.3 Attributable risk: intussusception and rotavirus

             vaccine 338

  8.6 Bibliographical notes and further material 341

Bibliography **343**

Index **355**

Preface

For several years after its publication in 1995, the self-controlled case series (SCCS) method met with a degree of scepticism. Gradually, it gained credence beyond its early core of advocates, especially among epidemiologists concerned with vaccine safety – the subject area in which the method was originally developed. Helped on by the increasing use of pre-existing databases of patient records in epidemiological research, the SCCS method also became more popular in non-vaccine pharmacoepidemiology.

Back in the early days, we spent much time presenting and popularising the SCCS method. Today, self-controlled methods are more widely accepted by epidemiologists, so this purpose has become less salient. Equally important, in our view, is the need to convey a better understanding of the method – and thus, hopefully, to motivate further methodological developments to extend its range of application and mitigate its limitations.

Over the past 20 years, we have provided practical advice to statisticians and epidemiologists who have approached us with queries about the method. Indeed several of these interactions have blossomed into long-term collaborations, and a few have motivated substantial methodological extensions. Enriched by this experience, we think that the time is now ripe to collect together a dispersed literature into a coherent narrative. Hence this book, and its associated R package SCCS.

We are greatly indebted to all those who contributed to the development of the method in various ways. Particular thanks are due to Elizabeth Miller and Stephen Evans for their early support and their unstintingly generous encouragement over many years. The long list of others to whom special thanks are due includes Rustam Al-Shahi Salman, Nick Andrews, Ruth Brauer, John Carlin, Bob Chen, Anne-Marie Connolly, Gisele Coutin-Marie, Bob Davis, Frank DeStefano, Caitlin Dodd, Ian Douglas, Philippe Duclos, Sylvie Escolano, Annie Fourrier-Réglat, Francesca Galeotti, Paul Gargiullo, François Haguinet, Steven Hawken, Mounia Hocine, Richard Hubbard, Pierre Joly, Piotr Kramarz, Ronny Kuhnert, Cécile Landais, Katherine Lee, Linda Lévesque, David Madigan, Yola Moride, Patrick Musonda, Danh Nguyen, Irene Petersen, Nicole Pratt, Catherine Quantin, Adrian Root, Dominique Rosillon, Martijn Schuemie, Liam Smeeth, Bart Spiessens, Julia Stowe, Therese Stukel, Laila Tata, Pascale Tubert-Bitter, Thomas Verstraeten, Charlotte Warren-Gash, Linda Wijlaars and Kumanan Wilson. The list is surely incomplete, and we apologise to anyone we have left out.

1

Introduction

1.1 Control and self-control in epidemiology

The Scottish physician James Lind is widely credited with conducting the first controlled clinical trial. In 1747, in his capacity as ship's surgeon on HMS Salisbury, Lind selected 12 crew members afflicted by scurvy, and allocated them in pairs to six treatments – one of which was daily consumption of two oranges and a lemon. A second pair received seawater; the rest were treated with a variety of other substances. Within a week, the patients taking the citrus fruit had fully recovered – though nearly a half century elapsed before the Royal Navy included lemon juice in its rations and eventually eradicated scurvy at sea (Dunn, 1997).

Lind's controlled trial is a seminal moment in the emergence of the scientific method and its application to medicine. Today, the judicious use of controls is a pervasive feature of modern epidemiological methods. Controls are used in an attempt to reveal causal mechanisms: ideally, by eliminating extraneous sources of systematic variation so that the experimental group and the control group differ in just one single respect, any differences that then emerge between the two groups can be ascribed to that single difference in initial conditions – or to chance. In epidemiology, the most rigorous application of this principle is in randomised controlled trials, the randomisation aiming primarily to ensure that the treatment and control groups are comparable in all respects other than the treatment allocation. However many questions in epidemiology cannot readily be addressed by randomised controlled trials. In particular, diseases that are very uncommon or require long durations of follow-up cannot realistically be investigated in this way, while some exposures cannot be applied experimentally for ethical reasons. Instead, the methods of observational epidemiology are used, notably traditional study designs such as cohort and case-control studies.

Control remains fundamental to the methodology of observational studies, but the absence of random allocation means that the exposure and control groups may differ in important respects. Any such differences must be adjusted for by statistical techniques, typically multiple regression, in an attempt to recreate the level playing field of the randomised clinical trial. Alternatively, causal inference methods can be applied, with the same aim.

However, the implementation or interpretation of all such methods requires

1

some prior knowledge of those confounding variables that could bias the comparison between treatment and control groups and hence yield erroneous inferences. Even when such variables are known, the precise causal pathways involved may not be, and hence attempts to allow fully for these variables by regression techniques may be only partly successful. For example, socioeconomic factors are known to be confounders in epidemiological investigations of many exposure and disease pairs. However, socioeconomic variables are often poorly measured. In addition, which aspect of social class is relevant in any particular setting, and hence what exactly should be measured, generally remains elusive. Likewise, analyses of clinical or administrative databases are limited by what data happen to be available, which may or may not include all relevant confounders. Indeed some potential confounders, such as genetic factors, are not realistically measurable.

Self-control offers a different approach to resolving this conundrum. Self-control is the use of a study subject as his or her own control, sampled at different times: individuals are matched with themselves, and constitute individual-level strata. Within such a scheme, all variables that are constant in time are necessarily identical within strata and thus, in certain circumstances, are completely controlled. This applies to time-invariant variables that are not even known to be confounders. Such variables could include, for example, genetic factors and, over suitable time scales, socioeconomic factors and underlying state of health. Time-varying confounders, on the other hand, are not controlled automatically, and must therefore be allowed for by other means.

1.2   Self-controlled methods

Self-controlled methods in epidemiology include the case-crossover method and the self-controlled case series method, the subject of this book. Both involve only cases, that is, individuals who have experienced the event of interest. The case-crossover method was introduced by Maclure (1991) to evaluate associations between transient exposures and acute health events. The self-controlled case series method was proposed by Farrington (1995) to study adverse health events potentially associated with vaccination. Both methods have been used more widely, notably in the study of adverse events potentially associated with pharmaceutical drugs.

The case-crossover method is a type of matched case-control design: the sampling scheme fixes the event times of the cases. Unlike standard case-control methods, in which controls are individuals selected among non-cases, the case-crossover design involves choosing control periods within the time line of the case. These control periods are defined in relation to the event time. In standard matched case-control designs, the event time of the case determines the index time in matched controls. In contrast, the self-controlled case series (or SCCS) method is derived from a Poisson model for the underlying retrospectively observed cohort, and the event times are not fixed by design, though only cases within the cohort are included in the analysis. However, both the case-crossover and the SCCS designs involve only within-person contrasts, rather than between-person contrasts or a combination of between and within-person contrasts as in standard cohort and case-control designs.

These features underpin the distinct properties of the cohort, case-control, case-crossover and SCCS designs. Table 1.1 exemplifies this typology, and how the methods relate to one another within it.

TABLE 1.1
Relationships between epidemiologic designs.

		Event times fixed by design	
		Yes	No
Within-person	Yes	Case-crossover	SCCS
contrasts only	No	Case-control	Cohort

Self-controlled methods are attractive, first, because time-invariant confounders can potentially be controlled automatically. This is particularly useful for studies conducted in administrative databases, in which relevant covariate information may be limited. In addition, a common feature of self-controlled methods is that non-cases are uninformative, and hence only cases are required. Indeed, this feature provided the original motivation for the development of the SCCS method. Requiring only cases reduces the sample size and simplifies data collection and checking, which can be focused entirely on those individuals experiencing the events of primary interest.

Self-controlled methods also suffer from limitations. For example, as for case-control methods, absolute event rates cannot be estimated directly. The extra control of time-invariant covariates comes at the cost of further assumptions. And finally, the association parameter that is the target of inference represents only the effect associated with within-individual variation in exposure. This may not represent the total effect of that exposure. For example, taking regular exercise has a beneficial effect in reducing the risk of cardiovascular disease. But an episode of energetic exercise may be associated with a short-term increase in risk. Self-controlled methods can only aspire to estimate the second, within-individual effect, which in SCCS analyses we refer to as the relative incidence.

1.3   Guide to contents

This book is about the analysis, application and design of the self-controlled case series method. It is written in the hope that it will prove useful to a range of audiences, including medical statisticians and epidemiologists. While its focus is practical, the book contains a mix of methodology and application, mathematical derivations and non-technical explanations from which the reader is invited to pick and choose. Material that is primarily of mathematical interest is grouped into starred sections which may be skipped entirely. Some other less technical sections can nevertheless be quite heavy on methodology: these end with an equation-free summary box, aimed at readers who wish to focus primarily on applications.

In Chapter 2, we provide an overview of the SCCS method, focusing on its application in epidemiology and sidestepping all technicalities. The SCCS method and its assumptions are described in greater detail in Chapter 3. Chapters 4 and 5 contain a detailed modelling guide for the standard SCCS model. Further SCCS models, and extensions of the SCCS framework, are described in Chapters 6 and 7. Finally, Chapter 8 covers aspects of the design and presentation of SCCS studies. In all chapters, the methods are illustrated by a wide range of applications in epidemiology.

The more technical starred sections of the book assume knowledge of basic statistical theory, and make use of statistical concepts that include Poisson processes, conditional probability, likelihood theory, and generalised linear models. However, where possible key derivations are preceded by heuristic motivation, often based on specific illustrations, that do not require any familiarity with this statistical material.

1.4   Computer package and data

Most of the examples in this book are implemented using the package SCCS within the R environment (R Core Team, 2015). R may be downloaded from the Comprehensive R Archive Network at `cran.r-project.org`. Instructions on how to download and install the R package SCCS, along with R code for the examples in this book, are available on the SCCS website at `sccs-studies.info`. This website also contains details of and code for other software to fit SCCS models. The R package SCCS is under constant development in an effort to improve it. This is also true of R itself, which is regularly updated with new releases, and of other R functions used in this book. The analyses in the book were run with the 64-bit build of R version 3.4.3. It is likely that, in the future, numerical results will differ from those in the book. Substantive updates and corrections will be posted on the SCCS website.

All data sets used in this book are available both within the R package SCCS and on the SCCS website. These data sets are based on real epidemiological studies. However, using the actual data from such studies is seldom possible owing to the ethical restrictions governing their use. Previously unpublished data sets relating to vaccines have been jittered (some dates moved randomly by a small amount) in order to protect patient confidentiality. The licensing conditions under which data are made available from major pharmacoepidemiology databases, such as the Clinical Practice Research Datalink and its predecessor the General Practice Research Database, and The Health Improvement Network, preclude making data publicly available. As it is essential for a book on the SCCS method to include examples from such databases, we have resorted to simulating data. The data on MMR vaccine and autism are also simulated. In these simulations, we have kept as close as possible to published accounts of the data. To maintain a degree of realism, the simulation models used to generate the data are not the same as those used to analyse them. The data are provided to illustrate the application of the SCCS method, and are not appropriate for substantive epidemiological investigations.

2

Epidemiological overview

This chapter provides an introduction to the SCCS method, focused on its epidemiological rather than statistical aspects. Our aim is to paint a broad overview of the method: its genesis, the epidemiological questions it can help to address, the ideas behind it, the data required, how it can be used, and the assumptions it is based on. To maintain momentum, much detail is omitted; this is remedied in subsequent chapters.

2.1 Genesis of the SCCS method

In 1992, a team of microbiologists and epidemiologists, along with a statistician, met in London to discuss a potential problem with the measles, mumps and rubella (MMR) vaccine, which had been introduced in the United Kingdom in 1988. Some time earlier, a signal had been picked up suggesting that mumps meningitis was occurring more frequently than expected following vaccination with MMR vaccines containing the Urabe mumps strain. In response, two investigations had been launched. In the first, cases of aseptic meningitis diagnosed from cerebrospinal fluid (CSF) samples were ascertained from public health laboratories. In the second, hospital discharges with a diagnosis of aseptic meningitis were obtained. Cases were sought aged 1–2 years, primarily in areas where MMR vaccines containing the Urabe strain were used. MMR vaccination history and vaccine type were then obtained for these cases. The meeting was convened to discuss these new data.

Of the 32 CSF-confirmed cases, 27 had received MMR vaccine during the second year of life. Of the 10 hospital cases, 9 had received MMR vaccine. The proportions vaccinated were unremarkable, since MMR vaccine uptake was high. More concerning were the temporal distributions of aseptic meningitis in relation to MMR vaccination. These are displayed in Figure 2.1. Thirteen of the 27 vaccinated CSF-confirmed cases and 5 of the 9 vaccinated hospital cases had onset within the 15–35 day period after MMR vaccine, which from studies in other countries was deemed to be the risk period (that is, the period potentially at higher risk owing to exposure) for vaccine-associated mumps meningitis. This degree of temporal clustering was highly suggestive of a causal link. Subsequently, public health authorities took action and replaced

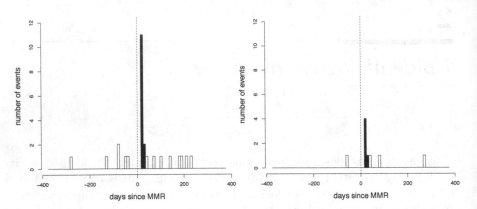

FIGURE 2.1
Distribution of intervals between aseptic meningitis diagnosis and MMR vaccination. Left: CSF-confirmed. Right: hospital cases. The vertical dashed lines represent time of MMR vaccination. The black bars represent cases occurring 15–35 days after MMR.

MMR vaccines containing the Urabe mumps strain with other MMR vaccines for which there was no evidence of an association.

At this stage, the association between MMR vaccination and aseptic meningitis could not readily be quantified, as the data comprised only cases, that is, children with aseptic meningitis. The condition was sufficiently rare that a cohort study was impractical. A case-control study would have faced the tricky problem of choosing appropriate controls when the population from which the cases were sampled was ill-defined. However, the cases alone clearly contained information on the strength of association, as represented by the degree of clustering revealed in Figure 2.1. The statistical problem was how to extract this information from the cases, and summarise it using a standard epidemiological measure such as a relative rate, relative risk or odds ratio.

This led to the development of the self-controlled case series (SCCS) method, first published in 1995, with these CSF data as the motivating example. Though the method was developed to use information only on cases, it turned out to have a very useful additional property: time-invariant confounders are adjusted for automatically, even if they are unknown or unmeasured.

2.2 Rationale for the SCCS method

In this section we briefly describe the rationale that lies at the heart of the SCCS method. First, we explore what types of epidemiological questions can be addressed from a randomly selected sample of cases, and what quantities may be estimated from such a case series. This provides some motivation for the SCCS method, which uses only cases, and helps throw light on how time-invariant confounders are controlled. Finally, we outline what data are required to apply the SCCS method.

2.2.1 Case series

A convenient way to introduce the SCCS method is to consider what epidemiological questions can be answered from data only on cases, that is, individuals who have experienced one or more events while under observation. The statistical methodology is then tailored to answer those questions.

It is not possible to estimate absolute rates or absolute risks from cases alone, as the population person-time denominators are unavailable. Thus, it is not possible to answer questions such as

Question 1

> *What is the risk of aseptic meningitis in*
> *the period 15–35 days after MMR vaccination?*

from case-only data. However, it is possible, in principle, to answer questions involving relative quantities, such as

Question 2

> *Given that an MMR-vaccinated child was diagnosed with*
> *aseptic meningitis in the second year of life, how much*
> *more likely is it that this diagnosis arose 15–35 days*
> *after vaccination rather than at some other time?*

The answer to Question 1 is an absolute rate or risk, for example 'one in 15 000 MMR doses'. The answer to Question 2 is a relative rate or risk, for example '10-fold higher'.

A key difference between the two questions is the formulation '*Given that an MMR-vaccinated child was diagnosed with aseptic meningitis in the second year of life*', which identifies Question 2 as a conditional one. This is important because, if the child had not had such a diagnosis, the rest of the question would not apply. Thus, non-cases play no role in answering this question.

The SCCS model reflects this conditionality principle, thus ensuring that the method is valid when applied to a sample of cases, or case series. In mathematical terms, the theory of the SCCS method is constructed around a conditional likelihood. Specifically, we condition on (that is, we fix) the number of events experienced by each case. This reflects the formulation of Question 2, which was conditioned on a child experiencing one event. The statistical model for the SCCS method is described in detail in Chapter 3.

The epidemiological parameters that are estimated in a SCCS study are relative incidences associated with exposure or age. We use the term relative incidence rather than relative rate, as in some circumstances the parameter of interest is a relative hazard rather than a relative rate. The term relative incidence is intended to cover both possibilities.

2.2.2 Self-control

The conditionality principle at the heart of the SCCS method implies that the method makes use of information solely on the relative timing of events within the period of observation of each case. This is also apparent from the way Question 2 was formulated. Thus, the analysis may be thought of as stratified by individuals: each case is a stratum of size 1. In this sense, the estimation of exposure and age effects is undertaken within cases: the method is self-controlled. In consequence, the impact of time-invariant covariates cannot be estimated in a SCCS study, as such covariates affect an individual's event rate equally at all times (under the assumptions of the SCCS model).

Figure 2.2 illustrates this feature. The figure represents the time lines of

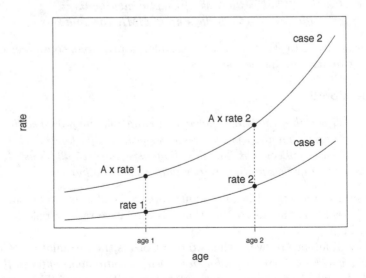

FIGURE 2.2
Two cases with proportional event rates: the rate ratios at ages 1 and 2 are the same for the two cases.

two cases with proportional event rates: at each time point the rate for case 2 is A times that for case 1. It follows that the within-individual rate ratios at ages 1 and 2 (that is, for each case, the rate at age 2 divided by the rate at age 1) are the same for cases 1 and 2, since the constant A cancels out. In consequence, within-individual comparisons provide no information on the constant A. Thus, a SCCS study cannot be used to quantify the effect of time-invariant covariates.

However, this turns out to be a bonus for estimating the effect of time-varying exposures, such as pharmaceutical drugs: it means that the SCCS method automatically adjusts for all time-invariant confounders that multiply the absolute rate by a constant. Modification of the exposure effect by time-invariant covariates, on the other hand, can be evaluated in SCCS models.

In epidemiological studies involving the collection of primary data, confounders must be known in advance so that information may be collected on them. In database studies, relevant covariate data are often limited or absent, and so confounder control based on the data available may be incomplete. The SCCS method circumvents these difficulties and, in principle, allows for full control of time-invariant confounders, even when these are unknown or unmeasured. Such confounders might include, for example, genetic factors, geographical location, or socioeconomic status. Over suitably short time scales, they might also include underlying state of health and behavioural factors.

Time-varying confounders, however, are not automatically controlled. These must be included explicitly in the SCCS model. The most common time-varying confounder is age, which is usually included in SCCS analyses as a matter of course. Calendar time effects, such as seasonal effects, may also be relevant in some applications.

2.2.3 Data requirements

In this section we provide a brief indication of the data required to conduct a SCCS study. A further example is provided in Chapter 3, Section 3.4. Full details on how to construct a SCCS dataset are given in Chapter 8, Section 8.1.

Most SCCS studies use age as the primary time line, though in some cases it is more appropriate to use calendar time. Which to choose depends on context. The choice of primary time line does not preclude adjusting for other temporal variation: thus, if age is chosen as the primary time line then adjustments for seasonal effects can also be made. For definiteness, we shall assume that age is the primary time line.

The minimum information required on each case to undertake a SCCS study is as follows: the age at which observation of the case began; the age at which it ended; the age (or ages) at which the event occurred; and the ages at which the exposure periods began and ended during the period of observation. One unusual feature of the SCCS method is that exposure information is required throughout the period of observation, including after the event: this is needed to answer Question 2 in Section 2.2.1. However, if exposure information is available only prior to the event, an extension of the SCCS method may be used. This is described in Chapter 7, Section 7.1.

For example, the first 10 lines of the data table for the aseptic meningitis cases confirmed from cerebrospinal fluid (CSF) samples, described in Section 2.1, are shown in Table 2.1. Each line corresponds to a different event. In these data, there is just one event per case. The columns represent variables; their names are typical of those used throughout this book. The first column, headed `case`, gives the case number. The second and third columns, headed `sta` and `end`, respectively, are the ages (in days) of start and end of observation for each case.

TABLE 2.1
Part of the data table for the study of MMR vaccine and aseptic meningitis confirmed from CSF.

case	sta	end	am	mmr
1	366	730	384	516
2	444	730	517	495
3	366	730	407	487
4	366	730	407	384
5	366	730	380	NA
6	366	730	584	NA
7	366	730	495	477
8	366	730	458	434
9	366	730	503	469
10	366	445	407	382
...	...	...	...	...

For 8 of the cases shown here, the observation period spans the whole second year of life: 366 to 730 days of age, inclusive. For case 2, the observation period is shorter: 444 to 730 days; similarly for case 10 it is 366 to 445 days. This is because, for these cases, the remainder of the second year of life fell outside the ascertainment period for the study: if events had occurred at ages 366 to 443 for case 2, or at ages 446 to 730 for case 10, these events would not have been ascertained, so these individuals would not have been featured as cases in our data set.

The fourth column, headed `am`, is the age at CSF-confirmed aseptic meningitis. Finally, column `mmr` gives age at MMR vaccination. For cases 5 and 6, this is missing (and coded NA): these cases were not exposed to the vaccine during their observation periods. Together with the risk period, which in this study is the period 15 to 35 days after MMR vaccine, this determines the start and end of exposure for each case. So for case 1 in Table 2.1, the period of exposure includes days 531 to 551 of age.

This completes the description of the data required for this particular study. In this study, some cases were unexposed, that is, they did not receive

MMR vaccine. It is not essential to include unexposed cases, but it can sometimes be helpful to do so. Applications with and without unexposed cases will be described in Chapter 4. In other applications, cases may experience more than one event, or more than one exposure during their observation period, and the structure of the data table is adapted to reflect this. These situations are dealt with in detail in Chapter 4. Applications of SCCS methodology to quantitative exposures require different data structures; these are described in Chapter 6, Sections 6.5 and 6.6.

Summary

- Conditional questions of the form 'given that an individual is a case...' may be answered using cases only.

- The SCCS method reflects this conditionality principle, and may be used to estimate relative rates from a sample of cases.

- Estimation is within-individuals, and in consequence time-invariant confounders are adjusted for automatically.

- The method requires data on event times, the period of observation, and the exposure history throughout this period.

2.3   Some illustrations

In this section we illustrate the use of the SCCS method using four examples from the epidemiological literature. We focus on the two key aspects of the method: its reliance only on cases, and confounder adjustment.

2.3.1   Using only cases

The potential benefits of basing an epidemiological study on cases only include simpler data handling, less onerous data checking, and in some cases, more timely results. Furthermore, the problem of selecting appropriate controls is sidestepped entirely. This is particularly useful when cases are ascertained from hospital records or disease registers for which the catchment population is ill-defined, thus making it more difficult to select suitable controls without introducing selection bias.

MMR vaccines and febrile convulsions
Live attenuated measles vaccines are known occasionally to cause febrile convulsions in children, typically in the second week after vaccination. After the introduction of the combined measles, mumps and rubella (MMR) vaccine in

the United States and the United Kingdom, studies were undertaken to quantify the risk of febrile convulsions associated with the measles component of
the new vaccines. Table 2.2 summarises their results.

TABLE 2.2
Two studies of MMR vaccination and febrile convulsions.

Study	Type	No. children	No. febrile convulsions	Risk period post-MMR	RI 95% CI
1	Cohort	679 942	487	8 - 14 days	2.83 1.44 – 5.55
2	SCCS	952 cases	1062	6 – 11 days	3.04 2.27 – 4.07

Study 1 (Barlow et al., 2001) was a cohort study of children undertaken
in the United States within the Vaccine Safety Datalink database. It involved
679 942 children (637 989 person-years of observation) under the age of 7 years,
of which 137 457 were vaccinated with the MMR vaccine. Within this cohort,
487 first febrile convulsions were validated by chart review. The analysis was
adjusted for age, sex, health maintenance organisation, calendar time and
receipt of DTP vaccine. The adjusted relative incidence (RI) for the 8–14 day
period after MMR was 2.83, 95% confidence interval (CI) (1.44, 5.55).

Study 2 (Farrington et al., 1995) was a SCCS study undertaken in the
United Kingdom using hospital admission data linked to vaccination records.
There were 1062 febrile convulsions (5 of these were coded as aseptic meningitis) in 952 children aged 12–24 months who were successfully linked to an
MMR vaccination record. All convulsions were included in the analysis. The
age-adjusted relative incidence for the 6–11 day period after MMR was 3.04,
95% CI (2.27, 4.07).

Despite some differences between the two studies, notably the post-
vaccination risk periods used, the results invite similar conclusions: MMR
vaccination is statistically significantly associated with a roughly 3-fold increase in the rate of febrile convulsions in the second week after vaccination.
The confidence intervals for the RI are narrower in the SCCS study: this reflects the greater number of events included in this study. The overall study
size, however, is strikingly smaller.

MMR vaccines and autism
In 1998 a paper published in *The Lancet* (since withdrawn) claimed that
MMR vaccination may be causally linked to autism, further suggesting a close
temporal association between the two events. In subsequent years, several
studies were undertaken to test this hypothesis. The results from three such
studies are presented in Table 2.3.

Study 1 (Taylor et al., 1999) was a SCCS study undertaken in the United

TABLE 2.3
Three studies of MMR vaccination and autism.

Study	Type	Sample size	RI or OR 95% CI
1	SCCS	357 cases	0.88
			0.40 – 1.95
2	Cohort	537 303 children,	0.92
		316 cases	0.68 – 1.24
3	Case-control	1294 cases,	0.86
		4469 controls	0.68 – 1.09

Kingdom. Children with autism aged under 16 years were identified from a variety of sources, and linked to computerised vaccination records. There were 357 cases of autism, of which 63 did not receive MMR vaccine. The original 1999 analysis used relatively short post-MMR risk periods, in line with the original hypothesis, which subsequently evolved. The analysis reported in Table 2.3 used an indefinite post-MMR risk period (Farrington and Whitaker, 2006). Thus, a child was regarded as being potentially at increased risk at all times after receiving MMR vaccine. The age-adjusted RI was 0.88, 95% CI (0.40, 1.95).

Study 2 (Madsen et al., 2002) was a retrospective cohort study undertaken in Denmark. The study included 537 303 children born between 1991 and 1998. Of these, 404 655 received MMR vaccine. The risk period included all time after MMR vaccination. The analysis was adjusted for age, calendar period, sex, birth weight, gestational age, mother's education, and socioeconomic status. There were 316 autism cases, leading to an adjusted relative incidence of 0.92, with 95% CI (0.68, 1.24).

Study 3 (Smeeth et al., 2004a) was a matched case-control study undertaken in the United Kingdom Clinical Practice Research Datalink. Cases were identified within age groups chosen to include all who might have received MMR vaccine. Cases and controls were matched by year of birth, sex and general practice; the analysis was adjusted for duration of GPRD record. The results in Table 2.3 relate to cases with a diagnosis of Pervasive Developmental Disorder; restricting the case definition to autism yielded similar results. The adjusted odds ratio (OR) for ever having received MMR vaccine was 0.86, 95% CI (0.68, 1.09).

The three studies yield similar results. In this specific context, it was important to obtain robust evidence quickly to limit the damage to the MMR vaccination programme: the original SCCS analysis was published in the year following publication of the hypothesis.

Note that the cohort study with 316 cases produces confidence intervals that are narrower than those obtained with the SCCS study with 357 cases:

the reason is that the SCCS method is less efficient when applied with long risk periods, as is the case here. The relative efficiency of the SCCS method and other epidemiological designs is discussed in Chapter 8, Section 8.3.

2.3.2 Controlling confounding

Although the original motivation for the SCCS method was to develop a valid epidemiological study design based only on cases, control of time-invariant confounders is a very useful property, and is often the main reason for undertaking a SCCS analysis, perhaps in addition to a more traditional analysis based on case-control or cohort methods. It is particularly useful for studies undertaken in pre-existing databases, where relevant covariate information may be limited.

Antidepressants and hip fracture
Antidepressant drugs have been associated with hip fracture; the association appears to be linked to the initiation of treatment with antidepressants. Hubbard et al. (2003) investigated this association in an elderly population using a matched case-control study, supplemented by a SCCS analysis based on the same cases, within the United Kingdom Clinical Practice Research Datalink (CPRD). Particular interest focused on distinguishing between two types of antidepressant drugs: tricyclic antidepressants (TCAs), and selective serotonin reuptake inhibitors (SSRIs). Some key results are in Table 2.4.

TABLE 2.4
Antidepressants and hip fracture: case-control and SCCS analyses.

Analysis	TCAs, 0–14 days		SSRIs, 0–14 days	
	OR or RI	95% CI	OR or RI	95% CI
Case-control	4.76	3.06 – 7.41	6.30	2.65 – 15.0
SCCS	2.30	1.82 – 2.90	1.96	1.35 – 2.83

Cases and controls were matched for age, sex, general practice and duration of the available CPRD record. The case-control analysis was also adjusted for history of falls and prescriptions for hypnotics and antipsychotics. Odds ratios were obtained for starting on an antidepressant between 0 and 14 days prior to hip fracture. In the SCCS analysis, which was adjusted for age, the risk period was 0–14 days after the start of an antidepressant. Other time intervals were also used, but are not reported here.

Both analyses found a statistically significant association between initiation of antidepressants and hip fracture, whatever type of antidepressant was used. However, the odds ratios (OR) from the case-control analysis are markedly higher than the relative incidences (RI) from the SCCS analysis, although the cases included were the same. Furthermore, the OR is higher for

SSRIs than for TCAs, whereas there is little difference between antidepressant type in the SCCS analysis.

As hip fracture is relatively uncommon, odds ratios and relative risks are equivalent, so OR and RI should be similar. The fact that they differ substantially suggests that the results of the case-control study may be affected, to some degree, by selection biases. Thus, persons at higher risk of hip fracture may be more likely to be prescribed antidepressants. Such an indication bias would inflate the odds ratios in the case-control study. Similarly, the contrasting results for TCAs and SSRIs may be due to physicians preferentially prescribing SSRIs to frail patients. Such a channelling bias would inflate the OR associated with SSRIs compared to that for TCAs. These biases are less likely to affect the SCCS analysis, insofar as patient frailty, over and above the effect of age, may be regarded as time-invariant over the course of the period of observation for each case, which in this study was on average 6 years.

Influenza vaccination and asthma exacerbations
This study was undertaken in children with asthma aged 1 to 6 years, to evaluate a possible association between receipt of the seasonal influenza vaccine and asthma exacerbations resulting in hospitalisation or an emergency department visit (Kramarz et al., 2000). The study was conducted using computerised medical records from four health maintenance organisations (HMO) in the United States. Retrospective cohort studies were undertaken during three influenza seasons; the cases from the cohorts were also analysed using SCCS. In both the cohort and SCCS analyses, the risk period included the 2 weeks immediately after influenza vaccination. Table 2.5 shows results from the 1995–96 influenza season.

TABLE 2.5
Influenza vaccination and asthma exacerbations: cohort and SCCS analyses.

Analysis	Sample size	RI	95% CI
Cohort, unadjusted	70 753 children with asthma	3.29	2.55 – 4.15
Cohort, adjusted	As above	1.39	1.08 – 1.77
SCCS	2075 cases	0.98	0.76 – 1.27

The unadjusted relative incidence is 3.29, with 95% CI (2.55, 4.15), suggesting a strong positive association between influenza vaccination and asthma. However, the analysis is prone to indication bias: children with more serious asthma are more likely to receive influenza vaccination. The adjusted cohort analysis includes adjustment for sex, age, calendar time, HMO and variables associated with underlying disease severity: prior use of β-agonists and cromolyn, prior hospitalisations, and emergency department visits for asthma. These adjustments produced a large drop in the RI, to 1.39, though it remained statistically significantly raised with 95% CI $(1.08, 1.77)$. The SCCS analysis, which adjusted for calendar time (this being the primary time line for analysis), produced a statistically non-significant RI of 0.98, 95% CI $(0.76, 1.27)$.

This example illustrates the difficulty of fully adjusting for confounders using proxy variables, and the potential benefit of a SCCS analysis, which sidesteps the problem.

2.4   Assumptions and alternatives

The SCCS model requires some assumptions, which are outlined in this section. However, extensions of the SCCS method are available when these assumptions are not met.

2.4.1   Assumptions of the SCCS method

The SCCS method is based on four assumptions:

A1 Events arise independently within individuals or, if non-recurrent, are uncommon.

A2 Occurrence of an event does not influence the subsequent period of observation.

A3 Occurrence of an event does not influence subsequent exposures.

A4 Exposures do not influence the ascertainment of events.

The first assumption is seldom problematic. Recurrences may be included in a SCCS analysis provided that they are not influenced by earlier events within the same individual. This might not be the case, for example, for myocardial infarction (MI): a first MI might increase the chance of a second. In this case, the SCCS study can proceed by including just the first event, provided that it is uncommon in the population of interest. This is often the case in practice.

The second assumption may be violated if the event is associated with high short-term mortality. For example, suppose that the event is stroke, which carries a relatively high short-term risk of death. As observation is curtailed at death, the period of observation depends on when the stroke occurred.

The third assumption will fail, for example, for studies involving exposure to a pharmaceutical drug when occurrence of the event is a contra-indication to treatment with that drug. An example is oral rotavirus vaccination and intussusception.

Finally, the fourth assumption is not specific to the SCCS method, but is included to avoid inappropriate use of the method. For example, events ascertained within a spontaneous adverse event reporting scheme should not be analysed with the SCCS method (unless suitably modified), since events are ascertained owing to a presumptive link with the exposure. Generally, the cases used in a SCCS study should comprise all or a random sample of the cases within a defined population, as would for example be used in a case-control study.

The rationale for the second and third assumptions relates to the conditionality principle upon which the SCCS method is based. All four assumptions are discussed in much greater detail in Chapter 3, Section 3.7.

2.4.2 What if the assumptions are not satisfied?

Failure to satisfy the assumptions does not necessarily mean that the results obtained using the SCCS method are invalid. For example, the assumption that events do not increase short-term mortality is violated when the event is MI. However, this was found to have no bearing on the results of a SCCS study of antipsychotics and MI (Brauer et al., 2015). Indeed, whatever the statistical method used, it is seldom the case that all assumptions are verified. For example, a key assumption of cohort and case-control methods is that all relevant confounders have been included in the model or allowed for in the design of the study. In practice, it is seldom possible to demonstrate that this has been achieved.

Whatever method is used, what matters primarily is that the results should not be overly sensitive to failure of assumptions – that is, the results should not be substantially biased if the assumptions are not met. Chapter 5 is devoted to verifying the assumptions of the SCCS model, and to investigating the sensitivity of the results to failure of assumptions.

When the results of a SCCS analysis are likely to be biased owing to assumptions not being met, one of several extensions of the SCCS method may be used. These are described in Chapter 7, and applied to several examples including those on stroke and intussusception mentioned in Section 2.4.1.

Many SCCS studies published in the epidemiological literature have used a traditional design, such as a cohort or case-control study, supplemented by a SCCS analysis of the cases from this study. Examples include the hip fractures and asthma studies described in Section 2.3.2. This is a fruitful approach. Different study designs require different assumptions, and comparing the results obtained using different methods can yield further insights into the substantive question of interest and the methodological strengths or limitations of the investigation.

Finally, there are occasions where the SCCS method is not applicable. For example, the SCCS method is not appropriate for studies of the potential association between developmental disorders in childhood and vaccination in infancy with vaccines containing thiomersal. Nor would it be suitable for investigations of lifelong exposures, such as the impact of diet on cancer incidence. The reason the SCCS method will not work in these settings is that the exposure does not vary within individuals over the age range at which events occur. The exposure, however, need not be transient, as illustrated in the MMR vaccine and autism example of Section 2.3.1. These issues, and the factors affecting the efficiency of the SCCS method, are discussed in Chapter 8.

Summary

- The SCCS method relies on the following four assumptions:

  A1 Events are uncommon or independent within subjects.

  A2 Events do not influence the subsequent period of observation.

  A3 Events do not influence subsequent exposures.

  A4 Exposures do not influence the ascertainment of events.

- If an assumption is not satisfied, an extension of the SCCS method may be used.

- Supplementing cohort or case-control methods by an analysis of cases using SCCS can be fruitful.

- The SCCS method is not appropriate when there is no variation in exposure within cases.

2.5 Bibliographical notes and further material

For more details of the studies on MMR vaccine and aseptic meningitis described in Section 2.1, see Miller et al. (1993). The SCCS model was first published by Farrington (1995). As explained in Section 2.1, the method was developed in order to use data available only on cases. Accordingly, it was originally called the case series method. The term self-controlled was added later to avoid confusion with case series arising from spontaneous reports or convenience samples, not all of which may validly be analysed with the SCCS method when case ascertainment is influenced by exposure history. Other accessible introductions to the SCCS method and its application include Whitaker et al. (2006) and Whitaker et al. (2009) in English, Hocine and Chavance (2010) in French and Pan et al. (2013) in Chinese.

A more detailed bibliography relating to the development of the SCCS method and related designs is deferred to Chapter 3, Section 3.9, so as to include connections to the wider statistical and epidemiological literatures, which will have become more apparent at that point.

3

The SCCS likelihood

Unlike other cohort-based epidemiological methods, the SCCS (self-controlled case series) method cannot readily be explained by reference to population rates, since only cases are sampled and consequently population rates are not estimated. In addition, the method has some features that are not shared with more standard epidemiological methods, and that therefore can appear unusual – for example, ignoring non-cases, automatically controlling multiplicative confounders, and requiring observation time after the event of interest has occurred. The reasons for these features only become apparent upon studying the SCCS likelihood. Therefore, this is where we have chosen to start.

To begin with, we describe the likelihood for the standard SCCS model, in which age and exposure effects are piecewise constant, that is, constant on intervals, because it is the most commonly used. We then move on to a more general form of the SCCS likelihood, its derivation from a cohort model, and the assumptions required for this derivation to work. The starred subsections within Section 3.7 and starred Section 3.8 are more mathematical and may be skipped.

3.1 Why start with the likelihood?

In a cohort analysis, absolute incidence rates in exposed and unexposed periods can be estimated directly by counting the number of events in each period and dividing by the total person time at risk within the cohort. Rates can then be contrasted, adjusting for age effects and covariates using suitable statistical models, yielding estimates of rate or hazard ratios with direct interpretations as ratios of absolute incidences. Similarly, in a case-control study, the odds ratio has a direct interpretation as the ratio of the odds of exposure in cases and controls.

With the SCCS method, as in a cohort study, our aim is to estimate the relative incidence – the common term we use to describe the intensity or rate ratio, for recurrent events, or hazard ratio, for non-recurrent events. However, only cases are sampled. Consequently, absolute incidence rates cannot be calculated directly as in a cohort analysis, since no population denominators are available. Nor are there any separate controls to compare with the cases. Thus, unlike standard epidemiological designs, there is no simple and intuitive estimator of the relative rate or odds ratio. Nor are descriptions of the method referring to comparisons of incidence rates in exposed versus unexposed periods within individuals wholly compelling, for the simple reason that incidence rates are not available.

Instead, estimates are derived indirectly from the likelihood. This is the probability or probability density of the available data on cases, expressed as a function of the relative incidence and other parameters. The parameter estimates are the values that maximise the likelihood; this estimation method is known as maximum likelihood.

Of course, cohort methods also make use of likelihoods – indeed maximum likelihood is the most commonly used estimation method in classical statistics. It is instructive to contrast the cohort and SCCS likelihoods. This will be done more formally in Section 3.8, but can also be described informally as follows. The cohort likelihood is the joint probability that each individual in the cohort experienced the observed temporal pattern of events, given that individual's exposure history. The SCCS likelihood, in contrast, is the joint probability that each individual experienced the observed temporal pattern of events, *given the observed number of events* and the exposure and observation history for that individual. The key difference is in italics: the SCCS likelihood conditions on the number of events observed for each individual. This implies that, in the SCCS method, information on the degree of association between exposure and event is obtained from the relative timing of events and exposures within individuals, rather than from marginal event counts, which are fixed by the conditioning.

Gaining some insight into the form of the SCCS likelihood, and how it is derived, is key to understanding the properties and the limitations of the method. The rest of this chapter is devoted to providing such insight.

3.2   Likelihood for the standard SCCS model

We shall assume to begin with that events for an individual i arise according to a non-homogeneous Poisson process with intensity rate function $\lambda_i(t|x_i, y_i)$ observed over an interval $(a_i, b_i]$, which we call the observation period. Observation periods may vary between individuals. Here t denotes age, x_i is the exposure and observation history for individual i up to the end of observation b_i and y_i is a vector of time-invariant covariates for individual i. Some further details of exposure and observation histories are provided in Section 3.8. The Poisson assumption will be relaxed later. We have assumed that the time line of primary interest is age, but it could just as well be calendar time: which is most appropriate is dependent on the context.

In the standard SCCS model, the intensities (or incidence rates, in epidemiological terminology) $\lambda_i(t|x_i, y_i)$ are assumed to be piecewise constant on age groups, and on non-overlapping exposure-related risk periods; these are intervals during which an individual is exposed. We shall assume that the relevant age range (chosen to include all the observation periods) is partitioned into $J + 1$ intervals, indexed by $j = 0, \ldots, J$. Exposure levels are similarly represented by age-varying step functions with up to $K + 1$ levels, varying from level $k = 0$ in the absence of exposure to risk levels $k = 1, \ldots, K$ in the presence of exposure. Several risk levels are allowed: for example, in pharmacoepidemiology, an individual might be regarded as unexposed $(k = 0)$ prior to taking the drug of interest. For a period after exposure to the drug, the individual may be at risk level $k = 1$. This might then be followed by a further period at some intermediate risk level $k = 2$, before returning to the reference risk level $(k = 0)$. Note that the same age groups are used for all cases, but the exposure step functions vary between individuals according to their exposure histories in x_i.

An illustration is provided in Figure 3.1. The top graph shows the time line of a case, indicated by the arrow. The observation period is denoted by the light grey bar below the time line. This is partitioned into three age groups, labelled $j = 0, 1, 2$, so $J = 2$. Above the time line, in darker grey, are the risk periods. There are two of these, both at the same risk level $k = 1$. So here, $K = 1$, and the exposure groups are labelled $k = 0, 1$. These age and exposure groups split the observation period into 7 distinct time intervals, indicated by the short vertical dotted lines.

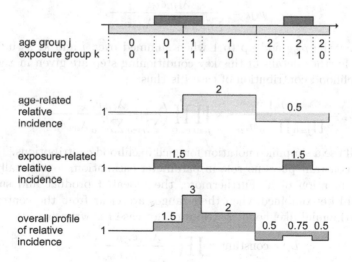

FIGURE 3.1
A case with piecewise constant intensity on age and exposure intervals (see text).

Let e_{ijk} denote the total duration (several non-adjacent time intervals may be involved) of observation time spent by individual i in age group j and at exposure level k. The intensity function for individual i is assumed to be constant within each such category (i, j, k):

$$\lambda_i(t|x_i, y_i) = \lambda_{ijk} \qquad \text{when individual } i \text{ at age } t \text{ is in age group } j$$
$$\text{and at exposure level } k.$$

For the case represented in Figure 3.1, the shape of the intensity function is displayed in the bottom graph. This shows the relative incidence, that is, the intensity relative to its value when $j = 0$ (age group 0) and $k = 0$ (the unexposed level). It is piecewise constant on the seven intervals defined on the top graph in Figure 3.1.

Suppose that a sample of N cases is available. Cases are individuals i, $i = 1, \ldots, N$, who have experienced $n_i \geq 1$ events over their observation period. The sample may be a random sample of cases, or all cases arising from an underlying cohort. Let n_{ijk} denote the number of events experienced by case i while observed in age group j and exposure group k. We now treat the number of events n_i for case i as fixed: this is called conditioning on n_i, and is the key statistical step in deriving the SCCS likelihood, as described informally in Chapter 2, Section 2.2.1. It then follows from the Poisson assumption that the event counts $\{n_{ijk} : j = 0, \ldots, J; k = 0, \ldots, K\}$ are distributed multinomial with index n_i and probabilities

$$p_{ijk} = \frac{\lambda_{ijk} e_{ijk}}{\sum_{r=0}^{J} \sum_{s=0}^{K} \lambda_{irs} e_{irs}}.$$

Note that the p_{ijk} add up to 1 when summed over j and k, as indeed they should. Further details of this key conditioning step are given in Section 3.8. The likelihood contribution of case i is thus:

$$L_i = \frac{n_i!}{\prod_{j=0}^{J} \prod_{k=0}^{K} n_{ijk}!} \times \prod_{j=0}^{J} \prod_{k=0}^{K} \left(\frac{\lambda_{ijk} e_{ijk}}{\sum_{r=0}^{J} \sum_{s=0}^{K} \lambda_{irs} e_{irs}} \right)^{n_{ijk}}.$$

We shall use a simplified notation for such likelihood contributions. The multinomial constant plays no role in parameter estimation, so we shall suppress explicit mention of it. Furthermore, the repeated product and summation signs will be combined when their ranges are clear from the context. Thus, the multinomial likelihood contribution for case i is written:

$$L_i = \text{constant} \times \prod_{j,k} \left(\frac{\lambda_{ijk} e_{ijk}}{\sum_{r,s} \lambda_{irs} e_{irs}} \right)^{n_{ijk}}. \tag{3.1}$$

Provided that events occur independently in different individuals, the overall likelihood is the product of the individual contributions L_i of the N cases:

$$L = \text{constant} \times \prod_{i=1}^{N} \prod_{j,k} \left(\frac{\lambda_{ijk} e_{ijk}}{\sum_{r,s} \lambda_{irs} e_{irs}} \right)^{n_{ijk}}. \tag{3.2}$$

This is the standard SCCS likelihood, which is of product multinomial form. Though derived under a Poisson assumption, it is also valid for non-recurrent events in the limit where these are rare, as will be shown in Section 3.8.

In this form, with separate parameters λ_{ijk}, the model is clearly over-parameterised. Parsimonious parameterisations of the standard SCCS model are discussed in Chapter 4. In the simplest such parameterisation,

$$\lambda_{ijk} = \phi_i \exp\left(\alpha_j + \beta_k\right),$$

with $\alpha_0 = \beta_0 = 0$. The parameters α_j and β_k describe the relative effects of age and exposure, respectively, on the log scale.

This model is illustrated in Figure 3.1. The relative effects of age and exposure are displayed in the two middle graphs, along with the values of the age-related relative incidence $\exp(\alpha_j)$ and the exposure-related relative incidence $\exp(\beta_k)$. These combine multiplicatively: the overall relative incidence profile is $\exp(\alpha_j + \beta_k) = \exp(\alpha_j) \times \exp(\beta_k)$, shown in the bottom graph. For example, on the third interval from the left, the age-related relative incidence is 2 and the exposure-related relative incidence is 1.5, so that the overall relative incidence on that interval is $2 \times 1.5 = 3$.

In this model, the parameters ϕ_i cancel out of Equation 3.2 and the SCCS likelihood just involves $J + K$ unknown parameters to be estimated. In fact it is more common to work with the log likelihood, which becomes:

$$l(\boldsymbol{\alpha}, \boldsymbol{\beta}) = \text{constant} + \sum_{i=1}^{N} \sum_{j,k} n_{ijk} \log\left\{\frac{\exp(\alpha_j + \beta_k)e_{ijk}}{\sum_{r,s} \exp(\alpha_r + \beta_s)e_{irs}}\right\} \qquad (3.3)$$

where $\boldsymbol{\alpha} = (\alpha_1, \ldots, \alpha_J)^T$ and $\boldsymbol{\beta} = (\beta_1, \ldots, \beta_K)^T$.

Some key features that emerge from the definition of the standard SCCS likelihood in Equation 3.2 are highlighted in the next section. A worked example is provided in Section 3.4.

Summary

- In the standard SCCS model, the incidence of events is assumed to be constant on pre-specified age and exposure categories.

- For each case, the distribution of events across age and exposure categories is multinomial.

- The likelihood for the standard SCCS model is the product of the contributions for each case, and is therefore product multinomial.

- In the simplest such model, the only parameters are those describing the relative effects of age and exposure.

3.3   Properties of the SCCS likelihood

First, note that only cases are required to calculate the likelihood in Equation 3.2. The N cases included in the SCCS likelihood can be thought of as arising from an underlying cohort: the non-cases in this cohort do not feature. Thus, the underlying cohort need not be observed, indeed it can be entirely notional. An example of a notional cohort is that which gives rise to hospital admissions: there is no need to define precisely the hospital catchment population to undertake a SCCS analysis based on hospital admissions. In addition, since only cases are involved, the collection, verification and preparation of the data for analysis is more straightforward.

Second, the SCCS likelihood involves ratios of intensities, and thus any time-invariant covariates that act multiplicatively on the intensity function will cancel out. Time-invariant here is taken to mean that the covariate for each case i does not vary over the observation period $(a_i, b_i]$. This feature was already in evidence in Equations 3.2 and 3.3, from which the constants ϕ_i cancelled out. More generally, if for some time-invariant covariate or random effect $\boldsymbol{y}_i$

$$\lambda_{ijk} = \phi_i h_i(\boldsymbol{y}_i) \times \nu_{ijk}$$

for some arbitrary constants ϕ_i and functions h_i, where the ν_{ijk} do not depend on $\boldsymbol{y}_i$, then the SCCS likelihood reduces to

$$L = \text{constant} \times \prod_{i=1}^{N} \prod_{j,k} \left(\frac{\nu_{ijk} e_{ijk}}{\sum_{r,s} \nu_{irs} e_{irs}} \right)^{n_{ijk}}, \qquad (3.4)$$

which does not feature the $\boldsymbol{y}_i$. In other words, time-invariant covariates or random effects acting multiplicatively on the intensity function are automatically eliminated from the likelihood, and therefore need not be included explicitly in a SCCS model. The main practical consequence of this property is that confounding by fixed multiplicative covariates is automatically adjusted for, even if such covariates are unmeasured, and indeed whether or not they are known to be confounders.

The ratio form of the SCCS likelihood is what underpins its self-controlled property. It also implies that only relative effects, rather than absolute incidence rates, are estimable. Note that this property applies only to main effects: interactions between time-invariant covariates and exposure variables do not cancel out and are estimable, as will be described in Chapter 4.

These two features – only requiring a case series, and self-control of multiplicative time-invariant confounders – are the key properties of the SCCS method, which motivated its name.

Third, the SCCS likelihood permits the inclusion of recurrent events: the number of events experienced by case i is n_i, which may be greater than 1. The form of the SCCS likelihood implies that recurrences must be independent within individuals. Thus, the same expression would be obtained if each case i were replicated n_i times, replicate $j = 1, \ldots, n_i$ featuring the jth event for case i.

Fourth, and finally, note that the SCCS likelihood 3.2 features the sums $\sum_{r,s} \lambda_{irs} e_{irs}$ for each case i in its denominator. Computation of these quantities requires information on the exposure histories over the entire observation periods $(a_i, b_i]$, including at ages *after* the occurrence of any events. Similarly, the intensities $\lambda(t|x_i, y_i)$ depend on the exposure and observation histories x_i over the entire observation periods $(a_i, b_i]$. This is a subtle point, but is critical to the conditioning argument used in deriving the likelihood. Some assumptions are needed for this argument to work. These assumptions were outlined in Chapter 2, Section 2.4 and are discussed in greater detail in Section 3.7.

Summary

- In the SCCS method, only cases are required. This simplifies data collection and verification.

- Any multiplicative covariate that does not vary over the observation period is automatically controlled for. This protects against confounding.

- The SCCS method can handle recurrent events provided that recurrences occur independently for each subject.

- The exposure history of each case over the entire observation period is required – both before and after any event.

3.4 Example: MMR vaccine and aseptic meningitis

In Chapter 2, Section 2.1, we described the application that motivated the development of the SCCS method. This was the association between measles, mumps and rubella (MMR) vaccines containing the Urabe mumps strain, and aseptic meningitis. Two studies were undertaken, both involving only cases. These studies suggested that events tended to cluster 15 to 35 days after MMR vaccination, which was defined to be the risk period of interest based on evidence from earlier studies. In the present section we illustrate the SCCS method using data from one of these two studies: the hospital study, undertaken in a health region where only Urabe-containing MMR vaccines were used.

Hospital admission records of all children with a diagnosis of aseptic meningitis (in fact, these were confirmed cases of viral meningitis) occurring on or between 1st October 1988 and 31st December 1991 in children aged between 1 and 2 years of age (that is, children aged 366 to 730 days) were obtained.

Linked MMR vaccination records for these children from 315 to 715 days of age were also available, so that each day in each child's observation period could be classified as exposed (if falling within the 15 to 35 day post-MMR risk period) or unexposed (otherwise).

There were 10 hospital admissions within the specified age and time boundaries, in 10 different children. Table 3.1 shows the data for these 10 cases.

TABLE 3.1
Aseptic meningitis study; ages are in days.

Case	First day of observation	First day of risk period	Last day of risk period	Day of event	Last day of observation
1	366	473	493	398	730
2	366	–	–	399	730
3	366	407	427	413	730
4	366	444	464	449	730
5	366	448	468	455	730
6	366	447	467	472	730
7	366	410	430	474	730
8	366	485	505	485	730
9	366	511	531	524	730
10	366	443	463	700	730

As it happens, the observation period for all 10 cases was 366 to 730 days inclusive (but note that this need not have been so). Case 2 was unexposed throughout the observation period; the other 9 cases experienced risk periods lasting 21 days. Of the 10 events, 5 occurred within a risk period, and 5 did not. Most events occurred early in the observation period, which suggests that the baseline incidence of aseptic meningitis (that is, the incidence in the absence of exposure to MMR vaccination) may vary with age. To keep matters simple, just two groups will be used in this example: ages 366–456 and ages 457–730 days, inclusive, so that each age group contains 5 events. The observation period for each case is split up into successive time intervals determined by changes in age group and exposure level, as shown in Figure 3.2 for the first case.

In Figure 3.2, the light grey bar below the time line represents the observation period, which starts on day 366 of age and ends on day 730. It is split into two age groups, with day 457 representing the first day of the second age group. The dark grey bar above the time line represents the risk period, which starts on day 473 of age and ends on day 493. Also indicated are the age at vaccination (at 458 days of age) and the age at event (398 days).

Thus, from age 366 to 456 (91 days), case 1 is in age group 0 and exposure group 0. From age 457 to 472, and from age 494 to 730 (a total of 253 days), case 1 is in age group 1 and exposure group 0. From age 473 to 493, case 1 is

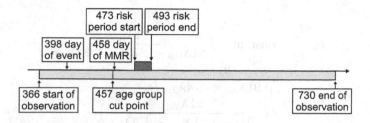

FIGURE 3.2

Observation period, risk period, age group boundary, age at MMR and age at event for case 1.

in age group 1 and exposure group 1. The unique event for case 1 occurs in age group 0 and exposure group 0.

In this example, e_{ijk} denotes the duration of observation time spent by case i in age group j ($j = 0$ for 366–456 days, $j = 1$ for 457–730 days) and exposure group k ($k = 0$ for unexposed, $k = 1$ for exposed), and n_{ijk} is the number of events for case i in each such period. Table 3.2 shows the values of e_{ijk} and n_{ijk} for case 1.

TABLE 3.2

Observation time and event count by age and exposure groups for case 1.

Case i	Age group j	Exposure group k	Duration e_{ijk}	Events n_{ijk}
1	0	0	91	1
1	0	1	0	0
1	1	0	253	0
1	1	1	21	0

The cumulative incidence rate for case 1 over the observation period is thus

$$\Lambda_1 = \sum_{r,s} \lambda_{1rs} e_{1rs} = 91\lambda_{100} + 0\lambda_{101} + 253\lambda_{110} + 21\lambda_{111},$$

and the SCCS likelihood contribution for case 1, from expression 3.1, is

$$
\begin{aligned}
L_1 &= \text{constant} \times \left(\frac{91\lambda_{100}}{\Lambda_1}\right)^1 \times \left(\frac{0\lambda_{101}}{\Lambda_1}\right)^0 \times \left(\frac{253\lambda_{110}}{\Lambda_1}\right)^0 \times \left(\frac{21\lambda_{111}}{\Lambda_1}\right)^0 \\
&= \text{constant} \times \frac{91\lambda_{100}}{91\lambda_{100} + 253\lambda_{110} + 21\lambda_{111}}.
\end{aligned}
$$

The contributions for the remaining 9 cases are obtained in the same way, yielding the following expression for the overall likelihood:

$$L = \text{constant} \times \left(\frac{91\lambda_{100}}{91\lambda_{100} + 253\lambda_{110} + 21\lambda_{111}} \right)$$

$$\times \left(\frac{91\lambda_{200}}{91\lambda_{200} + 274\lambda_{210}} \right)$$

$$\times \left(\frac{21\lambda_{301}}{70\lambda_{300} + 21\lambda_{301} + 274\lambda_{310}} \right)$$

$$\times \left(\frac{13\lambda_{401}}{78\lambda_{400} + 13\lambda_{401} + 266\lambda_{410} + 8\lambda_{411}} \right)$$

$$\times \left(\frac{9\lambda_{501}}{82\lambda_{500} + 9\lambda_{501} + 262\lambda_{510} + 12\lambda_{511}} \right)$$

$$\times \left(\frac{263\lambda_{610}}{81\lambda_{600} + 10\lambda_{601} + 263\lambda_{610} + 11\lambda_{611}} \right)$$

$$\times \left(\frac{274\lambda_{710}}{70\lambda_{700} + 21\lambda_{701} + 274\lambda_{710}} \right)$$

$$\times \left(\frac{21\lambda_{811}}{91\lambda_{800} + 253\lambda_{810} + 21\lambda_{811}} \right)$$

$$\times \left(\frac{21\lambda_{911}}{91\lambda_{900} + 253\lambda_{910} + 21\lambda_{911}} \right)$$

$$\times \left(\frac{267\lambda_{1010}}{77\lambda_{1000} + 14\lambda_{1001} + 267\lambda_{1010} + 7\lambda_{1011}} \right).$$

In the parameterisation $\lambda_{ijk} = \phi_i \exp(\alpha_j + \beta_k)$, with $\alpha_0 = \beta_0 = 0$, there are just two parameters to be estimated, α_1 and β_1. For case 1, for example,

$$L_1(\alpha_1, \beta_1) = \text{constant} \times \frac{91}{91 + 253\exp(\alpha_1) + 21\exp(\alpha_1 + \beta_1)},$$

and so the log likelihood for case 1 is:

$$l_1(\alpha_1, \beta_1) = \text{constant} - \log(91 + 253e^{\alpha_1} + 21e^{\alpha_1 + \beta_1}).$$

The overall log likelihood is:

$$
\begin{aligned}
l(\alpha_1, \beta_1) \;=\; & \text{constant} + 5\alpha_1 + 5\beta_1 \\
& - \log(91 + 253e^{\alpha_1} + 21e^{\alpha_1+\beta_1}) \\
& - \log(91 + 274e^{\alpha_1}) \\
& - \log(70 + 21e^{\beta_1} + 274e^{\alpha_1}) \\
& - \log(78 + 13e^{\beta_1} + 266e^{\alpha_1} + 8e^{\alpha_1+\beta_1}) \\
& - \log(82 + 9e^{\beta_1} + 262e^{\alpha_1} + 12e^{\alpha_1+\beta_1}) \\
& - \log(81 + 10e^{\beta_1} + 263e^{\alpha_1} + 11e^{\alpha_1+\beta_1}) \\
& - \log(70 + 21e^{\beta_1} + 274e^{\alpha_1}) \\
& - \log(91 + 253e^{\alpha_1} + 21e^{\alpha_1+\beta_1}) \\
& - \log(91 + 253e^{\alpha_1} + 21e^{\alpha_1+\beta_1}) \\
& - \log(77 + 14e^{\beta_1} + 267e^{\alpha_1} + 7e^{\alpha_1+\beta_1}).
\end{aligned}
$$

This log likelihood function defines a surface of height $l(\alpha_1, \beta_1)$ over the plane with coordinates (α_1, β_1). This likelihood surface is shown as a contour plot in Figure 3.3, with the constant in the log-likelihood function set to zero.

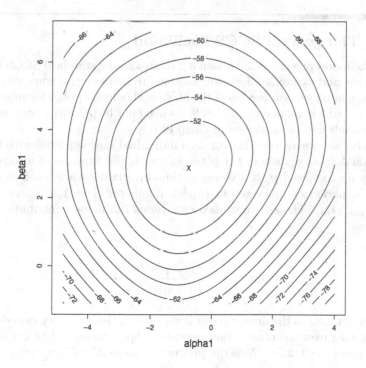

FIGURE 3.3
Contour plot for the log likelihood; × marks the maximum.

The maximum of the log likelihood is then -50.09. The estimates of the parameters α_1 and β_1 are the values that maximise the log likelihood. These values turn out to be $\hat{\alpha}_1 = -0.7577$ and $\hat{\beta}_1 = 2.8792$. Statistical software to obtain these estimates will be described in Chapter 4.

This worked example will be continued in Section 3.6, where we illustrate how the SCCS likelihood is derived from a cohort model.

We end the present section with some remarks about interval notation. In this and all other examples, and in the software, we describe age and time intervals, such as observation periods, age groups and risk periods, in the form [first day, last day]. This differs from the notation used in mathematical arguments, where intervals are written $(a, b]$, which denotes the set of values $\{t : a < t \le b\}$, and thus does not include a. The difference in notation arises because, in practical examples, time is discretised into integer units, typically days. From the formal point of view, $(a, b] = [a + 1, b]$ in discrete time. In mathematical arguments, where age and time are regarded as continuous, the $(a, b]$ notation is the most natural. In discrete time applications, however, it is far more convenient to specify an interval by its first and last days.

3.5   The general SCCS likelihood

The likelihood presented in Section 3.2 relates to the standard SCCS model in which age and exposure effects are assumed to be piecewise constant. Here we present a more general version of the likelihood, which applies for more general models in which age and exposure effects need not be piecewise constant. Some such models will be described in Chapter 6.

As before, we assume that for each individual i, events arise with intensity function $\lambda_i(t|x_i, \boldsymbol{y}_i)$ where t denotes age, x_i is the exposure and observation history up to b_i and $\boldsymbol{y}_i$ is a vector of time-invariant covariates. Suppose that case i experiences n_i events in $(a_i, b_i]$, numbered $j = 1, 2, \ldots, n_i$ at times $t_{i1}, t_{i2}, \ldots, t_{in_i}$. The self-controlled case series likelihood contribution of case i is then:

$$L_i = \text{constant} \times \frac{\prod_{j=1}^{n_i} \lambda_i(t_{ij}|x_i, \boldsymbol{y}_i)}{\left(\int_{a_i}^{b_i} \lambda_i(t|x_i, \boldsymbol{y}_i) dt \right)^{n_i}}.$$

The integral in the denominator is the cumulative intensity experienced by individual i over the observation period $(a_i, b_i]$. The overall SCCS likelihood for N cases $i = 1, 2, \ldots, N$ is the product of these N contributions:

$$L = \text{constant} \times \prod_{i=1}^{N} \frac{\prod_{j=1}^{n_i} \lambda_i(t_{ij}|x_i, \boldsymbol{y}_i)}{\left(\int_{a_i}^{b_i} \lambda_i(t|x_i, \boldsymbol{y}_i) dt \right)^{n_i}}. \tag{3.5}$$

The derivation of this likelihood will be presented in Section 3.8. It generalises the likelihood of Equation 3.2 since, if $\lambda_i(t|x_i, \boldsymbol{y}_i)$ is piecewise constant on age intervals $r = 0, \ldots, J$ and at different exposure levels $s = 0, \ldots, K$ within $(a_i, b_i]$, then, in the notation of Section 3.2,

$$\prod_{j=1}^{n_i} \lambda_i(t_{ij}|x_i, \boldsymbol{y}_i) = \text{constant} \times \prod_{r,s} \left(\lambda_{irs} e_{irs}\right)^{n_{irs}},$$

and

$$\int_{a_i}^{b_i} \lambda_i(t|x_i, \boldsymbol{y}_i) dt = \sum_{r,s} \lambda_{irs} e_{irs}.$$

All the properties of the standard SCCS likelihood described in Section 3.3 also hold of this more general version of the likelihood: only cases are required, time-invariant multiplicative covariates are automatically adjusted, and recurrences may be included. The main difference is that the general likelihood need not be product multinomial.

Summary

- A more general version of the SCCS likelihood is available, for which it need not be assumed that age and exposure effects are piecewise constant.

- This more general version of the likelihood shares the key properties of the standard SCCS likelihood, though it need not be product multinomial.

3.6 MMR vaccine and aseptic meningitis: derivation of the SCCS likelihood

For the remainder of this chapter, we consider the derivation of the SCCS likelihood from a cohort model, and the assumptions underpinning this derivation. The formal derivation is in Section 3.8. However the main ideas may be conveyed more directly using the worked example introduced in Section 3.4.

Recall that hospital admission records of all children with a diagnosis of aseptic meningitis occurring on or between 1st October 1988 and 31st December 1991 in children aged between 1 and 2 years of age (that is, children aged 366 to 730 days) were obtained. This yielded 10 cases. These 10 cases may be regarded as arising within the underlying cohort comprising all children within the study region aged between 366 and 730 days between 1st October 1988 and 31st December 1991. So, for example, a child born on 1st June

1990 would contribute an observation period of 214 days from age 366 days (reached on 1st June 1991) to 579 days inclusive (which falls on 31st December 1991). Suppose this child received MMR vaccine on 20th August 1991, aged 446 days of age. The risk period is defined to stretch from 15 to 35 days after this, namely from ages 461 to 481 inclusive. Admission to hospital for aseptic meningitis at any time within the observation period 366–579 days of age would have led to this child being classified as a case. As it happened, there was no such admission so this child is not a case.

We now consider the cohort likelihood contributions for this non-case, and for the first case listed in Table 3.1. The timelines for these two children, including the age group boundary at 457 days of age, are shown in Figure 3.4.

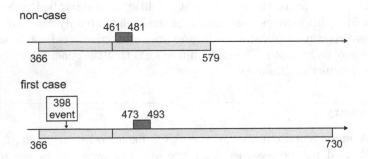

FIGURE 3.4
Timelines for a non-case and for case 1.

For simplicity, let us label the non-case $i = 0$ (and case 1 $i = 1$). The non-case spends 91 days unexposed in age group 0, 102 days unexposed in age group 1, and 21 days exposed in age group 1 (recall that age group 0 covers 366–456 days, age group 1 457–730 days). The cumulative incidence rate over the observation period for the non-case is therefore:

$$\Lambda_0 = 91\lambda_{000} + 0\lambda_{001} + 102\lambda_{010} + 21\lambda_{011}.$$

Since there were no events, the cohort likelihood contribution for the non-case is the Poisson probability

$$L_{c0} = \exp(-\Lambda_0).$$

This is also the marginal likelihood (or probability) L_{m0} of observing $n_0 = 0$ events, given this child's exposure and observation histories. The SCCS likelihood contribution for this child is the conditional probability of the observed event pattern, given the marginal total n_{i0}. This is:

$$
\begin{aligned}
L_0 &= \frac{L_{c0}}{L_{m0}} \\
&= \frac{\exp(-\Lambda_0)}{\exp(-\Lambda_0)} \\
&= 1.
\end{aligned}
$$

Thus this child, being a non-case, does not contribute (other than trivially) to the SCCS likelihood. The same argument applies to all non-cases in the cohort: their SCCS likelihood contributions are all equal to 1. In other words they contribute no information, and can be ignored.

Case 1, on the other hand, has the following cumulative incidence rate over the observation period 366–730 days, previously obtained in Section 3.4:

$$
\Lambda_1 = 91\lambda_{100} + 0\lambda_{101} + 253\lambda_{110} + 21\lambda_{111}.
$$

The event distribution for case 1 was shown in Table 3.2: 1 event during 91 non-exposed days in age group 0, and 0 events in the other periods. The cohort likelihood contribution for case 1 is the product of the Poisson probabilities for each interval. This is as follows:

$$
\begin{aligned}
L_{c1} &= 91\lambda_{100}\exp(-91\lambda_{100}) \times \exp(-0\lambda_{101}) \\
&\quad \times \exp(-253\lambda_{110}) \times \exp(-21\lambda_{111}) \\
&= 91\lambda_{100}\exp(-\Lambda_1).
\end{aligned}
$$

The marginal likelihood of observing $n_1 = 1$ event given case 1's exposure and observation history, on the other hand, is the Poisson probability

$$
\Lambda_{m1} = \Lambda_1 \exp(-\Lambda_1).
$$

The SCCS likelihood contribution for case 1 is the conditional probability of the observed event pattern, given the marginal total n_1. This is:

$$
\begin{aligned}
L_1 &= \frac{L_{c1}}{L_{m1}} \\
&= \frac{91\lambda_{100}\exp(-\Lambda_1)}{\Lambda_1 \exp(-\Lambda_1)} \\
&= \frac{91\lambda_{100}}{91\lambda_{100} + 253\lambda_{110} + 21\lambda_{111}},
\end{aligned}
$$

as specified in Equation 3.1, and as previously obtained in Section 3.4. The other 9 cases are dealt with in the same way. The overall SCCS likelihood is the product of the contributions for each of the 10 cases: the non-cases do not contribute and hence need not be sampled.

The arguments presented here require several assumptions. Events for each individual are assumed to arise in a Poisson process, which enables us to calculate Poisson probabilities. More subtly, conditioning on the number of events for each case should not affect the incidence, and hence the parameters we wish to estimate. These assumptions are considered in greater detail in Section 3.7. The general derivation of the SCCS likelihood presented in Section 3.8 involves similar steps as the special case described here. One benefit of using a more formal framework is that it helps to make explicit the assumptions required.

3.7   Assumptions of the SCCS method

The assumptions of the SCCS method have already been described informally in Chapter 2, Section 2.4. Stated slightly more precisely, they are as follows.

A1 Events are uncommon or arise in non-homogeneous Poisson processes.

A2 Events do not influence the length of observation periods.

A3 Events do not influence subsequent exposures.

A4 Exposures do not influence event ascertainment.

Assumptions 1 to 3 relate specifically to the SCCS method. Assumption 4 applies to other methods as well. In Chapter 2, Section 2.4 we described some situations in which the assumptions may fail. In this section we discuss these assumptions further, to explain in greater detail what they mean, why they are required, and when they might be violated. Methods for checking and sidestepping assumptions are described in Chapter 5. Extensions of the SCCS method developed to weaken assumptions are the subject of Chapter 7.

3.7.1   Assumption 1: Poisson or rare events

The assumption that events arise according to a non-homogeneous Poisson process within individuals, or alternatively that events are non-recurrent but uncommon, is required to ensure that the SCCS likelihood is of ratio form, that is, involves ratios of intensities; for non-recurrent events, this is a limiting property as the event becomes rare. The ratio form of the likelihood in turn ensures that time-invariant covariates that act multiplicatively on the intensity function (or the hazard, for non-recurrent events) factor out.

It cannot be assumed that time-invariant confounders cancel out of the likelihood if Assumption 1 is violated. A counter-example is described in Section 3.7.2. In practice, Assumption 1 is seldom restrictive. If the event of interest is uncommon, then $n_i = 1$ for most cases and any departure from the Poisson assumption will have little impact on results. Furthermore, Assumption 1 does not rule out clustering of events within individuals at higher risk. This is often represented in statistical models by a multiplicative time-invariant individual frailty U_i, with

$$\lambda_i(t|x_i, y_i, U_i) = U_i \nu_i(t|x_i, y_i)$$

where U_i is a non-negative random variable. The frailties U_i cancel out from the SCCS likelihood, just as fixed multiplicative covariates do.

One situation that Assumption 1 does not cater for is lack of independence of events within individuals. This arises, for example, if occurrence of an event increases the hazard of subsequent events, as might occur with repeated myocardial infarctions, or repeat hospital admissions within a single clinical episode.

3.7.2   A counter-example: negative binomial events*

Suppose that for the standard (piecewise-constant) SCCS model, events for individual i arise in successive intervals according to the generalised negative binomial distribution described by McCullagh and Nelder (1989), page 199. Thus, in the notation of Section 3.2, n_{ijk} has mean $\lambda_{ijk}e_{ijk}$ and variance $(1 + \theta_i^{-1})\lambda_{ijk}e_{ijk}$, for some positive θ_i. The probability mass function of n_{ijk} is

$$P(n_{ijk}|\theta_i, \lambda_{ijk}e_{ijk}) = \frac{\Gamma(n_{ijk} + \theta_i\lambda_{ijk}e_{ijk})\theta_i^{\theta_i\lambda_{ijk}e_{ijk}}}{n_{ijk}!\Gamma(\theta_i\lambda_{ijk}e_{ijk})(1 + \theta_i)^{n_{ijk}+\theta_i\lambda_{ijk}e_{ijk}}},$$

where Γ denotes the gamma function. The marginal total n_i is also generalised negative binomial, with the same dispersion parameter θ_i and mean $\sum_{r,s} \lambda_{irs}e_{irs}$. The conditional likelihood contribution for individual i given n_i is therefore

$$L_i = \text{constant} \times \prod_{j,k} \frac{\Gamma(n_{ijk} + \theta_i\lambda_{ijk}e_{ijk})}{\Gamma(\theta_i\lambda_{ijk}e_{ijk})} \times \frac{\Gamma(\theta_i \sum_{r,s} \lambda_{irs}c_{irs})}{\Gamma(n_i + \theta_i \sum_{r,s} \lambda_{irs}e_{irs})}.$$

Only when $n_i = 1$ (and trivially when $n_i = 0$, in which case L_i is constant) does this reduce to the SCCS likelihood contribution. For marginal counts $n_i > 1$, multiplicative factors in the λ_{ijk} do not cancel out.

3.7.3   Assumptions 2 and 3: validity of conditioning

Assumptions 2 and 3 relate to observation and exposure histories. We shall discuss these assumptions together. First, some new notation is needed. Let x_i^t denote the history of exposure and observation up to age t. Then $x_i = x_i^{b_i}$

---

* This section may be skipped.

is the history of exposure and observation up to the end of the observation period at age b_i. Further details of how exposure and observation histories are defined for SCCS models are given in Section 3.8.

. The distinction between x_i^t and x_i is important because, while the cohort model uses histories up to event age t, the SCCS model conditions on the observation and exposure history up to b_i, and therefore after the event. The SCCS model requires the following identity to be satisfied:

$$\lambda_i(t|x_i^t, \boldsymbol{y}_i) = \lambda_i(t|x_i, \boldsymbol{y}_i) \quad \text{for all } t \in (a_i, b_i], \tag{3.6}$$

This identity states that the incidence rate at age t is not altered by conditioning on the exposure and observation history up to b_i. The reason this is needed is so that the conditioning required to obtain the SCCS likelihood does not alter the quantities we wish to estimate. Assumptions 2 and 3 ensure that this condition is met, as will be shown below. First, we explain heuristically why the assumptions are needed.

Suppose first that Assumption 2 is not met, so that occurrence of an event influences the observation period. As an illustration, consider the extreme scenario in which observation necessarily stops some fixed time τ after the first event. Then conditioning on the observation period $(a_i, b_i]$ also fixes the first event time at $b_i - \tau$.

In consequence, the intensity conditional on the observation period must be zero at all times in $(a_i, b_i - \tau)$. This is because no event can occur prior to $b_i - \tau$: if an event did occur before then, observation would necessarily stop before b_i; but it ended at b_i. In contrast, without the conditioning, the hazard is not fixed in this way: an event can happen at any time t, after which observation terminates at $b_i = t + \tau$. Thus, conditioning on the observation period alters the intensity function in this hypothetical example, because fixing b_i also determines the event time. Incidentally, this also explains why it is incorrect to stop the observation process at the event time, which corresponds to setting $\tau = 0$. Realistic situations in which the event can influence the observation period include events with high short-term mortality, such as stroke.

Now suppose that Assumption 3 is not met, so that occurrence of an event influences the subsequent exposure process. Consider for example the extreme scenario in which occurrence of an event precludes any subsequent exposures. Suppose that case i is exposed at some age s_i in $(a_i, b_i]$. Conditioning on the exposure history, no event can occur before age s_i, so the conditional intensity must be zero on $(a_i, s_i]$, irrespective of what the intensity was in the absence of conditioning: again, conditioning alters the intensity function. Realistic situations in which the event can influence subsequent exposures include those in pharmacoepidemiology where occurrence of an event is a contra-indication to the drug exposure of interest. An example is intussusception and vaccination against rotavirus. Exposure variables satisfying Assumption 3 are sometimes called exogenous or external: see Kalbfleisch and Prentice (2002), pages 196–200.

Importantly, the direction of bias resulting from failure of Assumption 3 is often predictable. If occurrence of an event decreases the probability of subsequent exposures, and the SCCS method is applied without allowing for this, then the relative incidence will be biased upwards. This is because exposures will tend to occur prior to events, thus inducing bias in the direction of a positive association. If, on the other hand, occurrence of an event increases the probability of subsequent exposure, then the relative incidence will be biased downwards. The direction of bias resulting from failure of Assumption 2 is less easily predictable. The direction of the bias is influenced by the timing of exposures over the observation period.

In the more technical Section 3.7.4, it is shown how Assumptions 2 and 3 imply Equation 3.6. However, these technicalities, while necessary from the formal point of view, need not obscure what is really a rather straightforward requirement. In the SCCS method, we regard the exposure processes, the observation processes and the marginal event totals as fixed. Inference is based on the timing of events. One way to think of this inferential framework is to imagine the event history of each case being re-run over the same observation period, with the same exposures and the same total number of events. To avoid bias, the event times in such putative replications should be influenced only by those exposure and age effects we wish to estimate, irrespective of the conditioning involved.

3.7.4   A more formal demonstration*

We now show more formally how Assumptions 2 and 3 imply Equation 3.6. For simplicity we assume that the event is non-recurrent; for recurrent events, just suppress the condition $T \geq t$ in what follows, and interpret $T = t$ as meaning that an event occurred at t.

The hazard rate for individual i is formally defined as

$$P\{T \in [t, t + dt)|x_i^t, \boldsymbol{y}_i, T \geq t\} = \lambda_i(t|x_i^t, \boldsymbol{y}_i)dt, \tag{3.7}$$

where T is the event time. Let $x_i^t = \{x_{oi}^t, x_{ei}^t\}$ where x_{oi}^t is the observation history to age t and x_{ei}^t is the exposure history to age t for individual i.

Assumptions 2 and 3 may be stated formally as follows (we have suppressed the indices i to reduce clutter):

$$\text{A2} \quad : \quad P(x_o^u|x_e^u, x_o^t, \boldsymbol{y}, T = t) = P(x_o^u|x_e^u, x_o^t, \boldsymbol{y}, T \geq t) \quad \forall u \geq t; \tag{3.8}$$

$$\text{A3} \quad : \quad P(x_e^u|x_o^t, x_e^t, \boldsymbol{y}, T = t) = P(x_e^u|x_o^t, x_e^t, \boldsymbol{y}, T \geq t) \quad \forall u \geq t. \tag{3.9}$$

Note that Assumptions 2 and 3 are not symmetrical in their formal statements: thus, we allow the observation process to depend on the exposure process (as represented by the presence of x_e^u in Equation 3.8). For example, in a study of vaccine safety, it is acceptable to define the observation period as $(v - \tau_1, v + \tau_2]$ where v is age at vaccination. However, given the exposure history, the observation process must not depend on the event process.

---

* This section may be skipped.

Multiplying Equations 3.8 and 3.9 together, we obtain

$$P(x_o^u, x_e^u | x_o^t, x_e^t, \boldsymbol{y}, T = t) = P(x_o^u, x_e^u | x_o^t, x_e^t, \boldsymbol{y}, T \geq t) \quad \forall u \geq t. \quad (3.10)$$

Now by Bayes' Theorem, using the definition in Equation 3.7,

$$\lambda_i(t | x_i^u, \boldsymbol{y}_i) = \frac{P(x_i^u | x_i^t, \boldsymbol{y}_i, T = t) \times \lambda_i(t | x_i^t, \boldsymbol{y}_i)}{P(x_i^u | x_i^t, \boldsymbol{y}_i, T \geq t)}. \quad (3.11)$$

So if Assumptions 2 and 3 hold, combining Equations 3.10 and 3.11 with $x_i^t = \{x_{oi}^t, x_{ei}^t\}$ yields

$$\lambda_i(t | x_i^u, \boldsymbol{y}_i) = \lambda_i(t | x_i^t, \boldsymbol{y}_i) \quad \text{for all } u \geq t.$$

In particular, this holds for $u = b_i$, and hence the required condition 3.6 is satisfied.

3.7.5 Assumption 4: independent ascertainment

Assumption 4 states that the sampling process whereby cases are selected for inclusion in a SCCS study should not be influenced by the cases' exposure histories. This assumption differs from the other three in that it is shared by other study designs in epidemiology, including cohort and case-control studies. It is explicitly reaffirmed here because the SCCS method is so simple to apply to any collection of cases.

For example, in spontaneous reporting systems for potential drug-related adverse reactions, events of interest are reported when there is a suspicion that a drug may be the cause of the event. This is an instance where Assumption 4 is violated. While modified SCCS methods can sometimes be used in such circumstances, further assumptions are usually required: see Escolano et al. (2013).

Likewise, spurious effects may be generated by the way events are ascertained in some administrative databases. For example, in some databases medical histories are recorded retrospectively and post-dated to consultations at which drugs are prescribed, resulting in spurious associations between day of prescription and events. This is a further instance of a violation of Assumption 4. It serves to emphasise the importance of understanding the idiosyncracies of administrative databases before using the SCCS or indeed any other method of analysis.

Summary

- The SCCS method is based on the following four assumptions:

  A1 Events are uncommon or arise in Poisson processes.

  A2 Events do not influence the length of observation periods.

  A3 Events do not influence subsequent exposures.

  A4 Exposures do not influence event ascertainment.

- If Assumption 1 fails, time-invariant multiplicative confounders may not factor out of the likelihood.

- If Assumptions 2 or 3 fail, the relative incidence may be biased, because conditioning on observation periods or exposure histories alters the incidence function.

- If Assumption 3 fails, the direction of the bias is predictable.

- Assumption 4 is shared with other study designs. When applying the SCCS and other methods to data from administrative databases it is important to be aware of the idiosyncrasies of these databases.

3.8   Derivation of the SCCS likelihood*

In this section, the SCCS likelihood in Equation 3.5 is derived from a cohort model. As in Section 3.7.3, let x_i^t denote the history of exposure and observation up to age t. Then $x_i = x_i^{b_i}$ is the history of exposure and observation up to end of the observation period at age b_i.

The observation history to age t is a function on $(a_i, t]$ taking the value 1 when individual i is under observation and 0 when not. The observation history for $t \leq b_i$ is usually $(a_i, t]$, though in principle it could also consist of disjoint age or time intervals. The exposure history to age t is a set of functions on $(a_i, t]$, each representing a distinct exposure. Exposures can be quantitative or categorical. In the simplest standard SCCS model, there is a single categorical exposure, which may be represented as a time-varying factor.

We begin with a cohort of individuals labelled $i = 1, \ldots, M$ observed over age intervals $(a_i, b_i]$. These intervals are the observation periods, and may vary between individuals. Occurrences of the events of interest and exposure history up to b_i are recorded for each individual in the cohort. This cohort is

---

* This section may be skipped.

observed retrospectively, so the events and exposures for all individuals are known. Suppose that there are N cases, a case being an individual who has experienced one or more events within his or her observation period $(a_i, b_i]$. For simplicity, and without any loss of generality, we assume that the cases are listed first, and so are indexed by $i = 1, \ldots, N$. Each case experiences $n_i > 0$ events at times $t_{i1}, t_{i2}, \ldots, t_{in_i}$ in $(a_i, b_i]$, while $n_i = 0$ for the non-cases $i = N + 1, \ldots, M$. This notation is illustrated in Figure 3.5.

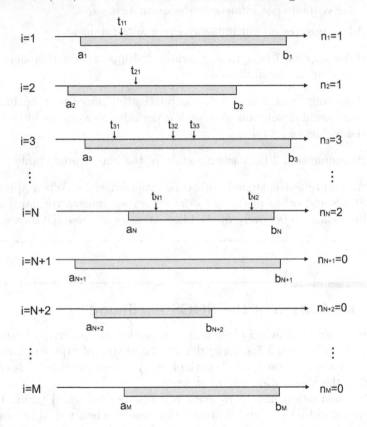

FIGURE 3.5
A cohort of size M and its N cases, showing observation periods and event times.

We suppose that Assumption 1 from Section 3.7 holds. To begin with assume that, for cohort member i, events arise in a non-homogeneous Poisson process with intensity function $\lambda_i(t|x_i^t, \boldsymbol{y}_i)$. The cohort likelihood for case $i = 1, \ldots, N$, with $n_i > 0$ events at times $t_{i1}, t_{i2}, \ldots, t_{in_i}$ in $(a_i, b_i]$, is then

$$L_{ci} = \prod_{j=1}^{n_i} \lambda_i(t_{ij}|x_i^{t_{ij}}, \boldsymbol{y}_i) \exp\left(-\int_{a_i}^{b_i} \lambda_i(s|x_i^s, \boldsymbol{y}_i)ds\right).$$

An individual $i = N+1, \ldots, M$ is a non-case and so experiences $n_i = 0$ events in $(a_i, b_i]$. The likelihood contribution for this non-case is

$$L_{ci} = \exp\left(-\int_{a_i}^{b_i} \lambda_i(s|x_i^s, \boldsymbol{y}_i)ds\right).$$

The overall likelihood for the entire cohort of cases and non-cases is thus:

$$L_c = \prod_{i=1}^{N}\prod_{j=1}^{n_i} \lambda_i(t_{ij}|x_i^{t_{ij}}, \boldsymbol{y}_i)\prod_{i=1}^{M}\exp\left(-\int_{a_i}^{b_i}\lambda_i(s|x_i^s, \boldsymbol{y}_i)ds\right). \tag{3.12}$$

The SCCS likelihood is derived from this cohort likelihood by conditioning, for each individual i, on the exposure and observation history x_i up to b_i, and the total number of events n_i observed for individual i. What is not conditioned upon is the set of event times $t_{i1}, t_{i2}, \ldots, t_{in_i}$ when $n_i > 0$.

As noted in Section 3.7.3, for inferences about the intensity functions $\lambda_i(x_i^t, \boldsymbol{y}_i)$ to be valid in the SCCS model, conditioning on the exposure and observation history x_i must not affect the intensities. Assumptions 2 and 3, stated in Section 3.7, imply the identity in Expression 3.6, namely:

$$\lambda_i(t|x_i^t, \boldsymbol{y}_i) = \lambda_i(t|x_i, \boldsymbol{y}_i) \quad \text{for all } t \text{ in } (a_i, b_i].$$

Thus, if these assumptions hold, we may replace x_i^t by x_i in Equation 3.12:

$$L_c = \prod_{i=1}^{N}\prod_{j=1}^{n_i} \lambda_i(t_{ij}|x_i, \boldsymbol{y}_i)\prod_{i=1}^{M}\exp\left(-\int_{a_i}^{b_i}\lambda_i(s|x_i, \boldsymbol{y}_i)ds\right). \tag{3.13}$$

The marginal probability, or likelihood, that individual i experiences n_i events, given the exposure and observation history, is

$$L_{mi} = \frac{1}{n_i!}\left(\int_{a_i}^{b_i}\lambda_i(s|x_i, \boldsymbol{y}_i)ds\right)^{n_i}\exp\left(-\int_{a_i}^{b_i}\lambda_i(s|x_i, \boldsymbol{y}_i)ds\right).$$

The marginal probability of the observed outcomes $n_i, i = 1, \ldots, M$ is the product of these terms, namely (since $n_i = 0$ for $i = N+1, \ldots, M$)

$$L_m = \prod_{i=1}^{N}\frac{1}{n_i!}\left(\int_{a_i}^{b_i}\lambda_i(s|x_i, \boldsymbol{y}_i)ds\right)^{n_i}\prod_{i=1}^{M}\exp\left(-\int_{a_i}^{b_i}\lambda_i(s|x_i, \boldsymbol{y}_i)ds\right). \tag{3.14}$$

The SCCS likelihood is obtained by dividing Equation 3.13 by Equation 3.14. Thus, dropping explicit mention of the constant term,

$$\frac{L_c}{L_m} = \text{constant} \times \prod_{i=1}^{N}\frac{\prod_{j=1}^{n_i}\lambda_i(t_{ij}|x_i, \boldsymbol{y}_i)}{\left(\int_{a_i}^{b_i}\lambda_i(s|x_i, \boldsymbol{y}_i)ds\right)^{n_i}}$$

which is the SCCS likelihood in Equation 3.5.

A consequence of this argument is that the non-cases drop out of the likelihood upon conditioning. The SCCS method is based on the relative timing of events and exposures, given the number of events. If there are no events, there is no information about such relative timings: non-cases are uninformative, and contribute 1 to the SCCS likelihood. The practical implication is that non-cases need not be sampled.

This derivation applies to events that arise in non-homogeneous Poisson processes within individuals, and are therefore potentially recurrent. Now suppose that the event of interest is non-recurrent, but rare. The $\lambda_i(t|x_i, \boldsymbol{y}_i)$ are then hazards rather than intensities. We assume that the M individuals in the underlying at-risk cohort have not experienced the event by the start of observation. Each case experiences a single event at age t_i in $(a_i, b_i], i = 1, \ldots, N$.

For t in $(a_i, b_i]$, let

$$S_i(a_i, t) = \exp\left(-\int_{a_i}^{t} \lambda_i(s|x_i, \boldsymbol{y}_i)ds \right)$$

denote the probability that individual i remains event-free at age t, given that he or she was event-free at the start of observation a_i. The cohort likelihood is

$$\begin{aligned}
L'_c &= \prod_{i=1}^{N} \lambda_i(t_i|x_i, \boldsymbol{y}_i) \exp\left(-\int_{a_i}^{t_i} \lambda_i(s|x_i, \boldsymbol{y}_i)ds \right) \\
&\quad \times \prod_{i=N+1}^{M} \exp\left(-\int_{a_i}^{b_i} \lambda_i(s|x_i, \boldsymbol{y}_i)ds \right) \\
&= \prod_{i=1}^{N} \lambda_i(t_i|x_i, \boldsymbol{y}_i) S_i(a_i, t_i) \prod_{i=N+1}^{M} S_i(a_i, b_i).
\end{aligned} \tag{3.15}$$

The marginal likelihood is

$$\begin{aligned}
L'_m &= \prod_{i=1}^{N} \left\{ \int_{a_i}^{b_i} \lambda_i(s|x_i, \boldsymbol{y}_i) S_i(a_i, s)ds \right\} \prod_{i=N+1}^{M} \exp\left(-\int_{a_i}^{b_i} \lambda_i(s|x_i, \boldsymbol{y}_i)ds \right) \\
&= \prod_{i=1}^{N} \left\{ 1 - S_i(a_i, b_i) \right\} \prod_{i=N+1}^{M} S_i(a_i, b_i).
\end{aligned} \tag{3.16}$$

The conditional likelihood is the ratio of Equations 3.15 and 3.16:

$$\frac{L'_c}{L'_m} = \prod_{i=1}^{N} \frac{\lambda_i(t_i|x_i, \boldsymbol{y}_i) S_i(a_i, t_i)}{\{1 - S_i(a_i, b_i)\}}.$$

This expression again only involves the N cases, but note that it is not the same as the SCCS likelihood L in Equation 3.5. However, it approximates to L since, by assumption, the event is rare. To see this, write

$$\lambda_i(t|x_i, \boldsymbol{y}_i) = \phi \nu_i(t|x_i, \boldsymbol{y}_i),$$

where ϕ is a positive constant and the functions $\nu_i(t|x_i, \boldsymbol{y}_i)$ are bounded on $(a_i, b_i]$, and consider the limit as ϕ tends to zero. In this limit, the intensity functions $\lambda_i(t|x_i, \boldsymbol{y}_i)$ tend to zero. Using the approximation $e^{-\epsilon} = 1 - \epsilon + O(\epsilon^2)$ for ϵ close to zero, it follows that

$$S_i(a_i, t) \simeq 1 - \int_{a_i}^{t} \lambda_i(s|x_i, \boldsymbol{y}_i)ds \quad \text{when } \phi \to 0.$$

So, in this limit, $S_i(a_i, t_i) \to 1$ and

$$\frac{\lambda_i(t_i|x_i, \boldsymbol{y}_i)}{1 - S_i(a_i, b_i)} \to \frac{\nu_i(t_i|x_i, \boldsymbol{y}_i)}{\int_{a_i}^{b_i} \nu_i(s|x_i, \boldsymbol{y}_i)ds} = \frac{\lambda_i(t_i|x_i, \boldsymbol{y}_i)}{\int_{a_i}^{b_i} \lambda_i(s|x_i, \boldsymbol{y}_i)ds}.$$

Thus in the limit as $\phi \to 0$,

$$\frac{L'_c}{L'_m} = \prod_{i=1}^{N} \frac{\lambda_i(t_i|x_i, \boldsymbol{y}_i)}{\int_{a_i}^{b_i} \lambda_i(s|x_i, \boldsymbol{y}_i)ds},$$

which is equivalent to the SCCS likelihood in Equation 3.5 with $n_i = 1$ and $t_i = t_{i1}$ for $i = 1, \ldots, N$. Thus, for non-recurrent events, the SCCS likelihood is valid in the limit in which the event is rare, which is usually the case in practice.

3.9 Bibliographical notes and further material

The standard SCCS model was proposed by Farrington (1995) as an epidemiological method for assessing the safety of vaccines; its genesis is described in Chapter 2, Section 2.1. The general SCCS likelihood appeared in Farrington and Whitaker (2006). The SCCS method brings together statistical theory on conditional Poisson inference, and self-controlled and case-only cohort methods from epidemiology. These three strands have numerous antecedents.

Andersen (1970) elucidated the properties of conditional likelihoods, with an example showing how incidental parameters can be eliminated by conditioning on the sum of Poisson counts. A close connection is to the work of Cox (1972) on modulated Poisson processes: Cox's conditional likelihood for a modulated Poisson process is identical to a SCCS likelihood for a single individual. Hausman et al. (1984) applied this idea in econometrics to the analysis of panel data; see also Lancaster (2000).

The use of self-controls in the context of cohort studies was discussed by Ray and Griffin (1989). Their suggestion was to compare incidence rates shortly after a point exposure to incidence rates at later periods after the exposure, controlling for age and potential confounders. When there are no age effects, this effectively reduces to the SCCS method as the estimator of the relative incidence involves only cases.

Aalen et al. (1980) proposed a method to analyse the cases arising within a cohort. This approach was developed further by Prentice et al. (1984), who suggested using a proportional hazards model on case-only data. Feldmann (1993a,b) developed a case-only method specifically for the investigation of adverse drug reactions. This coincides with the SCCS method when the event is rare and the baseline hazard is constant. The SCCS method was also derived by Becker et al. (2004), with further development in Becker et al. (2006).

Like the SCCS method, the case-crossover method of Maclure (1991) is a case-only method with self-controls. Maximum likelihood estimation for this method is described in Marshall and Jackson (1993), and design issues are discussed in Mittleman et al. (1995). Unlike the SCCS method, it is a case-control method, with referents selected from the case's own history. The method requires exposures to be exchangeable (Vines and Farrington, 2001). This implies that the probability of exposure must be constant over time, a condition that is relaxed in the case-time-control method of Suissa (1995), further investigated by Jensen et al. (2014). Case-crossover methods are useful in evaluating associations between transient exposures and acute events, and need not require information on post-event exposures.

The case-crossover method has also been used in environmental epidemiology, notably to study the health impacts of air pollution. The nomenclature in this area is a little tangled: thus, the time-stratified case-crossover method of Lumley and Levy (2000) is actually a SCCS method, event times being regarded as random rather than fixed as they are in standard case-crossover designs. The 'full-stratum' version (but not other versions) of the bidirectional case-crossover method of Navidi (1998) is a special case of the time-stratified case-crossover design, and therefore is also a SCCS method. These connections are elucidated in Whitaker et al. (2007) and Armstrong et al. (2014), and are discussed further in Chapter 6, Section 6.6. Several other case-only designs in epidemiology are discussed in Greenland (1999) and Farrington (2004).

4

The standard SCCS model

In the standard SCCS model, the observation period for each case is partitioned into non-overlapping segments on which the age and exposure effects are assumed to be constant. A version of the model was briefly described in Chapter 3, Section 3.2. In this chapter we consider this model in detail. Other models will be considered in Chapter 6.

The bulk of the chapter is devoted to fitting the standard SCCS model using the R package SCCS, illustrated with numerous practical examples, starting from Section 4.3. In this section, SCCS analyses with one exposure per case are described. In subsequent sections more complex settings are introduced: repeated exposures in Section 4.4, multiple exposure types in Section 4.5, model comparison in Section 4.6, interactions and effect modification in Section 4.7, indefinite and extremal risk periods in Section 4.8, and seasonal effects in Section 4.9.

Section 4.6.2 on combining multinomial categories and Section 4.10, in which the parameterisation of the model is described more formally, are starred to indicate that they may be skipped.

Chapter 4 may be regarded as the first half of a modelling guide for the standard SCCS model, to be completed in Chapter 5. In the present chapter, we focus on data structures and model fitting, and present some graphical displays to guide this process. In the next chapter, we will turn to checking the validity of the assumptions and modelling choices, with further graphical displays for this purpose.

4.1 Proportional incidence models

The SCCS likelihood is defined in terms of the intensity (or hazard) function $\lambda_i(t|x_i, \boldsymbol{y}_i)$ for cases $i = 1, \ldots, N$. We now turn to statistical models for this function, our primary focus being applications in epidemiology. In keeping with epidemiological terminology, we shall refer to the intensity function as the incidence rate.

All the models considered in this book are proportional incidence models. These are built up by multiplying together separate components for age, exposure and covariate effects. Thus, in conceptual terms,

Incidence rate = Baseline × Age effect × Exposure effect × Covariate effect.

In mathematical notation, the proportional incidence model is of the form:

$$\lambda_i(t|x_i, \boldsymbol{y}_i) = \phi_i \psi(t|\boldsymbol{y}_i) \rho(t|x_i, \boldsymbol{y}_i) h_i(\boldsymbol{y}_i).$$

The constants ϕ_i are absolute incidence rates at some reference age, describing the baseline incidence. The function $\psi(t|\boldsymbol{y}_i)$ represents the age effect at age t for individual i, relative to that reference age. The relative age effect may depend on the time-invariant covariates $\boldsymbol{y}_i$. The function $\rho(t|x_i, \boldsymbol{y}_i)$ represents the relative incidence associated with exposure. This depends on the exposure history in x_i for individual i, and may also depend on the time-invariant covariates $\boldsymbol{y}_i$. The functions h_i specify the main effect of the time-invariant covariates $\boldsymbol{y}_i$ on the incidence rate, as distinct from any interactions with age effects or time-varying exposures.

The constants ϕ_i and the time-invariant effects $h_i(\boldsymbol{y}_i)$ cancel out of the SCCS likelihood, as previously described in Chapter 3. These quantities are not estimated in the SCCS model, and so will not be considered further. For this reason, we leave them unspecified and focus on the time-varying kernel of the incidence rate function:

$$\nu(t|x_i, \boldsymbol{y}_i) = \psi(t|\boldsymbol{y}_i) \rho(t|x_i, \boldsymbol{y}_i). \tag{4.1}$$

In its simplest form, this model may be written:

Incidence rate kernel = Age effect × Exposure effect.

In the standard SCCS model, age and exposure effects are assumed to be piecewise constant. Age effects take different levels on pre-defined age groups. The age groups and levels are common to all cases. Exposures are discrete, switching on and off or between a restricted set of levels during an individual's observation period. They might represent, for example, treatment period on pharmaceutical drugs, the durations of which may vary between patients, or washout periods following treatments. They might also represent risk intervals following point exposures, such as vaccinations. Quantitative exposures (those measured on a continuous scale) will be discussed in Chapter 6. The age and exposure levels are represented by parameters, the values of which are estimated by maximising the SCCS likelihood.

The simplest such model assumes there is a single exposure type and no interactions with time-invariant covariates. The incidence rate kernel is piecewise constant, taking values that depend only on age parameters α_j representing the age effect at levels $j = 0, \ldots, J$, and exposure parameters β_k representing the exposure effect at levels $k = 0, \ldots, K$.

In this simple model, the incidence rate kernel at age t takes the value

$$\nu_{ijk} = \exp(\alpha_j) \times \exp(\beta_k) = \exp(\alpha_j + \beta_k)$$

when t lies within an interval at level j for age and level k for exposure for case i. The parameters α_j and β_k are log relative incidences, relative to the reference level 0, with $\alpha_0 = \beta_0 = 0$. Thus, there are $J + K$ parameters to be estimated.

Generally, the exposure-related parameters β_k are of primary interest, and hence provide the focus of inference. The log relative incidence parameter β_k has the following interpretation: the incidence rate is multiplied by $\exp(\beta_k)$ when the individual is at exposure level k, relative to the incidence rate when at the reference level 0, over and above any age effect. Thus, if $\beta_k = 0$ there is no effect at exposure level k. The exposure is associated with an increase in incidence if $\beta_k > 0$, and with a decrease in incidence if $\beta_k < 0$. The age parameters α_j have a similar interpretation. Thus, the incidence at age level j is the incidence at the reference level 0, multiplied by $\exp(\alpha_j)$. Further details of this parameterisation may be found in Section 4.10.

Summary

- All SCCS models considered are proportional incidence models, in which the different components (of age, exposure, covariates) are combined multiplicatively.

- Time-invariant quantities cancel out of the SCCS likelihood, so we focus on the incidence rate kernel which involves only time-varying effects.

- The simplest such model is of the form

    Incidence rate kernel = Age effect × Exposure effect.

- In the standard SCCS model, age and exposure effects are assumed to be piecewise constant, and so the incidence rate kernel is also piecewise constant.

4.2   Fitting the standard SCCS model

The simple model $\nu_{ijk} = \exp(\alpha_j + \beta_k)$ described in Section 4.1 defines a log-linear model with model formula

Age + Exposure.

The model can be elaborated further to include interactions with time-invariant covariates y_i, several exposures (and interactions between them), and seasonal as well as age effects. All these features will be exemplified in subsequent sections.

The first step in fitting the model is to reshape the data (a practical illustration is provided in Section 4.3.2). Each individual's observation period is split into distinct segments E_{ijk} of length e_{ijk}, on which the incidence rate kernel for individual i is constant at age level j and exposure level k. The boundaries of the segments E_{ijk} are determined by the cutpoints used to define the age and exposure groups. The number of events n_{ijk} in each segment for individual i is also obtained. Let n_i denote the array $\{n_{ijk}, j = 0, \ldots, J; k = 0, \ldots, K\}$, for $i = 1, \ldots, N$, N being the number of cases. The standard SCCS model is then

$$n_i \sim \text{Multinomial}(n_i; p_i),$$

this denoting the multinomial distribution with index n_i and probability array p_i with elements

$$p_{ijk} = \frac{\nu_{ijk} e_{ijk}}{\sum_{r,s} \nu_{irs} e_{irs}}.$$

The model can be fitted directly with software for conditional Poisson or product multinomial models. Alternatively, some other models commonly used in epidemiology can be coaxed into a form suitable for our purposes. We briefly describe two such options.

The first method is to use the so-called Poisson trick, whereby an associated Poisson model is fitted with an extra individual-level factor γ with levels $i = 1, \ldots, N$ (McCullagh and Nelder, 1989, page 212). This associated model has a logarithmic link and offsets $\log(e_{ijk})$ and is defined as follows:

$$n_{ijk} \sim P(\nu_{ijk} e_{ijk}),$$
$$\log(\nu_{ijk}) = \alpha_j + \beta_k + \gamma_i.$$

This model can be fitted with any software for generalised linear models. The parameters γ_i are needed to constrain the marginal totals to their observed values, but are of no intrinsic interest. In large data sets, γ is high-dimensional and so it is desirable to use a fitting algorithm with an absorption facility, so that the incidental parameters γ_i are not estimated explicitly.

A second approach is to note that the likelihood contribution for each event, say

$$\frac{\nu_{ijk} e_{ijk}}{\sum_{r,s} \nu_{irs} e_{irs}}, \tag{4.2}$$

is of the same form as that of a case-control set in a $1 : M_i$ matched case-control study (Breslow and Day, 1980, page 248). The 'case' is a case interval, namely the interval in which the event occurred; the 'controls' are the M_i non-empty control intervals within the observation period $(a_i, b_i]$ in which the event did not occur. Software to fit conditional logistic regression models can thus be adapted to fit the standard SCCS model. Indeed, software to fit the

Cox proportional hazards model can also be adapted to this purpose, the form of Expression 4.2 being similar to that of a partial likelihood contribution, the risk set now playing the role of the matched case-control set (Cox and Oakes, 1984, page 92). This is the approach taken in R package SCCS.

Summary

- The first step in fitting the standard SCCS model is to reshape the data, by splitting each observation period into non-overlapping intervals in which the age and exposure effects are constant.

- The standard SCCS model is a log-linear product multinomial model. Several techniques can be used to fit the model using standard statistical software.

4.3 The R package SCCS: standard SCCS model

To download R and the R package SCCS, see Chapter 1, Section 1.4. The standard model is fitted using the single function standardsccs. This function reshapes the data and fits the model.

All data sets should include an individual identifier (in the function standardsccs this is argument indiv), the age at event (argument aevent), the age at start of observation (astart), and the age at end of observation (aend). Variables describing the exposures – which take different forms depending on the application – and time-invariant covariates will be described where they arise. If calendar time is the time line of interest, ages are replaced by times from a reference date. In most of the applications described in this book, ages or times are in days; other choices may be appropriate depending on context, but must be specified as integers.

In the examples in this section, each case is exposed once. The data comprise one line per event. In Section 4.4, two different data formats will be described to handle more general situations in which there are repeat exposures.

4.3.1 A single point exposure: MMR vaccine and ITP

These data were collected to investigate the association between measles, mumps and rubella (MMR) vaccine and idiopathic thrombocytopaenic purpura (ITP). Cases were obtained from hospital admissions and linked to vaccination records. All admissions to these hospitals occurring in children aged 366 to 730 days – that is, the second year of life – between specified dates in

1991 and 1994 (which varied between hospitals) were identified. The data are based on those published in Miller et al. (2001).

The data comprise 44 ITP admissions in 35 children. The observation period for each of the 35 children is determined by the age and time boundaries used to select the cases. For example, in one hospital the calendar time period of data collection was 1st October 1991 to 30th September 1994; the observation periods for cases from that hospital, on a scale of age in days, stretch from the maximum of 366 and age (in days) on 1st October 1994, to the minimum of 730 days and age (in days) on 30th September 1994. (The choice of observation periods is discussed more generally in Chapter 8.) Five cases had two events, and one case had five events. The data for the first six cases are shown in Table 4.1.

TABLE 4.1
The first 6 cases from the MMR vaccine and ITP study; ages are in days.

Case	Age at event	Age at first day of observation	Age at last day of observation	Age at MMR vaccination	Sex
1	691	454	730	670	1
2	722	366	730	868	2
3	442	366	730	540	1
4	429	366	730	378	2
5	414	366	730	710	1
5	418	366	730	710	1
6	708	439	730	487	1

Case 5 in Table 4.1 had two events, at ages 414 and 418 days. Case 2 was vaccinated at 868 days, after the end of observation, and so is unexposed in the observation period.

The risk period was taken to be the six-week period after MMR vaccination (if the child received MMR vaccine), that is, the period 0 to 42 days inclusive post-MMR, day 0 denoting the day MMR vaccine was administered. To investigate in more detail the risk profile, the period was also split into 3 two-week risk periods: 0 to 14, 15 to 28, and 29 to 42 days post-MMR. These risk periods are shown in Figure 4.1.

In this study, ITP cases not at risk from MMR during the observation period were included. These cases contribute to the estimation of the age effect, which was assumed to be constant on the 2-month intervals [366, 426], [427, 487], [488, 548], [549, 609], [610, 670] and [671, 730] days; the age group boundaries are shown in Figure 4.1.

The case identifier (taking the same value for events within the same individual) is case. The start and end of the observation periods are in variables sta and end, while the age at ITP is in variable itp. The exposure information

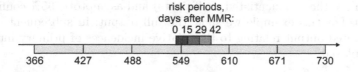

FIGURE 4.1
Observation period, age group boundaries and risk periods for the ITP and MMR study.

available is the age at MMR vaccination, in variable mmr. The fixed covariate sex is also available (coded 1 for boys, 2 for girls).

The package SCCS includes all the data sets used in this book. The data for this application are in data frame itpdat. The standard SCCS model is specified as follows.

```
library(SCCS)
itp.mod1 <- standardsccs(event~mmr+age, indiv=case, astart=sta,
            aend=end, aevent=itp, adrug=mmr, aedrug=mmr+42,
            expogrp=c(0,15,29), agegrp=c(427,488,549,610,671),
            data=itpdat)
```

The entry

event~mmr+age

specifies the model formula, in standard R syntax. The individual identifier is indicated by indiv=case. The ages at which the observation periods begin and end are defined by the pair

astart=sta, aend=end.

The age at event is specified by aevent=itp. The exposure groups are defined by the triple

adrug=mmr, aedrug=mmr+42, expogrp=c(0,15,29).

The variable adrug specifies the age at MMR vaccine, while aedrug is the end of drug-related exposure. The vector expogrp defines the exposure periods: the convention used throughout is to specify the first day of each risk period in relation to adrug. The risk periods are assumed to be contiguous, the final one ending at aedrug. The vector agegrp specifies the first day of each age group except the first (which is the earliest age at start of observation); it defaults to NULL if no age groups are required, in which case there is effectively a single age group covering all observation periods. Finally, the data frame from which the variables are chosen is specified by the data argument.

The output, which is stored in itp.mod1, includes the estimated parameters and their standard errors, as well as the corresponding relative incidences

(which are the exponentiated coefficients) and asymptotic 95% confidence intervals. For this example we show the full output; in subsequent examples,
only edited output relating to the relative incidences of primary interest will
be displayed.

```
> itp.mod1
Call:
coxph(formula = Surv(rep(1, 392L), event) ~ mmr + age +
    strata(indivL) + offset(log(interval)), data =
    chopdat, method = "exact")

  n= 392, number of events= 44

        coef exp(coef) se(coef)       z Pr(>|z|)
mmr1  0.2692    1.3089   0.7529   0.357   0.7207
mmr2  1.7841    5.9540   0.4388   4.065 4.79e-05 ***
mmr3  0.9556    2.6002   0.6375   1.499   0.1339
age2 -0.4209    0.6565   0.4075  -1.033   0.3017
age3 -1.5584    0.2105   0.6448  -2.417   0.0156 *
age4 -1.2329    0.2915   0.5756  -2.142   0.0322 *
age5 -0.9266    0.3959   0.5356  -1.730   0.0836 .
age6 -0.9123    0.4016   0.5360  -1.702   0.0887 .
---
Signif. codes:  0 *** 0.001 ** 0.01 * 0.05 . 0.1   1

     exp(coef) exp(-coef) lower .95 upper .95
mmr1    1.3089     0.7640   0.29922    5.7253
mmr2    5.9540     0.1680   2.51922   14.0717
mmr3    2.6002     0.3846   0.74536    9.0709
age2    0.6565     1.5233   0.29538    1.4591
age3    0.2105     4.7513   0.05948    0.7447
age4    0.2915     3.4311   0.09432    0.9006
age5    0.3959     2.5259   0.13857    1.1311
age6    0.4016     2.4902   0.14046    1.1482

Rsquare= 0.075    (max possible= 0.399 )
Likelihood ratio test= 30.45  on 8 df,    p=0.0001757
Wald test             = 34.63  on 8 df,    p=3.129e-05
Score (logrank) test = 49.14   on 8 df,    p=5.977e-08
```

The output of primary interest lies in the second table of results. The rows
labelled mmr1, mmr2 and mmr3 corresponds to the three risk periods. The first
column (under exp(coef)) gives the relative incidence; the last two columns
give the lower and upper 95% confidence limits. The remaining rows of this
table, labelled age2 to age6, correspond to the age effects relative to the first
age group.

The estimated relative incidence is raised in the 0–42 day period after MMR vaccination, significantly so in the second and third week after receiving the vaccine, when the relative incidence (RI) is 5.95, 95% confidence interval (CI) (2.52, 14.1). The age-specific relative incidence appears to decline with age after the first 2-month period (the reference period) before increasing again slightly.

To obtain the average relative incidence over the 0–42 day post-MMR risk period, we combine the three risk periods into one and refit the SCCS model (from now on, only edited output will be displayed):

```
itp.mod2 <- standardsccs(event~mmr+age, indiv=case, astart=sta,
          aend=end, aevent=itp, adrug=mmr, aedrug=mmr+42,
          agegrp=c(427,488,549,610,671), data=itpdat)
```

This yields:

```
> itp.mod2
......
      exp(coef) exp(-coef) lower .95 upper .95
mmr1    3.2262      0.310    1.53197    6.7941
```

Thus the relative incidence over the 0–42 day period post-MMR is 3.23, with 95% CI (1.53, 6.79).

4.3.2   Reshaping the MMR vaccine and ITP data

Before the SCCS model can be applied, the data first need to be reshaped as described in Section 4.2. The function `standardsccs` automatically reshapes the data, so there is usually no need to delve into this aspect of the analysis. Nevertheless, in this section we give some brief details of how this is done for the MMR vaccine and ITP data from Section 4.3.1.

Briefly, the observation period of each case is split up into successive intervals on which the age and exposure effects are constant. The reshaped data comprise the interval lengths indexed by the levels of the age and exposure variables, and the number of events in each interval. The reshaping is done by the R function `formatdata` within the R package SCCS. This function produces a new data frame with a row for each time interval (the original data comprised a row for each event). The function uses a similar syntax to `standardsccs`, but without the model formula.

For example, `formatdata` is applied to the MMR vaccine and ITP data as follows:

```
itp.dat1 <- formatdata(indiv=case, astart=sta, aend=end,
          aevent=itp, adrug=mmr, aedrug=mmr+42,
          expogrp=c(0,15,29), agegrp=c(427,488,549,610,671),
          data=itpdat)
```

The new data frame `itp.dat1` comprises 12 variables and 392 rows. Owing to space constraints we present only 9 of these 12 variables (the three not displayed are expanded versions of `aevent`, `astart` and `aend`), and limit the output to 19 rows of data. The leftmost column should be ignored (it numbers the intervals; the missing numbers correspond to intervals of zero length, which have been removed).

```
> itp.dat1
    indivL event eventday lower upper interval age mmr indiv
3        1     0      691   454   487       34   2   0     1
4        1     0      691   488   548       61   3   0     1
5        1     0      691   549   609       61   4   0     1
6        1     0      691   610   669       60   5   0     1
7        1     0      691   670   670        1   5   1     1
8        1     0      691   671   684       14   6   1     1
9        1     1      691   685   698       14   6   2     1
10       1     0      691   699   712       14   6   3     1
11       1     0      691   713   730       18   6   0     1
......
475     44     0      411   366   382       17   1   0    35
476     44     0      411   383   397       15   1   1    35
477     44     1      411   398   411       14   1   2    35
478     44     0      411   412   425       14   1   3    35
479     44     0      411   426   426        1   1   0    35
480     44     0      411   427   487       61   2   0    35
481     44     0      411   488   548       61   3   0    35
482     44     0      411   549   609       61   4   0    35
483     44     0      411   610   670       61   5   0    35
484     44     0      411   671   730       60   6   0    35
```

The first 9 rows correspond to the exposure and event history of the first case (`indiv=1`), who experienced a single event. The last 10 rows correspond to the last case (`indiv=35`), who also experienced a single event. The new variables `lower` and `upper` specify the endpoints of each interval, and `interval` its duration. The variable `event` is an indicator variable showing which interval contains the event; and variables `age` and `mmr` contain the age and exposure levels corresponding to each interval.

Thus, for example, the first interval for the first case is [454, 487] days, which does not contain an event, is at age level 2, and exposure level 0 (unexposed). The last interval for the last case is [671, 730] days, does not contain an event, is at age level 6 and exposure level 0.

Individuals with several events are replicated; the new variable `indivL` counts events, not individuals, and thus takes values 1 to 44 (the number of events) rather than 1 to 35 (the number of cases).

4.3.3   Extended exposures: antidepressants and hip fracture

In the MMR and ITP example, the risk periods were determined by the point exposure resulting from receipt of the MMR vaccine. In other situations, the risk periods are determined by the treatment, the duration of which will generally vary between individuals. The present example uses 1000 simulated cases similar to the data in Hubbard et al. (2003). The exposure is the first period of treatment with an antidepressant and the outcome is first hip fracture. The risk periods are defined as follows. Each period on drug is split into three risk periods: an initial period of 0–14 days (0 days being the start of treatment) to represent the acute risk associated with treatment initiation, followed by an intermediate risk period of 15–42 days. A third risk period then stretches from day 43 until the end of treatment. At the end of the treatment period, there are two washout periods of 91 days each before the risk is assumed to return to baseline. These washout periods are intended to capture residual effects of the drug after its withdrawal, but also reflect uncertainty in the precise end of exposure. Thus, we use 5 relative incidence parameters: 3 for the period on drug, and 2 for the washout periods. These choices are illustrated in Figure 4.2.

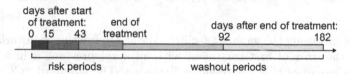

FIGURE 4.2
Risk and washout periods for the antidepressants and hip fracture data.

There are 1000 cases, in data frame `hipdat`. When dealing with moderately large data sets it is useful to visualise the observation periods, or other aspects of the data, in a suitable plot. The following code produces the plot in Figure 4.3.

```
par(mar=c(4.1,4.1,1,1), cex.lab=1.4)
os <- order(hipdat$sta)
plot(c(min(hipdat$sta/365.25),max(hipdat$end/365.25)), c(1,
    length(hipdat$case)), type="n", xlab="age (years)",
    ylab="case rank")
segments(hipdat$sta[os]/365.25, hipdat$case,
        hipdat$end[os]/365.25, hipdat$case)
```

The observation periods span the age range 72 to 87 years, with much variation in their starting points and durations. A simple way to choose the age bands is to use the quantiles of the age at event (rounded to integer days) via the `quantile` function; we define 20 age groups in this way. The washout periods

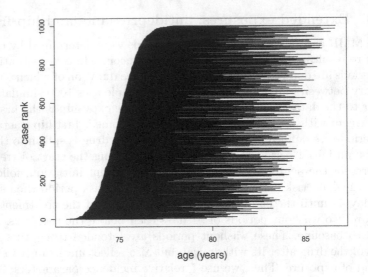

FIGURE 4.3
Distribution of the observation periods for the hip fracture data.

are specified using the washout facility. Age at hip fracture is in variable frac. Age at the start of first treatment with an antidepressant is in ad, and the age at the end of this treatment is in endad. The standard SCCS model is specified as follows.

```
ageq <- floor(quantile(hipdat$frac, seq(0.05,0.95,0.05),
        names=F))
hip.mod1 <- standardsccs(event~ad+age, indiv=case, astart=sta,
            aend=end, aevent=frac, adrug=ad, aedrug=endad,
            expogrp=c(0,15,43), washout=c(1,92,182),
            agegrp=ageq, data=hipdat)
```

The two washout periods are [endad+1, endad+91] and [endad+92, endad+182]. The entries in the washout vector are the days at the start of each interval, counted from aedrug, and the end of the final washout period.

The edited output for the five risk periods is:

```
> hip.mod1
......
      exp(coef) exp(-coef) lower .95 upper .95
ad1     2.1477    0.4656    1.2594    3.663
ad2     1.8472    0.5414    1.2013    2.840
ad3     1.5164    0.6595    1.2583    1.827
ad4     1.2527    0.7983    0.9263    1.694
ad5     1.0273    0.9734    0.7368    1.432
```

The five relative incidences are given by ad1 to ad5. In the $[0, 14]$-day risk period, $RI = 2.15$, 95% CI $(1.26, 3.66)$. In the $[15, 42]$-day risk period, $RI = 1.85$, 95% CI $(1.20, 2.84)$. Thus, the risk of a hip fracture is significantly increased in the 0–14 and 15–42 day periods after first receiving an antidepressant. The relative incidence remains significantly above 1 for the rest of the treatment period: $RI = 1.52$, 95% CI $(1.26, 1.83)$. It drops to values not statistically significantly different from 1 during the washout periods.

4.4 Data formats for repeated exposures

In both the ITP and the hip fracture examples, each case was exposed once, and the exposure periods were contiguous. Very commonly, there may be repeat exposures, corresponding for example to multiple doses of the same vaccine, or repeat treatment periods with the same drug. To handle these more general settings, we use one of two data formats, specified within the function standardsccs by the argument dataformat. The two options are dataformat="stack" (the default) and dataformat="multi".

Suppose that there is just one type of exposure, that may be repeated several times; in Section 4.5 we will consider several different types of exposure. In the stack format, repeat exposures are stacked into one single column, and for each event there are as many rows of data as repeat exposures. In the multi format, on the other hand, repeat exposures are specified by multiple sets of columns – one set for each repeat – and there is one row of data per event.

For example, suppose that individual i has start of observation a, end of observation b, event at t, and two exposure periods $[c_1, d_1]$ and $[c_2, d_2]$. In data format stack, individual i appears as two rows in the data set, one for each exposure; entries unrelated to the exposure are repeated:

```
indiv   astart   aend   aevent   expo   endexpo
......
  i       a        b       t       c1       d1
  i       a        b       t       c2       d2
......
```

In data format multi, on the other hand, individual i appears as one row in the data set:

```
indiv   astart   aend   aevent   expo1   endexpo1   expo2   endexpo2
......
  i       a        b       t       c1        d1       c2        d2
......
```

Format stack is particularly useful when the number of repeated exposures is large, which makes it awkward to accommodate them as separate variables. A typical application is to intermittent treatments for chronic conditions. Format `multi` may be used when there is a small number of repeated exposures, and when a dose effect of the exposures may be present. This format is useful when there are successive doses of a drug, as for multi-dose vaccines. Under data format `multi`, the model is specified using only the variable name for the first exposure period; this will be described in Section 4.4.2. Occasionally, the risk periods may overlap: for example, the risk period after one dose may end after the next dose. The convention used in data format `"multi"` is that the most recent exposure period takes precedence, and the parameterisation of the SCCS model is adjusted accordingly.

If an individual experiences more than one event, the information for each recurrence is entered as additional rows. Thus, for example, if individual i described above has two events at times t_1 and t_2, these appear as four rows under format `stack`:

indiv	astart	aend	aevent	expo	endexpo
. . . . . .
i	a	b	t1	c1	d1
i	a	b	t1	c2	d2
i	a	b	t2	c1	d1
i	a	b	t2	c2	d2
. . . . . .

and as two rows under format `multi`:

indiv	astart	aend	aevent	expo1	endexpo1	expo2	endexpo2
. . . . . .
i	a	b	t1	c1	d1	c2	d2
i	a	b	t2	c1	d1	c2	d2
. . . . . .

The variable `indiv` is used to keep track of which events occur within which individuals.

4.4.1 Intermittent treatments: NSAIDs and GI bleeds

This example uses data in format `stack`, the default format. Non-steroidal anti inflammatory drugs (NSAIDs) are known to increase the risk of gastrointestinal (GI) bleeds. The data in this example are a subset of a simulated data set to be described in Section 4.5.2. This subset includes 838 cases of a first GI bleed. Exposure to NSAIDs is intermittent: these cases had a total 2920 such exposures, of different durations. Only cases with at least one exposure are included. In Chapter 5, we will discuss the validity of the assumptions for these data.

The data are in data frame `gidat`. This being in format `stack`, the information on the exposure periods is stacked in two columns: `ns`, containing the age at start of exposure, and `endns`, containing the age at the end of the period of exposure. These exposure periods constitute the risk periods. Age at first GI bleed is in `bleed`. The variable `case` identifies the distinct cases (the numbering is not consecutive as the data are extracted from a larger data set).

Plots of the observation periods and risk periods may be obtained from the following code; for the former, we first need to remove duplicated starts and ends of the observation periods which inevitably arise for repeated exposures in data format `stack`; this is done using R function `duplicated`.

```
par(mfrow=c(1,2), mar=c(4.1,4.1,1,1), cex.lab=1.4)
usta <- gidat$sta[duplicated(gidat$case)==0]
uend <- gidat$end[duplicated(gidat$case)==0]
os <- order(usta)
plot(c(min(usta)/365.25,max(uend)/365.25), c(1,length(os)),
     type="n", xlab="age (years)", ylab="case rank")
segments(usta[os]/365.25, 1:length(os), uend[os]/365.25,
         1:length(os))
os2 <- order(gidat$ns)
plot(c(min(gidat$ns)/365.25, max(gidat$endns)/365.25), c(1,
     length(os2)), type="n", xlab="age (years)", ylab=
     "exposure rank")
segments(gidat$ns[os2]/365.25, 1:length(os2),
         gidat$endns[os2]/365.25, 1:length(os2))
```

The plots are shown in Figure 4.4. NSAID exposures are generally brief, longer exposures are more frequent at older ages. The observation periods last

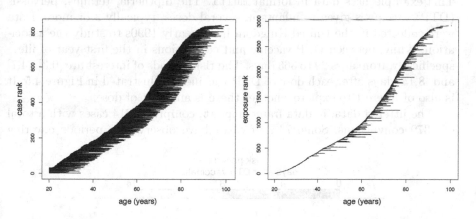

FIGURE 4.4
GI bleed data. Left: observation periods. Right: exposures to NSAIDs.

between 6 months and 15 years, much less than the span of the data. We shall use 40 age groups, based on the quantiles of the age at GI bleed. Note that rows relating to multiple exposures need to be removed for this purpose:

```
ageq <- floor(quantile(gidat$bleed[duplicated(gidat$case)==0],
       seq(0.025,0.975,0.025), names=F))
```

The default factor level for the age factor is the first, lowest age group. This being a rather atypical age group, we change the reference level to the middle age group (level 21); this does not alter the exposure effects. With this age group as reference, the standard SCCS model is fitted as follows (specifying dataformat="stack" is not strictly necessary as this is the default).

```
gi.mod1 <- standardsccs(event~ns+relevel(age,ref=21),
           indiv=case, astart=sta, aend=end, aevent=bleed,
           adrug=ns, aedrug=endns, agegrp=ageq,
           dataformat="stack", data=gidat)
```

This produces the following results.

```
> gi.mod1
......
          exp(coef) exp(-coef) lower .95 upper .95
ns1        2.02466     0.4939    1.64957    2.4850
```

The relative incidence is 2.02, 95% CI (1.65, 2.49). Thus, NSAIDs are associated with a twofold increase in GI bleeds.

4.4.2   Multiple vaccine doses: convulsions and DTP vaccine

This example uses data in format multi. The diptheria, tetanus, pertussis (DTP) vaccine is given to infants in several doses, typically 3 or more. Data were collected in the United Kingdom in the early 1990s to study the association, if any, between DTP vaccine and convulsions in the first year of life – specifically, from ages 29 to 365 days. The risk periods of interest are [0,3], [4,7] and [8,14] days after each dose of DTP vaccine, as illustrated in Figure 4.5. It is also of interest to explore whether there is an effect of dose.

The jittered data, in data frame dtpdat, comprise 1214 cases with a total of 1379 convulsions. Some 73% of cases have observation periods covering

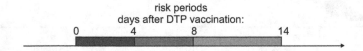

FIGURE 4.5
Risk periods for DTP vaccine and convulsions.

the whole period 29 to 365 days, so the histogram of ages at convulsion in Figure 4.6 is informative about the trend with age – which is increasing from about 6 months of age. DTP vaccinations, on the other hand, occur mainly in the first six months of life. The age at event is in variable conv. The ages

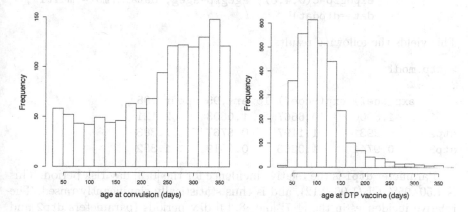

FIGURE 4.6
Left: age at convulsion. Right: age at DTP vaccine (3 doses combined).

at DTP vaccination are in three separate variables, called dtp for the first dose, dtpd2 for the second dose and dtpd3 for the third dose. Not all children received all 3 doses.

Figure 4.6 is obtained as follows. The R function duplicated is used to obtain the ages at DTP vaccination in cases; these are numbered in variable case. It is needed because a case can experience several convulsions.

```
par(mfrow=c(1,2), mar=c(4.1,4.1,1,1), cex.lab=1.4)
hist(dtpdat$conv, breaks=seq(29,369,20), xlab=
    "age at convulsion (days)", main=NULL)
uni <- (duplicated(dtpdat$case)==0)
vac <- c(dtpdat$dtp[uni==1],dtpdat$dtpd2[uni==1],
    dtpdat$dtpd3[uni==1])
hist(vac, main=NULL, xlab="age at DTP vaccine (days)")
```

In view of the strong age dependence of both events and exposures, careful control of age is required. We shall use 12 roughly 4-weekly age groups. The exposure information is entered in function standardsccs as the array cbind(dtp,dtpd2,dtpd3). However, the model formula is specified as event~dtp+age – thus, the exposure is called by the name of the first dose. The default model under data format multi assumes common exposure parameters at each dose. There are three exposure periods after each dose, so there are three parameters, common to each dose. The model is specified as follows.

```
ageg <- c(57,85,113,141,169,197,225,253,281,309,337)
dtp.mod1 <- standardsccs(event~dtp+age, indiv=case, astart=sta,
           aend=end, aevent=conv, adrug=cbind(dtp,dtpd2,
           dtpd3), aedrug=cbind(dtp+14,dtpd2+14,dtpd3+14),
           expogrp=c(0,4,8), agegrp=ageg, dataformat="multi",
           data=dtpdat)
```

This yields the following results.

```
> dtp.mod1
......
      exp(coef) exp(-coef) lower .95 upper .95
dtp1    1.5000     0.6667    1.0608     2.121
dtp2    0.8931     1.1197    0.5767     1.383
dtp3    0.9741     1.0266    0.7019     1.352
```

Parameter dtp1 is the relative incidence for the $[0, 3]$ day risk period. This is 1.50, 95% CI $(1.06, 2.12)$, and is thus statistically significantly raised. The relative incidences in the $[4, 7]$ and $[8, 14]$ day periods (parameters dtp2 and dtp3, respectively) are 0.89 and 0.97, and are both statistically non significant.

This model assumes that there is no dose effect, so that the relative incidences in each dose-related risk period are the same for all three doses – with a common parameter for each risk period. Setting sameexpopar = F allows a separate dose-specific parameter to be fitted at each dose (the default is sameexpopar = T). We now alter the model to allow different parameter values at different doses.

```
dtp.mod2 <- standardsccs(event~dtp+age, indiv=case, astart=sta,
           aend=end, aevent=conv, adrug=cbind(dtp,dtpd2,
           dtpd3), aedrug=cbind(dtp+14,dtpd2+14,dtpd3+14),
           expogrp=c(0,4,8), agegrp=ageg, dataformat="multi",
           sameexpopar=F, data=dtpdat)
```

This yields:

```
> dtp.mod2
......
      exp(coef) exp(-coef) lower .95 upper .95
dtp1    1.5678     0.6379    0.8741     2.812
dtp2    0.8499     1.1766    0.3914     1.845
dtp3    1.2519     0.7988    0.7513     2.086
dtp4    1.3495     0.7410    0.7282     2.501
dtp5    0.6128     1.6318    0.2506     1.499
dtp6    0.9051     1.1048    0.5128     1.598
dtp7    1.5984     0.6256    0.9114     2.803
dtp8    1.2274     0.8147    0.6501     2.318
dtp9    0.7716     1.2959    0.4212     1.414
```

There are now 9 exposure parameters: one for each risk period, for each of the three doses. The three parameters corresponding to the $[0, 3]$ day risk periods are labelled dtp1, dtp4, dtp7. Their values are similar, so there is little evidence of a dose effect. The parameters for the $[4, 7]$ day risk periods are labelled dtp2, dtp5, dtp8, and those for the $[8, 14]$ day risk periods are dtp3, dtp6, dtp9.

Inspection of the parameter estimates suggests that there is little evidence of any effect other than in the $[0, 3]$ day risk period, and little evidence of any variation with dose (a more formal procedure will be described in Section 4.6). Accordingly, we simplify the model to include only this risk period, and fit it without the dose effect, that is, with the default setting sameexpopar = T:

```
dtp.mod3 <- standardsccs(event~dtp+age, indiv=case, astart=sta,
             aend=end, aevent=conv, adrug=cbind(dtp,dtpd2,
             dtpd3), aedrug=cbind(dtp+3, dtpd2+3,
             dtpd3+3), agegrp=ageg, dataformat="multi",
             sameexpopar=T, data=dtpdat)
```

which yields:

```
> dtp.mod3
......
     exp(coef) exp(-coef) lower .95 upper .95
dtp1    1.5187     0.6585    1.0795     2.137
```

In conclusion, there is a marginally significant effect in the risk period $[0, 3]$ days after DTP vaccination, $RI = 1.52$, 95% CI $(1.08, 2.14)$, and little evidence of a dose effect.

Note finally that we chose to name the first DTP dose dtp rather than dtp1 and the second and third DTP doses dtpd2 and dtpd3 rather than dtp2 and dtp3 in order to avoid confusion with the parameters, which are labelled dtp1, dtp2... . We shall use a similar convention with other multi-dose vaccines.

4.5 Multiple exposure types

In some circumstances, several exposures of different types (as distinct from repeated exposures of the same type) may be associated with the event of interest. It may then be advisable to include these different exposure types simultaneously in the model. For both data formats, the additional exposure types are included as additional columns. For the stack format, missing values NA are used as padding when the number of exposures for different types differ. For example, suppose that there are two exposure types expo1 and expo2, and that individual i with a single event at age t experiences two episodes $[c_j, d_j]$, $j = 1, 2$, of the first exposure type, and three episodes $[e_k, f_k]$, $k = 1, 2, 3$, of the second exposure type. In data format `stack`, the data for individual i will then be as follows:

```
indiv  astart  aend  aevent  expo1  endexpo1  expo2  endexpo2
......
  i      a      b     t       c1      d1        e1      f1
  i      a      b     t       c2      d2        e2      f2
  i      a      b     t       NA      NA        e3      f3
......
```

We consider examples in both data formats.

4.5.1 Exposures of several types: convulsions, Hib and MMR vaccines

In this example, there is at most one instance of each exposure for each case, so the two data formats coincide (and we use the default format). The vaccine against *Haemophilus influenzae* type B (Hib) is administered to babies, with a further booster dose in the second year of life. The present data concern the possible association between Hib vaccination and convulsions in children aged 366 to 730 days of age. However, this is also the age range at which measles, mumps and rubella (MMR) vaccine is given, which has a well-known association with convulsions. To investigate the association, if any, between Hib booster vaccine and convulsions, it is therefore necessary to allow for the effect of MMR vaccine, which may be given at the same time as or in close temporal proximity to Hib vaccine. Thus, both exposure types must be modelled simultaneously.

The jittered data include 2435 convulsions in 2201 children, and are in data frame `condat`. Variables `conv`, `mmr`, `hib` are the ages at convulsion, MMR vaccine and Hib vaccine, respectively. Most observation periods cover the whole second year, so the histogram at age of event shown in Figure 4.7 is informative about the age effect – which is declining. We shall use 20-day age groups, and risk periods [0,7] and [8,14] days after the Hib vaccine. The model is specified as follows.

```
ageg <- seq(387,707,20)
con.mod1 <- standardsccs(event~hib+age, indiv=case, astart=sta,
            aend=end, aevent=conv, adrug=hib, aedrug=hib+14,
            expogrp=c(0,8), agegrp=ageg, data=condat)
```

This produces the following results.

```
> con.mod1
......
      exp(coef) exp(-coef) lower .95 upper .95
hib1    0.9170    1.0905    0.5174    1.6253
hib2    1.6833    0.5941    1.0648    2.6610
```

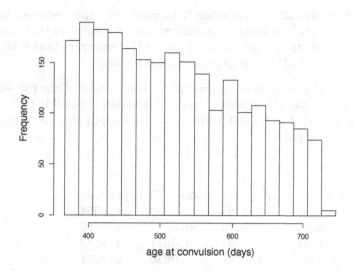

FIGURE 4.7
Age at convulsion for 2201 children aged 366 to 730 days.

The relative incidence in the [8, 14] day risk period is statistically significantly raised: 1.68 with 95% CI (1.06, 2.66). However, 212 of the 542 Hib vaccines administered were given on the same day as the MMR vaccine. We investigate the impact of the MMR vaccine, using the same risk periods [0, 7] and [8, 14].

```
con.mod2 <- standardsccs(event~mmr+age, indiv=case, astart=sta,
            aend=end, aevent=conv, adrug=mmr, aedrug=mmr+14,
            expogrp=c(0,8), agegrp=ageg, data=condat)
```

This yields:

```
> con.mod2
......
      exp(coef) exp(-coef) lower .95 upper .95
mmr1    1.0952    0.9131     0.8470    1.4162
mmr2    2.4257    0.4123     2.0081    2.9301
```

There is a strong effect in the [8, 14] day risk period: relative incidence 2.43, 95% CI (2.01, 2.93). This may affect the Hib results. In consequence, we need to allow for the MMR-related exposures in the model for Hib vaccine. Thus, the model should contain both the exposure related to Hib vaccination, and the exposure related to MMR vaccination. The required model formula is of the form:

$$hib + mmr + age.$$

This is implemented as follows.

```
con.mod3 <- standardsccs(event~hib+mmr+age, indiv=case, astart=
            sta, aend=end, aevent=conv, adrug=cbind(hib,mmr),
            aedrug=cbind(hib+14,mmr+14), expogrp=list(c(0,8),
            c(0,8)), agegrp=ageg, data=condat)
```

Note the use of a list to define `expogrp`: the kth element of the list defines the risk periods for the kth exposure type. This makes it possible to specify different risk periods for Hib and MMR vaccines, if required. This code produces the following output.

```
> con.mod3
......
      exp(coef) exp(-coef) lower .95 upper .95
hib1    0.8958     1.1163     0.4999    1.6054
hib2    1.0663     0.9378     0.6630    1.7150
mmr1    1.1061     0.9041     0.8511    1.4373
mmr2    2.4101     0.4149     1.9830    2.9291
```

The relative incidences for MMR are little different from those in model `con.mod2`. However, the relative incidence for Hib vaccine in the risk period [8, 14] days has changed compared to that obtained in model `con.mod1`. From being significantly raised, it is now close to 1: relative incidence 1.07, 95% CI (0.66, 1.72). We conclude that there is little evidence of an association between Hib vaccine and convulsions in the second week after vaccination with the booster dose, though there is an association with MMR vaccine.

4.5.2 Multiple exposures of several types: NSAIDs, antidepressants and GI bleeds

In Section 4.4.1, the association between non-steroidal anti-inflammatory drugs (NSAIDs) and gastro-intestinal bleeding (GI bleeds) was discussed. It has been suggested that some classes of antidepressants (ADs) are also associated with GI bleeds.

To investigate this, we use simulated data on 1000 persons aged 20 to 100 years with a first GI bleed, similar to those described in Tata et al. (2005). The exposures are of two types: NSAIDs and ADs. Each exposure is recurrent, with up to 10 different periods on drug for each drug type. The data are in data frame `addat`, in the default data format `stack`. Variables `bleed`, `ns`, `ad` contain the ages at GI bleed, NSAID prescription and AD prescription, respectively. Of the 1000 cases, 838 were exposed to NSAIDs and 502 to ADs; 340 were exposed to both NSAIDs and ADs. The ages at and durations of NSAID exposures have already been shown in Figure 4.4; the corresponding plot for AD exposures is shown in Figure 4.8.

Periods on ADs are spread throughout the age range. Most are very brief, though there are clusters of longer treatment periods in middle and later age. As for the NSAIDs analysis in Section 4.4.1, we shall use 40 age groups defined

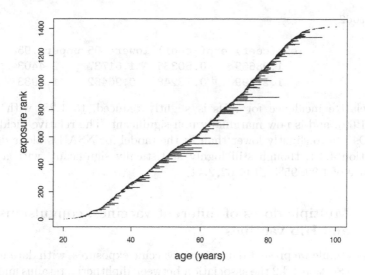

FIGURE 4.8
Age and duration of exposure to antidepressants.

by the quantiles of age at GI bleed. The SCCS model with AD exposure alone
is specified as follows.

```
ageq <- floor(quantile(addat$bleed[duplicated(addat$case)==0],
        seq(0.025,0.975,0.025), names=F))
ad.mod1 <- standardsccs(event~ad+relevel(age,ref=21),
            indiv=case, astart=sta, aend=end, aevent=bleed,
            adrug=ad, aedrug=endad, agegrp=ageq, data=addat)
```

This gives:

```
> ad.mod1
......
            exp(coef) exp(-coef) lower .95 upper .95
ad1          1.36490    0.73265   1.03222    1.8048
```

Thus, ADs are marginally significantly associated with GI bleeds: the relative
incidence is 1.36, 95% CI (1.03, 1.80) in an analysis with just ADs.

The analysis with both ADs and NSAIDS is specified as follows.

```
ad.mod2 <- standardsccs(event~ns+ad+relevel(age,ref=21),
            indiv=case, astart=sta, aend=end, aevent=bleed,
            adrug=cbind(ns,ad), aedrug=cbind(endns,endad),
            agegrp=ageq, data=addat)
```

This model produces the following results.

```
> ad.mod2
......
           exp(coef) exp(-coef) lower .95 upper .95
ns1          1.98669    0.50335   1.61737    2.4403
ad1          1.27799    0.78248   0.96452    1.6933
```

The relative incidence for ADs is slightly reduced, to 1.28, with 95% CI (0.96, 1.69), and is now marginally non-significant. The relative incidence for NSAIDs is also slightly lower than in the model for NSAIDs alone described in Section 4.4.1, though still highly statistically significant, with a relative incidence of 1.99, 95% CI (1.62, 2.44).

4.5.3 Multiple doses of different vaccines: convulsions, DTP and Hib vaccines

In this example we present data on two vaccine exposures, with data in format multi. In Section 4.4.2 the association between diphtheria, tetanus and pertussis (DTP) vaccination and convulsions in the first year of life was discussed. In the present example, our focus is still on DTP vaccine, but we also include exposures related to primary vaccination with the vaccine against *Haemophilus influenzae* type b (Hib) which, like DTP vaccine, is administered in three doses during the first year of life.

The data comprise 1213 cases with 1378 convulsions (one fewer than in the DTP data of Section 4.4.2: one case with incorrect Hib vaccine information was deleted). The jittered data are in data frame hibdat; conv is the age at convulsion. The ages at the three doses of DTP vaccine are in dtp, dtpd2, dtpd3. The ages at the three doses of Hib vaccine are in hib, hibd2, hibd3.

The numbers of DTP vaccinated cases are 1068, 1036, 950 for doses 1, 2 and 3 respectively. For Hib vaccine, the numbers are 662, 615, 550. Figure 4.9 shows the scatterplot of age at Hib and age at DTP vaccines, all doses combined, for cases with both vaccines. The strong diagonal indicates that many DTP and Hib vaccines are given on the same day. For those that are not, Hib vaccines tend to be given later. (Since these data were collected, the DTP and Hib antigens have been combined into a single vaccine.) We shall use different risk periods for the two vaccines. For DTP vaccine the risk periods are [0, 3], [4, 7] and [8, 14] days after each dose. For Hib vaccine we use risk periods [0, 7] and [8, 14] after each dose. The age groups are as in Section 4.4.2.

Recall from Section 4.4.2 that the relative incidence was raised in the [0, 3] day period after DTP, with little evidence of a dose effect: in model dtp.mod1, RI = 1.50, 95% CI (1.06, 2.12). To two decimal places, the same result is obtained in the present data set.

We shall first of all fit a SCCS model in which it is assumed that the effect is the same at all doses of each vaccine. Thus, there are 5 vaccine-related parameters: 3 for the common effect of DTP, and 2 for the common effect of Hib vaccine. This model is specified as follows.

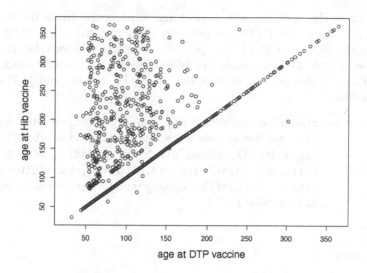

FIGURE 4.9
Scatterplot of ages at Hib and DTP vaccines, all doses combined.

```
ageg <- c(57,85,113,141,169,197,225,253,281,309,337)
hib.mod1 <- standardsccs(event~dtp+hib+age, indiv=case, astart=
            sta, aend=end, aevent=conv, adrug=list(cbind(dtp,
            dtpd2,dtpd3),cbind(hib,hibd2,hibd3)), aedrug=
            list(cbind(dtp+14,dtpd2+14,dtpd3+14),cbind(hib+14,
            hibd2+14,hibd3+14)),expogrp=list(c(0,4,8),c(0,8)),
            agegrp=ageg, dataformat="multi", data=hibdat)
```

Note that the exposure information is now specified using lists. The first elements of lists **adrug**, **aedrug** and **expogroup** relate to the first exposure type, namely DTP vaccine, and the second elements of the lists relate to the second exposure type, namely Hib vaccine. For **adrug** and **aedrug**, the various doses within each exposure type are entered as an array with dose 1 in the first column, dose 2 in the second, and so on.

This model yields the following results.

```
> hib.mod1
......
      exp(coef) exp(-coef) lower .95 upper .95
dtp1    1.3822     0.7235    0.9240    2.0678
dtp2    0.8232     1.2147    0.5080    1.3341
dtp3    1.2778     0.7826    0.8757    1.8645
hib1    1.1526     0.8676    0.7990    1.6627
hib2    0.5514     1.8135    0.3384    0.8985
```

Here, **dtp1** refers to the relative incidence (RI) in the $[0,3]$ risk period, **dtp2** is the RI in the $[4, 7]$ day risk period and dtp3 is the RI in the $[8, 14]$ day risk period after any DTP vaccine dose. Similarly, hib1 and hib2 are the RIs for the $[0, 7]$ and $[8, 14]$ day periods after any Hib vaccine dose. None of the exposure effects are statistically significant. We simplify the model by restricting the risk periods to $[0, 3]$ days for DTP vaccine and $[0, 7]$ days for Hib vaccine:

```
hib.mod2 <- standardsccs(event~dtp+hib+age, indiv=case, astart=
            sta, aend=end, aevent=conv, adrug=list(cbind(dtp,
            dtpd2,dtpd3), cbind(hib,hibd2,hibd3)), aedrug=
            list(cbind(dtp+3,dtpd2+3,dtpd3+3),cbind(hib+7,
            hibd2+7,hibd3+7)), agegrp=ageg, dataformat="multi",
            data=hibdat)
```

This yields:

```
> hib.mod2
......
     exp(coef) exp(-coef) lower .95 upper .95
dtp1    1.4472    0.6910    0.9907     2.114
hib1    1.1037    0.9061    0.7946     1.533
```

The DTP vaccine-associated relative incidence in the $[0, 3]$ day period, when exposure due to Hib vaccine is included in the model, is 1.45, 95% CI $(0.99, 2.11)$, which is marginally statistically non-significant. To check whether there is a dose effect of DTP vaccine in this risk period, we now specify sameexpopar=c(F,T). This signifies that for the first exposure type (namely the three DTP doses) we set sameexpopar=F and so fit dose-specific parameters for the three doses, while for the second exposure type (the three Hib vaccine doses) we retain the default sameexpopar=T and fit a common parameter for the three doses. The model is specified as follows.

```
hib.mod3 <- standardsccs(event~dtp+hib+age, indiv=case, astart=
            sta, aend=end, aevent=conv, adrug=list(cbind(dtp,
            dtpd2,dtpd3), cbind(hib,hibd2,hibd3)), aedrug=
            list(cbind(dtp+3,dtpd2+3,dtpd3+3),cbind(hib+7,
            hibd2+7,hibd3+7)), sameexpopar=c(F,T), agegrp=
            ageg, dataformat="multi", data=hibdat)
```

This yields:

```
> hib.mod3
......
     exp(coef) exp(-coef) lower .95 upper .95
dtp1    1.4722    0.6792    0.8094     2.678
dtp2    1.3177    0.7589    0.6989     2.484
dtp3    1.5460    0.6468    0.8624     2.772
hib1    1.1034    0.9063    0.7944     1.533
```

Note that the meanings of `dtp1`, `dtp2` and `dtp3` have changed. They now represents the effects of doses 1, 2 and 3 of the DTP vaccine, in the [0, 3] day risk period after each dose, respectively. These are 1.47 at dose 1, 1.32 at dose 2 and 1.55 at dose 3. These values are similar, suggesting there is no dose effect. We conclude that the evidence for a DTP effect is weak, and that there is little indication of variation with dose.

4.5.4 Overlapping risk periods: convulsions and DTP

In this section we discuss in a little more detail how overlapping risk periods are handled. Consider two exposures, labelled 1 and 2, experienced by the same individual. Exposure 1 occurs in interval $[c_1, d_1]$ and exposure 2 in $[c_2, d_2]$. An overlap occurs if, for example, $c_1 < c_2 < d_1 < d_2$: the risk periods then overlap in $[c_2, d_1]$. This is represented graphically in Figure 4.10.

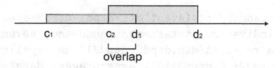

FIGURE 4.10
Overlapping risk periods for distinct exposures.

Suppose that β_1 is the log relative incidence associated with exposure 1, and β_2 is the log relative incidence associated with exposure 2. Under the standard parameterisation used in format `stack`, with exposures 1 and 2 entered in distinct columns, the combined effect of these exposures in the overlap $[c_2, d_1]$ is $\beta_1 + \beta_2$. However, if exposures 1 and 2 are adjacent doses of the same drug, then in format `multi` a different parameterisation is used: precedence is given to the most recent dose. Thus, for the scenario represented in Figure 4.10, the combined exposure effect in the overlap $[c_2, d_1]$ is β_2, since the most recent dose is exposure 2. This convention is also used for overlapping risk periods of the same exposure with data in either format.

The two conventions produce different results when there are overlaps between doses. To illustrate this, consider once more the data on convulsions and DTP vaccine (and Hib vaccine, though we shall not use these) described in Section 4.5.3. The minimum separation between adjacent doses of the vaccine is 6 days: thus, for risk periods of 6 days or more post-vaccination, there will be overlaps. We take the risk period [0, 14] days after each DTP dose, and the same age groups as in Section 4.5.3. Using data format `multi` with `sameexpopar=F` to allow dose-specific parameters , the model is as follows:

```
ageg  <- c(57,85,113,141,169,197,225,253,281,309,337)
hib.mod4 <- standardsccs(event~dtp+age, indiv=case,
          astart=sta, aend=end, aevent=conv, adrug=
```

```
        cbind(dtp,dtpd2,dtpd3), aedrug=
        cbind(dtp+14,dtpd2+14,dtpd3+14), agegrp=
        ageg, dataformat="multi", sameexpopar=F,
        data=hibdat)
```

This yields:

```
> hib.mod4
......
      exp(coef) exp(-coef) lower .95 upper .95
dtp1    1.2288     0.8138    0.8352     1.808
dtp2    0.9438     1.0595    0.6314     1.411
dtp3    1.1145     0.8973    0.7755     1.602
```

Now suppose we use data format stack, and enter the three DTP doses as different exposure types:

```
hib.mod5 <- standardsccs(event~dtp+dtpd2+dtpd3+age,
            indiv=case, astart=sta, aend=end, aevent=conv,
            adrug=list(dtp,dtpd2,dtpd3), aedrug=list(dtp+14,
            dtpd2+14,dtpd3+14), agegrp=ageg, dataformat=
            "stack", data=hibdat)
```

This now yields:

```
> hib.mod5
......
        exp(coef) exp(-coef) lower .95 upper .95
dtp1      1.2275     0.8146    0.8344     1.806
dtpd21    0.9405     1.0632    0.6293     1.406
dtpd31    1.1144     0.8974    0.7755     1.601
```

The parameter names are different from those obtained using data format multi as the exposures are treated as being of different types, rather than doses of the same type. More importantly, the numerical values differ slightly: this is entirely due to the different conventions used in treating overlaps.

If we were to repeat this analysis with the risk period $[0,3]$ days, for example, the two models would yield identical results. This is because there are no overlaps, since the minimum separation between doses is 6 days.

4.6 Comparing models: likelihood ratio tests

Likelihood ratio tests are used to test null hypotheses $\theta_1 = \cdots = \theta_k = 0$, where the θ_j are parameters of the model. They may also be used to test null hypotheses of the form $\theta_1 = \cdots = \theta_k$, which is equivalent to $\theta_2 - \theta_1 =$

$0, \ldots, \theta_k - \theta_1 = 0$. This is achieved by fitting nested models M_1 (the reduced model) and M_2 (the full model) with p_1 and p_2 parameters, where $M_1 \subset M_2$ and $p_1 < p_2$. (Model M_1 is nested within model M_2 if setting $p_2 - p_1$ parameters to zero in model M_2 yields model M_1.) The likelihood ratio test statistic is

$$\text{LRT} = -2\{\log(L_1) - \log(L_2)\},$$

where L_1 is the maximised likelihood for the reduced model M_1 and L_2 is the maximised likelihood for the full model M_2. Under the null hypothesis that the true model is M_1, LRT has approximately a chi-squared distribution on $p_2 - p_1$ degrees of freedom in large samples.

This applies only to models that are nested one within the other. In the case of SCCS models, some care is needed when testing null hypotheses of the form $\theta_1 = \cdots = \theta_k$. If the reduced model is obtained by combining categories (such as risk periods, for example), the reduced model is no longer strictly nested within the full model, since the multinomial categories have changed. However, combining categories in this way only affects the constant multiplier of the multinomial likelihood: provided an appropriate correction factor is applied, the likelihood ratio test can still validly be used. The details are given in Section 4.6.2, which is starred and may be skipped. The function lrtsccs in package SCCS automatically applies this correction factor. The use of this function is described in Section 4.6.1.

4.6.1   Comparing models: ITP and MMR vaccine

We return to the example on MMR vaccine and idiopathic thrombocytopaenic purpura (ITP) described in Section 4.3.1. Consider the following sequence of four SCCS models.

```
itp.mod1 <- standardsccs(event~mmr+age, indiv=case, astart=sta,
             aend=end, aevent=itp, adrug=mmr, aedrug=mmr+42,
             expogrp=c(0,15,29), agegrp=c(427,488,549,610,671),
             data=itpdat)
itp.mod2 <- standardsccs(event~mmr+age, indiv=case, astart=sta,
             aend=end, aevent=itp, adrug=mmr, aedrug=mmr+42,
             agegrp=c(427,488,549,610,671), data=itpdat)
itp.mod3 <- standardsccs(event~age, indiv=case, astart=sta,
             aend=end, aevent=itp, adrug=mmr, aedrug=mmr+42,
             expogrp=c(0,15,29), agegrp=c(427,488,549,610,671),
             data=itpdat)
itp.mod4 <- standardsccs(event~mmr, indiv=case, astart=sta,
             aend=end, aevent=itp, adrug=mmr, aedrug=mmr+42,
             expogrp=c(0,15,29), agegrp=c(427,488,549,610,671),
             data=itpdat)
```

Models itp.mod1 and itp.mod2 are the same as those fitted in Section 4.3.1. Model itp.mod1 is the full model with both exposure and age effects. The other three are reduced models: in `itp.mod3` the exposure effect is omitted from the model formula (which is equivalent to assuming that the relative incidence is 1 for the three post MMR vaccine risk groups), in `itp.mod4` the age effect is omitted (equivalent to assuming that there is no age effect), while in `itp2` the three risk groups [0, 14], [15, 28] and [29, 42] are collapsed into one, which corresponds to the null hypothesis $\beta_1 = \beta_2 = \beta_3$. Models `itp.mod3` and `itp.mod4` are nested within `itp.mod1`. The corresponding likelihood ratio tests may be undertaken as follows.

```
> lrtsccs(itp.mod1,itp.mod3)
   test df    pvalue
 13.43  3 0.003793
```

The likelihood ratio test statistic for the null hypothesis that there is no exposure effect is 13.43 on 3 degrees of freedom, $p = 0.0038$. Thus, the exposure effect is highly statistically significant.

```
> lrtsccs(itp.mod1,itp.mod4)
   test df  pvalue
 10.28  5 0.06768
```

The age effect, on the other hand, is marginally statistically non-significant, with $\chi^2(5) = 10.28$, $p = 0.068$.

The reduced model `itp.mod2` is not strictly speaking nested within the full model `itp.mod1`, as the three risk groups have been merged into one. This is taken into account by the R function `lrtsccs`, which produces a valid likelihood ratio test for these models.

```
> lrtsccs(itp.mod1,itp.mod2)
   test df  pvalue
 4.865  2 0.08782
```

Here we have $\chi^2(2) = 4.87$, $p = 0.088$. Thus there is little evidence against the null hypothesis that the relative incidence is the same in all three risk periods.

Note finally that the order in which the models are specified in `lrtsccs` is immaterial.

4.6.2   Combining multinomial categories*

To make matters definite, suppose that the null hypothesis is $\beta_k = \beta_l$ for $0 \leq k, l \leq K$. Let M_1 denote the reduced model with the same multinomial categories as the full model M_2, and let M_1' denote the collapsed reduced model with exposure categories k and l combined into a single new category labelled

---

* This section may be skipped.

m. Thus, $\lambda_{ijk} = \lambda_{ijl} = \lambda_{ijm}$ in the reduced models. Also, $e_{ijm} = e_{ijk} + e_{ijl}$ and $n_{ijm} = n_{ijk} + n_{ijl}$.

The multinomial likelihood contributions L'_{ijm} of the new exposure category m in the collapsed reduced model M'_1 and of exposure categories k and l in the reduced original model M_1 are related as follows:

$$
\begin{aligned}
L'_{ijm} &= \left(\frac{\lambda_{ijm}e_{ijm}}{\sum_{r,s}\lambda_{irs}e_{irs}}\right)^{n_{ijm}} \\
&= \frac{e_{ijm}^{n_{ijm}}}{e_{ijk}^{n_{ijk}}\,e_{ijl}^{n_{ijl}}} \times \left(\frac{\lambda_{ijk}e_{ijk}}{\sum_{r,s}\lambda_{irs}e_{irs}}\right)^{n_{ijk}} \times \left(\frac{\lambda_{ijl}e_{ijl}}{\sum_{r,s}\lambda_{irs}e_{irs}}\right)^{n_{ijl}} \\
&= \text{constant} \times L_{ijk} \times L_{ijl}.
\end{aligned}
$$

The multinomial likelihood contributions thus differ only by a constant term, and hence the overall likelihoods for models M_1 and its collapsed version M'_1 are proportional, that is, $L'_1 = cL_1$. The same constant multiplier applies to the null models with all age and exposure parameters set to zero: $L_0 = cL_0$. The likelihood ratio test statistic may therefore be written as follows:

$$
\begin{aligned}
\text{LRT} &= -2\{\log(L_1) - \log(L_2)\} \\
&= \left[-2\{\log(L'_1) - \log(L'_0)\}\right] - \left[-2\{\log(L_2) - \log(L_0)\}\right].
\end{aligned}
$$

This involves the full model M_2 and the collapsed reduced model M'_1, and their null counterparts. The full model M_2 and the collapsed reduced model M'_1 can be compared using the likelihood ratio test in this way. The R function lrtsccs makes use of this identity to obtain the likelihood ratio test statistic.

4.7 Interactions: effect modification and stratification

In the examples considered so far, all model formulas have been of the form

Age + Exposure(s).

Others are of course possible. In particular, while time-invariant multiplicative covariates factor out of the SCCS likelihood, we can still examine their impact as effect modifiers on the association between exposure and event, via the interaction between the covariate and the exposure variable. This would involve fitting a model with model formula

Age + Exposure + Exposure.Covariate

where Exposure.Covariate is the interaction term between the covariate and the exposure variable. Note that the main effect of the covariate is not included in the model formula, since it cannot be estimated in a SCCS model as it drops out of the likelihood.

Interactions between one or more time-invariant covariates and the age effect can also be included in the model. When the covariate is a factor, the model is then stratified by the levels of the covariate. The model formula is then

Age + Exposure + Age.Covariate

Finally, if there are several time-varying exposures, we might be interested in the interaction between them. This is represented by the model formula

Age + Exposure$_1$ + Exposure$_2$ + Exposure$_1$.Exposure$_2$.

Combinations of these models may also be used.

Models with these model formulas can be parameterised in several ways. Which parameterisation is preferable depends on context. For example, suppose that the covariate is a factor. The model formula

Age + Exposure + Exposure.Covariate

can be fitted in two different ways. Using the crossing operator * as in `Age + Exposure*Covariate` returns the interaction terms, which indicate the amount by which the covariate modifies the effects of exposure. Using the nesting operator / as in `Age + Covariate/Exposure` returns the exposure effect at each level of the covariate.

4.7.1   Interactions: sex, ITP and MMR vaccine

The incidence of idiopathic thrombocytopaenic purpura (ITP) is known to depend on gender, being more common in males. This raises two questions: might sex be an effect modifier for the association between MMR vaccine and ITP? And might the age-related incidence of ITP be different in males and females? To answer these questions we continue the example of Sections 4.3.1 and 4.6.1. We fit models with suitable interaction terms.

We begin with effect modification. We define a new model `itp.mod5` with the interaction between sex and exposure. Sex is coded 1 for males and 2 for females, and is entered in the model as a factor.

```
itp.mod5 <- standardsccs(event~factor(sex)*mmr+age, indiv=case,
            astart=sta, aend=end, aevent=itp, adrug=mmr, aedrug=
            mmr+42, expogrp=c(0,15,29), agegrp=c(427,488,549,
            610,671), data=itpdat)
```

The likelihood ratio test of the null hypothesis that the interaction terms are zero is as follows; `itp.mod1` defined in Sections 4.3.1 and 4.6.1 is the reduced model with no interactions.

```
> lrtsccs(itp.mod1,itp.mod5)
    test df pvalue
  0.5973  3 0.8971
```

The *p*-value being 0.90, there is little evidence to reject the null hypothesis that the interaction terms are zero. The model parameters are as follows.

```
> itp.mod5
. . . . . .
```

	exp(coef)	exp(-coef)	lower .95	upper .95
factor(sex)2	NA	NA	NA	NA
mmr1	1.0336	0.9675	0.13439	7.9494
mmr2	4.7702	0.2096	1.53093	14.8635
mmr3	2.8557	0.3502	0.62508	13.0465
age2	0.6723	1.4875	0.29844	1.5144
age3	0.2185	4.5758	0.06123	0.7801
age4	0.3008	3.3246	0.09601	0.9423
age5	0.4070	2.4570	0.14124	1.1728
age6	0.4193	2.3848	0.14459	1.2161
factor(sex)2:mmr1	1.8165	0.5505	0.09525	34.6442
factor(sex)2:mmr2	1.7478	0.5722	0.31114	9.8178
factor(sex)2:mmr3	0.8139	1.2286	0.05873	11.2801

The first row in this portion of the output shows the main effect of sex: this is not estimable in a SCCS model, hence all entries are missing. R also produces a warning message (not shown) relating to this. Then come the three main effects of exposure: the values in column `exp(coef)` are the relative incidences in males. These are followed by the main effects of age. Finally, the last three rows are the interactions between sex and exposure. The values in column `exp(coef)` are the amounts by which the exposure effect in males must be multiplied to get the exposure effect in females. None of these interactions are individually significant, in line with the result of the likelihood ratio test: we conclude that there is little evidence of gender-related effect modification.

We now turn to the interaction between sex and age. The issue here is whether we ought to stratify the analysis by sex, so that the age effect is allowed to be different in males and females. Thus, it is convenient to use the parameterisation giving relative age effects within males and females (rather than the effect modification). Accordingly we specify the model with the nesting operator /.

```
itp.mod6 <- standardsccs(event~mmr+factor(sex)/age, indiv=case,
            astart=sta, aend=end, aevent=itp, adrug=mmr, aedrug=
            mmr+42, expogrp=c(0,15,29), agegrp=c(427,488,549,
            610,671), data=itpdat)
```

The parameters of the model `itp.mod6` are as follows.

```
> itp.mod6
......
                      exp(coef) exp(-coef) lower .95 upper .95
mmr1                  1.326e+00  7.539e-01   0.29977     5.869
mmr2                  5.846e+00  1.711e-01   2.42032    14.121
mmr3                  2.524e+00  3.961e-01   0.71085     8.965
factor(sex)2                NA         NA        NA        NA
factor(sex)1:age2     9.383e-01  1.066e+00   0.32695     2.693
factor(sex)2:age2     3.915e-01  2.554e+00   0.10160     1.509
factor(sex)1:age3     1.357e-01  7.368e+00   0.01622     1.136
factor(sex)2:age3     3.118e-01  3.208e+00   0.06472     1.502
factor(sex)1:age4     2.745e-01  3.643e+00   0.05542     1.360
factor(sex)2:age4     3.368e-01  2.969e+00   0.06952     1.632
factor(sex)1:age5     7.854e-01  1.273e+00   0.23885     2.583
factor(sex)2:age5     3.204e-09  3.121e+08   0.00000       Inf
factor(sex)1:age6     4.782e-01  2.091e+00   0.11729     1.950
factor(sex)2:age6     3.425e-01  2.920e+00   0.07068     1.659
```

Note first that the relative incidences associated with MMR vaccination
(shown in the first three rows of this output) are only marginally affected
by stratifying the age effect, compared to those of model `itp.mod1` from Section 4.3.1. The last 10 rows show the age effect, stratified by sex. The relative
age effect in girls in age group 5 is 0.0000 because there are no events in this
category. Figure 4.11 displays the stratified age effect.

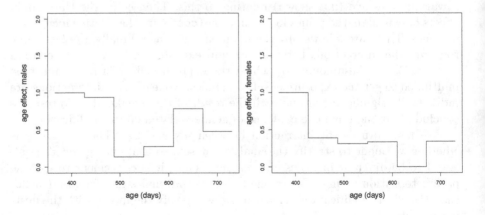

FIGURE 4.11
Relative age effects for ITP data, stratified by sex. Left: males. Right: females.

   This plot is obtained using the following code:

```
par(mfrow=c(1,2), mar=c(4.1,4.1,1,1), cex.lab=1.4)
am<-c(1,itp.mod6$coef[c(5,7,9,11,13),2],itp.mod6$coef[13,2])
```

```
af<-c(1,itp.mod6$coef[c(6,8,10,12,14),2],itp.mod6$coef[14,2])
age<-c(366,427,488,549,610,671,730)
plot(age, am, type="s", ylim=c(0,2), xlab="age (days)",
    ylab="age effect, males")
plot(age, af, type="s", ylim=c(0,2), xlab="age (days)",
    ylab="age effect, females")
```

The likelihood ratio test of the null hypothesis of no interaction between sex and age is as follows.

```
> lrtsccs(itp.mod1,itp.mod6)
  test df pvalue
 7.384  5 0.1936
```

Thus there is little evidence to reject the null hypothesis that there is no interaction between age and sex, since $p = 0.19$. All in all, it would appear that stratifying the analysis by sex is not necessary.

4.7.2 Interactions between exposures: GI bleeds, NSAIDs and antidepressants

In Section 4.5.2, simulated data were used to illustrate the effects of non-steroidal anti-inflammatory drugs (NSAIDs) and antidepressants (ADs) on gastro-intestinal (GI) bleeds. For NSAIDs, the relative incidence was 1.99 and highly statistically significant; for ADs it was 1.28 and marginally non-significant. It has been suggested, however, that the effect of ADs can be higher when taken in conjunction with an NSAID. Thus, the interaction between these drugs is of interest.

The baseline model includes the exposure effects of both NSAIDs and ADs, but no interaction; this was model ad.mod2 in Section 4.5.2. For completeness, here it is again, along with edited output.

```
> ageq <- floor(quantile(addat$bleed[duplicated(addat$case)==0],
          seq(0.025,0.975,0.025), names=F))
> ad.mod2 <- standardsccs(event~ns+ad+relevel(age,ref=21),
            indiv=case, astart=sta, aend=end, aevent=bleed,
            adrug=cbind(ns,ad), aedrug=cbind(endns,endad),
            agegrp=ageq, data=addat)
> ad.mod2
......
        exp(coef) exp(-coef) lower .95 upper .95
ns1       1.98669    0.50335   1.61737    2.4403
ad1       1.27799    0.78248   0.96452    1.6933
```

We now include the interaction between the two exposures, starting with the effect modification parameterisation.

```
ad.mod3 <- standardsccs(event~ns*ad+relevel(age,ref=21),
            indiv=case, astart=sta, aend=end, aevent=bleed,
            adrug=cbind(ns,ad), aedrug=cbind(endns,endad),
            agegrp=ageq, data=addat)
```

This yields (the interaction term is at the bottom of the output table):

```
> ad.mod3
......
          exp(coef) exp(-coef) lower .95 upper .95
ns1         2.14232    0.46678   1.72896    2.6545
ad1         1.48872    0.67172   1.09600    2.0222
......
ns1:ad1     0.54922    1.82076   0.31654    0.9529
```

The interaction is 0.55, 95% CI $(0.32, 0.95)$. As the confidence interval excludes 1, the interaction is statistically significant, as confirmed by the likelihood ratio test:

```
> lrtsccs(ad.mod2,ad.mod3)
  test df  pvalue
 4.701  1 0.03015
```

In the absence of ADs, the relative incidence associated with NSAIDs is 2.14, 95% CI $(1.73, 2.65)$. In the absence of NSAIDs, the relative incidence associated with ADs is 1.49, 95% CI $(1.10, 2.02)$. Thus, both drugs, on their own, are significantly positively associated with GI bleeds. The interaction term is 0.55; this being less than 1, it corresponds to an inhibitory effect. The relationship between the relative incidences is as follows:

$$RI_{\text{NSAID+AD}} = RI_{\text{NSAID}} \times RI_{\text{AD}} \times RI_{\text{Interaction}}.$$

Thus, we have

$$RI_{\text{NSAID+AD}} \quad = \quad 2.14232 \times 1.48872 \times 0.54922$$
$$\simeq \quad 1.75.$$

Thus, the relative incidence associated with both NSAIDs and ADs is higher than with ADs alone, but not as high as if no interaction were present, in which case, from ad.mod2, it would be $1.99 \times 1.28 \simeq 2.54$. The inhibitory effect of the interaction is represented graphically in Figure 4.12.

In the presence of NSAIDs, do ADs significantly increase the risk of a GI bleed over and above the risk level associated with NSAIDs? This may be answered directly using the alternative parameterisation:

```
ad.mod4 <- standardsccs(event~ns/ad+relevel(age,ref=21),
            indiv=case, astart=sta, aend=end, aevent=bleed,
            adrug=cbind(ns,ad), aedrug=cbind(endns,endad),
            agegrp=ageq, data=addat)
```

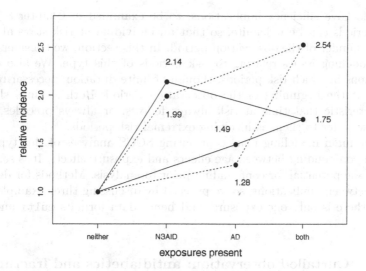

FIGURE 4.12
Relative incidences: models with (full lines) and without (dashes) interaction.

This yields (again, the interaction terms are at the end of the output table):

```
> ad.mod4
.....
           exp(coef) exp(-coef) lower .95 upper .95
ns1          2.14232    0.46678   1.72896     2.6545
......
ns0:ad1      1.48872    0.67172   1.09600     2.0222
ns1:ad1      0.81764    1.22304   0.49213     1.3585
```

The last term is the relative incidence associated with ADs, in the presence of NSAIDs. It is 0.82, 95% CI (0.49, 1.36): the effect is not statistically significant. We conclude that, when taken alone, both NSAIDs and ADs increase the risk of a GI bleed. When taken together, there is no evidence that the risk associated with ADs is greater than that associated with NSAIDs alone: if anything, the risk appears to be reduced.

4.8 Indefinite and extremal risk periods

A common misconception about SCCS studies is that risk periods must be of short duration and transient. They need not be either, though exposures do need to be time-varying. Long risk periods are perfectly acceptable, though they do have efficiency implications, to be examined in Chapter 8. In fact, risk periods can be indefinite, so that an individual at risk stays at risk for the remainder of the observation period. In this section, we consider some of the modelling issues relating to risk periods of this type. We also consider situations in which risk periods, though of finite duration, necessarily always occur at the beginning of the observation period. Both settings share the characteristic that time at risk always follows, or always precedes, control time: we refer to them as involving extremal risk periods.

The main modelling issue confronting SCCS analyses of this type is potential confounding between age effects and exposure effects. It is sensible to assess the potential for confounding prior to analysis. Methods for doing this vary between applications, so we proceed by discussing three examples. In all three there is only one exposure, and hence data formats `multi` and `stack` coincide.

4.8.1   Curtailed observation: antidiabetics and fractures

If it is not known what the risk profile is likely to be after the end of a treatment period, one option is to curtail the observation period at the end of treatment: this circumvents having to make any assumption about the level of risk following the end of treatment. We present an instance of such a design, using 2000 simulated events based on Douglas et al. (2009). This was an investigation of the association between treatment with thiazolidinedione antidiabetic drugs and fractures. A single risk period was used, comprising the period from initiation of treatment until 60 days after the first interruption of treatment for more than 60 days. The risk and observation periods are shown in Figure 4.13.

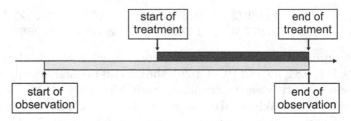

FIGURE 4.13
Observation and risk periods for the antidiabetics and fracture study.

Curtailing the observation period at a time determined by the exposure history is perfectly acceptable in SCCS studies (see Chapter 3, Section 3.7). However, care is required to ensure that age effects are fully allowed for in the analysis. The risk period always follows the control period: since the incidence of fractures increases with age, failure to control for age effects will bias the relative incidence upwards.

In this example, separating the effects of age and exposure is further complicated by the fact that only cases with exposure to the drug were sampled. The data are in data frame `adidat`; variable `frac` is the age at first fracture, variable `adi` is the age at the start of first antidiabetic treatment. We shall use age groups defined by 40 quantiles of `frac`. To ensure that age and exposure effects can be separated, we need to check that there is both exposed and unexposed time within each age group. A visual check is provided by Figure 4.14, which is obtained as follows.

```
ageq <- quantile(adidat$frac, seq(0.025,0.975,0.025), names=F)
par(mar=c(4.1,4.1,1,1), cex.lab=1.4)
vals <- c(min(adidat$sta),ageq,max(adidat$end))/365.25
plot(adidat$adi/365.25, adidat$frac/365.25, xlim=
    c(min(adidat$sta)/365.25,max(adidat$end)/365.25),
    xlab="age at drug (years)", ylab="age at event (years)",
    pch=16, cex=0.5)
abline(v=vals, lty=2)
```

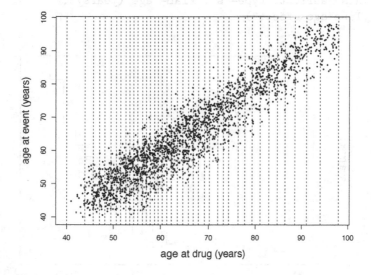

FIGURE 4.14
Scatterplot of age at fracture and age at drug for antidiabetics data. Vertical dashed lines denote the age group boundaries.

Figure 4.14 shows that each age group contains values of `adi` and hence both exposed and unexposed observation time. Thus, the data contain the information required to separate the effects of age and exposure.

The overall effect of exposure to this class of antidiabetics is obtained as follows.

```
adi.mod1 <- standardsccs(event~adi+age , indiv=case,
            astart=sta, aend=end, aevent=frac, adrug=
            adi, aedrug=end, expogrp=0, agegrp=ageq,
            data=adidat)
```

The results are as follows:

```
> adi.mod1
......
           exp(coef) exp(-coef) lower .95 upper .95
adi1          1.5569     0.6423    1.3504     1.795
```

Thus the relative incidence is 1.56, with 95% CI (1.35, 1.80).

The age-specific relative incidence is relatively steady to age 70 then increases sharply. It is shown in Figure 4.15, obtained using the following code.

```
par(mar=c(4.1,4.1,1,1), cex.lab=1.4)
acoef <- as.vector(adi.mod1$coef[2:40,2])
aeffect <- c(1,acoef,acoef[39])
plot(vals, aeffect, type="s", xlab="age (years)",
     ylab="age effect")
```

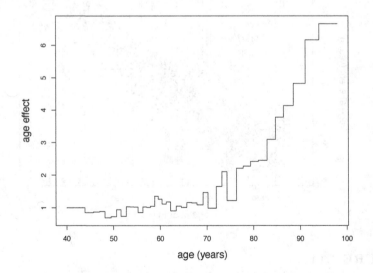

FIGURE 4.15

Estimated relative age effect for fracture in antidiabetics data.

Also of interest is whether the relative incidence varies with time since the beginning of treatment. To investigate this we introduce additional cutpoints to obtain the relative incidences at intervals roughly corresponding to 0–1, 1–2, 2–3, 3–4, 4–5, 5–6 and 6+ years after the beginning of treatment.

```
exint <- c(0,366,731,1096,1461,1826,2191)
adi.mod2 <- standardsccs(event~adi+age, indiv=case,
            astart=sta, aend=end, aevent=frac, adrug=
            adi, aedrug=end, expogrp=exint, agegrp=ageq,
            data=adidat)
```

This gives the following results.

```
> adi.mod2
......
        exp(coef) exp(-coef) lower .95 upper .95
adi1      1.2932    0.7733     1.0808    1.5475
adi2      1.4454    0.6918     1.1762    1.7762
adi3      1.9328    0.5174     1.5528    2.4059
adi4      2.6115    0.3829     2.0649    3.3027
adi5      2.7269    0.3667     2.0873    3.5625
adi6      2.3144    0.4321     1.6850    3.1788
adi7      1.5988    0.6255     1.1559    2.2113
```

The relative incidence increases up to 4–5 years after the beginning of treatment, then declines. This age variation may be investigated further using a likelihood ratio test.

```
> lrtsccs(adi.mod1,adi.mod2)
  test df   pvalue
 58.25  6 1.02e-10
```

Since $p < 0.0001$, the variation of the relative incidence with time since start of treatment is highly statistically significant.

4.8.2   Indefinite risk periods: MMR vaccine and autism

In the applications considered so far, the events of interest have generally been acute, with a clearly defined time of onset. The SCCS method can also, in some circumstances, be used with conditions that develop gradually, and to which a time of onset can at best only be ascribed notionally. For such conditions, using short risk periods is not sensible: long or indefinite risk periods are needed, that allow time for the condition of interest to emerge and be diagnosed. Indefinite risk periods are also suitable if it is hypothesised that the risk of the event is increased at all times after the beginning of the exposure.

Autism and its potential association with MMR vaccine provides an instance of such a setting. The present example uses simulated data based on Taylor et al. (1999); an analysis using indefinite risk periods is presented in Farrington et al. (2001). The data, in data frame autdat, include age at MMR vaccination, in variable mmr, and age at autism diagnosis, in variable diag, for 350 cases of autism.

The observation periods used in the present example span ages from 275 days (9 months) to 5730 days (15.7 years) of age. Unlike the antidiabetics example of Section 4.8.1, age at exposure (median 1.2 years) generally precedes age at event (median 3.2 years), as shown in Figure 4.16.

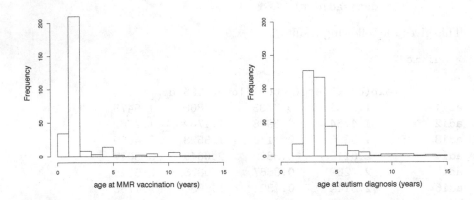

FIGURE 4.16
Age distributions for MMR and autism data. Left: MMR vaccination. Right: autism diagnosis.

Key to separating the effects of age and time since MMR in these data is the presence of 64 unvaccinated autism cases. The inclusion of 42 cases vaccinated after the second year of life, under the MMR vaccination catch-up programme, also helps. In view of the substantial age variation in MMR and autism diagnosis, it is sensible to use a fine partition of age. We shall use 40 quantiles of diag.

```
ageq <- quantile(autdat$diag, seq(0.025,0.975,0.025), names=F)
aut.mod1 <- standardsccs(event~mmr+age, indiv=case, astart=sta,
            aend=end, aevent=diag, adrug=mmr, aedrug=end,
            expogrp=0, agegrp=ageq, data=autdat)
```

This yields

```
> aut.mod1
......
        exp(coef) exp(-coef) lower .95 upper .95
mmr1      1.051     0.95157     0.5176     2.133
```

Thus there is little evidence of an association: the relative incidence is 1.05, with 95% CI $(0.52, 2.13)$. It is also of interest to investigate the variation of the relative incidence with time since MMR vaccination. This is achieved by the following code, where cutpoints have been included to split the risk intervals into 0–2, 2–4, 4–6 and 6+ years since vaccination.

```
exint <- c(0,731,1461,2191)
aut.mod2 <- standardsccs(event~mmr+age, indiv=case, astart=sta,
            aend=end, aevent=diag, adrug=mmr, aedrug=end,
            expogrp=exint, agegrp=ageq, data=autdat)
```

This produces the following results.

```
> aut.mod2
......
          exp(coef) exp(-coef) lower .95 upper .95
mmr1       1.0497    0.95261    0.5152    2.139
mmr2       0.8987    1.11271    0.3987    2.026
mmr3       0.7765    1.28785    0.2586    2.332
mmr4       1.1800    0.84747    0.3317    4.198
```

Thus there is little evidence of a statistically significant effect in any of these periods since MMR vaccination.

The autism data provide an opportunity to demonstrate the benefit of including unexposed cases in SCCS models when age and exposure effects are likely to be confounded. This is the case with the present data, owing to the positive correlation in vaccinated cases between time since vaccination and age, which is mitigated but not eliminated by the presence of some late vaccinees.

To this end, we refit the model with time since MMR vaccination, using subset to select only vaccinated cases:

```
aut.mod3 <- standardsccs(event~mmr+age, indiv=case, astart=sta,
            aend=end, aevent=diag, adrug=mmr, aedrug=end,
            expogrp=exint, agegrp=ageq,
            data=subset(autdat,mmr>0))
```

This yields:

```
> aut.mod3
......
          exp(coef) exp(-coef) lower .95 upper .95
mmr1       1.5059    0.66404    0.61946   3.661
mmr2       1.4322    0.69822    0.47842   4.287
mmr3       2.6981    0.37063    0.51315   14.186
mmr4       8.1960    0.12201    0.88158   76.199
```

The estimates, though still not statistically significantly greater than 1, are higher than those obtained from model aut.mod2, and also much less precise, as shown by the width of the confidence intervals. The contrast is particularly striking for the later times since vaccination. The reason for the difference is that, when unvaccinated cases are excluded, there is little information to distinguish between the effects of age and time since vaccination, particularly at older ages and longer times since vaccination. Including unvaccinated cases increases the information available on age effects. This in turn reduces confounding, and improves the estimation of vaccine effects.

4.8.3 Initial risk periods: NRT and MI

In this final example on extremal risk periods we consider an application where the risk period is always at the start of the observation period – and furthermore, in which all individuals are exposed. The exposure is the initiation of nicotine replacement therapy (NRT), and the outcome is the first myocardial infarction. Smokers who experience a myocardial infarction may be encouraged to follow a course of NRT, thus violating an assumption of the SCCS method. Starting the observation period at NRT initiation of sidesteps this problem. Another issue is MI-related mortality: this will be discussed in Chapter 7.

The data are in data frame **nrtdat**. The observation period stretches from the age on the day the NRT started (variable **nrt**), to 365 days after that date (variable **end**), even if the patient record ends sooner. There are 141 simulated cases, aged between 39 and 82 years, based on data from Hubbard et al. (2005a). Interest is focused on the relative incidence of MI in the period immediately following the initiation of NRT. Accordingly we use four 1-week risk periods: 0–7, 8–14, 15–21, and 22–28 days after **nrt**. The risk intervals and observation periods are represented schematically in Figure 4.17.

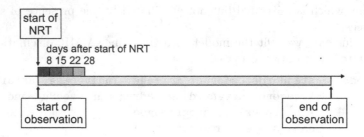

FIGURE 4.17
Observation and risk periods for MI and NRT initiation study.

The risk periods always precede the control period. In addition, the observation periods are short (1 year) in relation to the age range of the data (43 years), as shown in Figure 4.18. This graph is obtained using the following R code.

```
par(mar=c(4.1,4.1,1,1), cex.lab=1.4)
perm <- order(nrtdat$nrt, nrtdat$end, nrtdat$mi)
s <- nrtdat$nrt[perm]/365.25
e <- nrtdat$end[perm]/365.25
t <- nrtdat$mi[perm]/365.25
v <- 1:length(t)
plot(t, v, xlab="age (years)", ylab="case number", type="p",
    pch=16, cex=0.5)
segments(s,v,e,v)
```

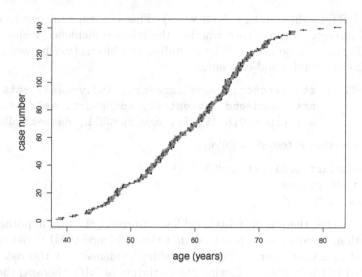

FIGURE 4.18
Observation periods (lines) and ages at event (points) for 141 MI cases.

If we were to use age intervals of, say, 5 years, most observation periods would be entirely contained within a single age band. The age adjustment would therefore have little impact on the results – for most cases, the age effect would be time-invariant over the observation period. Provided the incidence of MI does not vary much over a 1-year period, it is reasonable not to fit any age effect. In this case, the model is defined as follows.

```
nrt.mod1 <- standardsccs(event~nrt, indiv=case, astart=nrt,
            aend=end, aevent=mi, adrug=nrt, aedrug=nrt+28,
            expogrp=c(0,8,15,22), agegrp=NULL, data=nrtdat)
```

This yields

```
> nrt.mod1
......
      exp(coef) exp(-coef) lower .95 upper .95
nrt1    1.685     0.5935    0.6893     4.119
nrt2    1.926     0.5193    0.7877     4.708
nrt3    1.155     0.8655    0.3677     3.631
nrt4    1.155     0.8655    0.3677     3.631
```

The relative incidences **nrt1** and **nrt2**, which correspond to the first two weeks following the initiation of NRT therapy, are elevated but far from statistically significant.

The variable **cage** contains the centred age at NRT, in years (the mean age at NRT in these data is 58.8 years). This is a time-invariant covariate. It is of interest to investigate whether the relative incidence varies with age at NRT: this can be achieved by including the interaction between `cage` (a continuous variable) and exposure.

```
nrt.mod2 <- standardsccs(event~cage*nrt, indiv=case, astart=
            nrt, aend=end, aevent=mi, adrug=nrt, aedrug=nrt+28,
            expogrp=c(0,8,15,22), agegrp=NULL, data=nrtdat)
```

The interaction is tested as follows.

```
> lrtsccs(nrt.mod1,nrt.mod2)
  test df pvalue
 0.3826  4 0.9839
```

Since $p = 0.98$, there is very little evidence to reject the null hypothesis of no interaction. In conclusion, provided that the incidence of MI varies little over a period of a year, there is little compelling evidence that the risk of MI is increased in the 4 weeks following the initiation of NRT therapy, though the confidence intervals are wide, which suggests low power.

SCCS studies with identical short observation periods defined in relation to point exposures have sometimes been called self-controlled risk interval studies (Baker et al., 2015). When such studies are analysed without the inclusion of age effects, conditioning on numbers of events within cases turns out to be largely optional: identical maximum likelihood estimates and standard errors are obtained regardless of the conditioning. These designs are discussed in Chapter 8.

4.9   SCCS analyses with temporal effects

So far, all SCCS models have used age as the time line of interest. In this section, we consider situations where temporal variation, such as a seasonal effect, is important. In some circumstances, notably when both the exposure and the event incidences vary seasonally, and the observation period is relatively short, age effects can be disregarded and the analysis can be couched wholly in terms of calendar time, with seasonal variation taking the place of age variation. This is the situation considered in the first example, in Section 4.9.1.

In other circumstances, both age and calendar time effects may be relevant. In this case, the SCCS model must be augmented to include the effect of season as well as age on the baseline incidence. In the simplest such model, in which the effects of age and time are taken to be independent, the age-related relative incidence is of the form

$$\psi(t|t_{0i}) = \psi(t)\sigma(t + t_{0i}),$$

where t_{0i} is the date of birth of individual i, measured using some time origin common to all individuals. Thus, $t + t_{0i}$ is the calendar time at which individual i reaches age t. The function $\psi(t)$ is, as before, the age-specific relative incidence function common to all individuals. The function $\sigma(s)$ represents the relative incidence associated with calendar time s. If the temporal effects of interest are seasonal, $\sigma(s)$ is a periodic function with period one year.

Seasonal effects may be handled within the framework of the standard SCCS model by modelling seasonal variation as piecewise constant. Thus, a further set of cutpoints is introduced, which partitions the observation periods into time intervals on which the seasonal effect is constant. This is illustrated in Figure 4.19 for a single case, born on 18th April (of 2014).

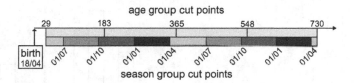

FIGURE 4.19
Schematic representation of age and seasonal cutpoints.

The observation period for this case is $[29, 730]$ days. There are four age groups (roughly 5 months for the first and 6 months for the other three), and quarterly season groups with start dates in *ddmm* format (1st January, 1st April, 1st July and 1st October). The date of birth is needed to calculate the age of the case at the seasonal group cutpoints. These seasonal cutpoints partition the observation period of this case into nine intervals. The seasonal factor has four levels, and thus three free parameters. Other seasonal groups may be used, according to the context. For monthly seasonal effects, for example, a seasonal factor with 12 levels (and 11 free parameters) would be required, corresponding to monthly cutpoints.

The SCCS model is now fitted with a model formula of the form

$$\texttt{Exposure + Age + Season.}$$

A vector of season group boundaries in *ddmm* format must be specified. A variable giving the date of birth of each case, in the format *ddmmyyyy*, is required to convert seasonal cutpoints into ages for each case. All ages (start and end of the observation period, age at event, ages at exposure, age group boundaries) must be given as days since birth. The syntax for the function `standardsccs` is described, along with an example, in Section 4.9.2.

4.9.1 Calendar time: GBS and influenza vaccine

This application relates to the possible association between influenza vaccine and Guillain–Barré syndrome (GBS), using data from Galeotti et al. (2013).

The study was undertaken in Italy during the 2010–2011 influenza season, which was deemed to last from 1st October 2010 to 15th May 2011. A sample of 174 cases of GBS with onset within this period was collected. Of these cases, 52 received the seasonal influenza vaccine.

The data, which have been jittered, are in data frame `gbsdat`; `flu` is the time of influenza vaccination and `gbs` is the time of GBS onset. Times are counted from 1st October 2010, which is day 1. The latest vaccination occurred on day 107. Both influenza vaccination and GBS are seasonal, as suggested by Figure 4.20. Thus, a SCCS analysis should adjust for season.

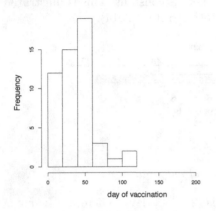 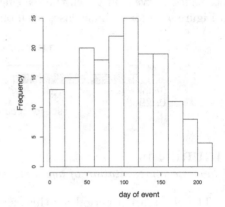

FIGURE 4.20
Numbers vaccinated (left) and GBS cases (right) by day of observation.

The observation period stretches from 1st October 2010 (day 1) to 15th May 2011 (day 227). It is unlikely that the incidence of GBS will vary much with age over such a short period. Thus in this example, the primary time line is calendar time, rather than age, though it is still called `age` in the model. The risk period is taken to be 0–42 days after vaccination. We shall control for season in calendar months October to March, and a final category 1st April to 15th May. The code for the model is as follows.

```
seas   <- cumsum(c(31,30,31,31,28,31))
gbs.mod1 <- standardsccs(event~flu+age, indiv=case, astart=sta,
              aend=end, aevent=gbs, adrug=flu, aedrug=flu+42,
              expogrp=0, agegrp=seas, data=gbsdat)
```

Note that season is entered in the model formula as `age`; the partition of the observation period in `agegrp` is defined by `seas`. This model yields:

```
> gbs.mod1
......

        exp(coef) exp(-coef) lower .95 upper .95
flu1      2.5825     0.3872    1.4161    4.7096
```

Thus, the relative incidence is 2.58 with 95% CI (1.42, 4.71). (The validity of the assumptions underpinning this estimate will be discussed in Chapter 5.) The model without any season effect is

```
gbs.mod2 <- standardsccs(event~flu, indiv=case, astart=sta,
                aend=end, aevent=gbs, adrug=flu, aedrug=flu+42,
                expogrp=0, agegrp=seas, data=gbsdat)
```

yielding the following result and likelihood ratio test

```
> gbs.mod2
......
        exp(coef) exp(-coef) lower .95 upper .95
flu1        2.899      0.345     1.666     5.044

> lrtsccs(gbs.mod1,gbs.mod2)
   test df    pvalue
  35.33  6 3.719e-06
```

The effect of season is highly statistically significant ($p < 0.0001$ in the likelihood ratio test) though the estimated relative incidence is little affected by the inclusion of seasonal effects in the model.

Variable sage gives the age of each case, in years, on 1st October 2010. The age range is wide, stretching from 19 to 96 years, so it is of interest to investigate whether age at the start of observation – a time-invariant continuous covariate – is an effect modifier for the association between influenza vaccination and GBS. The interaction model is as follows.

```
gbs.mod3 <- standardsccs(event~sage*flu + age, indiv=case,
                astart=sta, aend=end, aevent=gbs, adrug=flu,
                aedrug=flu+42, expogrp=0, agegrp=seas, data=gbsdat)
```

This yields the following likelihood ratio test.

```
> lrtsccs(gbs.mod1,gbs.mod3)
   test df pvalue
  0.1208  1 0.7282
```

Thus, since $p = 0.73$, there is little evidence that age at start of observation is an effect modifier.

4.9.2   Seasonal SCCS model: OPV and intussusception

In this example, the time line of primary interest is age, but calendar seasonal effects also need to be taken into account. The exposure is vaccination with the oral polio vaccine (OPV), and the outcome is intussusception in children under 1 year of age. The data were collected in Cuba; the study was published as Galindo-Sardiñas et al. (2001).

The jittered data are in data frame `intdat` and are in data format `multi`. Age at intussusception is in variable `intus`. The oral polio vaccine is administered in two doses in Cuba. The ages at OPV are in `opv` and `opvd2`. We shall use three risk periods: 0–14, 15–28 and 29–42 days after each dose. Age is controlled in 30-day intervals with a final interval of 35 days. The SCCS model with age effect is as follows.

```
age <- seq(30,330,30)
int.mod1 <- standardsccs(event~opv+age, indiv=case, astart=sta,
            aend=end, aevent=intus, adrug=cbind(opv,opvd2),
            aedrug=cbind(opv+42,opvd2+42), expogrp=c(0,15,29),
            agegrp=age, dataformat="multi", data=intdat)
```

This model assumes a common effect at each dose. The exposure estimates are as follows.

```
> int.mod1
......
      exp(coef) exp(-coef) lower .95 upper .95
opv1    1.349    0.74108    0.8960    2.032
opv2    1.148    0.87134    0.7263    1.813
opv3    1.435    0.69710    0.9302    2.212
```

The relative incidences are 1.35, 1.15 and 1.44 for the risk periods 0–14, 15–28 and 29–42 days after either dose, respectively. All are greater than one, though none are statistically significant.

However, in Cuba, the two OPV doses are administered in national campaigns that take place mainly, though not exclusively, during the months of February to April. The seasonal distribution of OPV in the 273 cases in the study is shown in Figure 4.21. Also shown is the seasonal distribution of the 273 intussusceptions. These figures were obtained with the following code; variable `dob` is the date of birth, in format *ddmmyyyy*.

```
par(mfrow=c(1,2), mar=c(4.1,4.1,1,1), cex.lab=1.4)
bdate <- as.Date(formatC(intdat$dob, width=8, format="d",
         flag="0"), "%d%m%Y")

mopv <- factor(c(months(bdate+intdat$opv, abbreviate=T),
           months(bdate+intdat$opvd2, abbreviate=T)),
           levels=c("Jan","Feb","Mar","Apr","May",
           "Jun","Jul","Aug","Sep","Oct","Nov","Dec"), ordered=T)
barplot(table(mopv), xlab="Month of vaccination (both doses)")

mevent <- factor(months(bdate+intdat$intus, abbreviate=T),
           levels=c("Jan","Feb","Mar","Apr","May",
           "Jun","Jul","Aug","Sep","Oct","Nov","Dec"), ordered=T)
barplot(table(mevent), xlab="Month of event")
```

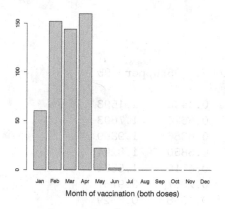
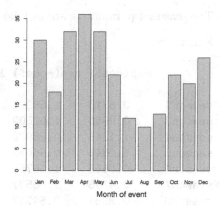

FIGURE 4.21
Seasonal distribution of OPV vaccinations (left) and intussusceptions (right).

The vaccinations are highly seasonal; the intussusceptions less so, though there is some clustering of events in the first half of the year. Thus, there is a possibility of seasonal confounding: it is advisable to control for season, as well as age.

We now describe how the function `standardsccs` may be used to fit a seasonal (calendar time) effect as well as an age effect. As previously noted, all age variables must be specified as days of age since birth. (This is the case for the OPV and intussusception data.) Two additional arguments are supplied to the function `standardsccs`. First, the date of birth of each case, in format *ddmmyyyy*, is specified in argument `dob`. Second, the cutpoints for the season groups are specified in argument `seasongrp` in format *ddmm*, these representing the first days of each season group. The seasonal effect is a factor, the reference level being the time interval starting at the earliest date in `seasongrp`.

For the OPV and intussusception data, we shall control for season in calendar months. Thus we define:

```
month <- c(0101,0102,0103,0104,0105,0106,0107,0108,0109,0110,
           0111,0112)
```

This will generate a 12-level factor, and thus 11 additional seasonal parameters. The model with OPV-associated exposure effects, and both age and season effects, is fitted with the model formula `opv+age+season`, as follows.

```
int.mod2 <- standardsccs(event~opv+age+season, indiv=case,
               astart=sta, aend=end, aevent=intus, adrug=
               cbind(opv,opvd2), aedrug=cbind(opv+42,opvd2+42),
               expogrp=c(0,15,29), agegrp=age, seasongrp=month,
               dob=dob, dataformat="multi", data=intdat)
```

The seasonal parameters are as follows:

```
> int.mod2
  .....
          exp(coef) exp(-coef) lower .95 upper .95
  .....
season2     0.6313    1.58392    0.3438    1.1593
season3     0.9950    1.00502    0.5624    1.7603
season4     1.1245    0.88930    0.6386    1.9800
season5     1.0345    0.96662    0.5850    1.8294
season6     0.8565    1.16754    0.4710    1.5574
season7     0.4795    2.08537    0.2357    0.9757
season8     0.3934    2.54217    0.1858    0.8329
season9     0.4977    2.00920    0.2513    0.9857
season10    0.8030    1.24528    0.4487    1.4373
season11    0.7677    1.30265    0.4267    1.3812
season12    0.9445    1.05880    0.5536    1.6112
```

The earliest date in `seasongrp` is 0101, January 1st, so the reference level is January. Parameter `season2` corresponds to February, parameter `season3` to March, etc. With this parameterisation, statistically significant seasonal effects are obtained for July to September: in these months the relative incidence is significantly lower than in January.

The vaccine exposure effects, adjusted for both age and season, are now as follows:

```
        exp(coef) exp(-coef) lower .95 upper .95
opv1     1.1479    0.87118    0.7123    1.8497
opv2     0.9450    1.05823    0.5607    1.5926
opv3     1.1521    0.86795    0.6999    1.8965
```

All three estimates are closer to 1 than with model `int.mod1`. Thus, there is some confounding by season, though this will not alter the interpretation of the results.

Models `int.mod2` and `int.mod1` are nested, so the statistical significance of the seasonal effect may be evaluated using a likelihood ratio test:

```
> lrtsccs(int.mod1,int.mod2)
    test df  pvalue
  18.41 11 0.07254
```

Thus the seasonal effect as a whole is marginally statistically non-significant. We may also fit a dose-specific seasonal model:

```
int.mod3 <- standardsccs(event~opv+age+season, indiv=case,
            astart=sta, aend=end, aevent=intus, adrug=
            cbind(opv,opvd2), aedrug=cbind(opv+42,opvd2+42),
            expogrp=c(0,15,29), agegrp=age, seasongrp=month,
```

```
            dob=dob, dataformat="multi", sameexpopar=F,
            data=intdat)
```

The relative incidences associated with each dose of OPV are now as follows:

```
> int.mod3
.....
          exp(coef) exp(-coef) lower .95 upper .95
opv1        1.0404     0.96116    0.5477    1.9763
opv2        0.7154     1.39791    0.3360    1.5229
opv3        1.1392     0.87778    0.6043    2.1476
opv4        1.2499     0.80007    0.6721    2.3245
opv5        1.2123     0.82490    0.6289    2.3368
opv6        1.2138     0.82385    0.6069    2.4275
```

None of these parameters are statistically significantly different from 1, nor is there much evidence of a dose effect. This may be verified with a likelihood ratio test:

```
> lrtsccs(int.mod3,int.mod2)
   test df pvalue
   1.328  3 0.7225
```

We may thus conclude that, having controlled for both age and season effects, there is little evidence of any association between OPV and intussusception, and little evidence of a dose effect.

Note finally that the syntax described above enables other season groups to be defined. Cuba is a tropical country with a rainy season from May to October and a dry season from November to April. This rainy/dry seasonality is reflected by the following seasonal groups:

```
rainydry <- c(0105,0111)
```

The model with these seasonal groups (and common vaccine effects at each dose) is then

```
int.mod4 <- standardsccs(event~opv+age+season, indiv=case,
            astart=sta, aend=end, aevent=intus, adrug=
            cbind(opv,opvd2), aedrug=cbind(opv+42,opvd2+42),
            expogrp=c(0,15,29), agegrp=age, seasongrp=rainydry,
            dob=dob, dataformat="multi", data=intdat)
```

The vaccine effects are similar to those obtained without any seasonal effect (model `int.mod1`). The seasonal effect is as follows:

```
> int.mod4
.....
       exp(coef) exp(-coef) lower .95 upper .95
.....
season2     1.266    0.79001    0.9516     1.684
```

The earliest date in `seasongrp` is 0105, so the reference level is the rainy season, May to October. Parameter `season2` now corresponds to the dry season, November to April. The relative incidence for the dry season (relative to the rainy season) is 1.27 which, with 95% CI $(0.95, 1.68)$, is not statistically significantly different from 1.

In any specific application, the choice of season groups should depend on context.

4.10   Parameterisation of the standard SCCS model*

In this section we describe more formally the parameterisation of the standard SCCS model. The material in this section is primarily for use in later starred sections. We begin by describing in more detail the simple version of the standard model introduced in Section 4.1.

In this simple model, there are no time-invariant covariates y_i, and there is a single type of exposure. All individuals share the same age effect $\psi(t)$. Only the effects for ages t lying within the observation period $(a_i, b_i]$ of at least one of the N cases need to be specified. Thus, we partition the age interval $(a, b]$ where $a = \min\{a_i : i = 1, \ldots, N\}$ and $b = \max\{b_i : i = 1, \ldots, N\}$ into $J + 1$ disjoint intervals $(c_j, c_{j+1}], j = 0, \ldots, J$ with $c_0 = a$ and $c_{J+1} = b$. The age effect is assumed to be piecewise constant on these intervals. It is represented by a single age-dependent factor $u(t)$ with $J + 1$ levels, parameterised by the vector $\boldsymbol{\alpha}$, level j corresponding to interval $(c_j, c_{j+1}]$. Thus the relative age effect is the step function

$$\psi(t) = \exp\{u(t)^T \boldsymbol{\alpha}\} = \exp(\alpha_j) \quad \text{for } t \text{ in } (c_j, c_{j+1}].$$

The parameter corresponding to the reference level is set to zero. We shall generally assume that the reference age level is level 0, corresponding to the age group $(c_0, c_1]$, so $\alpha_0 = 0$ and the parameters to be estimated are $\alpha_1, \ldots, \alpha_J$. These are log relative incidences, relative to the reference age category.

Exposures are handled in a similar way to age effects, but with the difference that their timing typically varies between cases, since it depends on the exposure history in x_i. We suppose that the exposure takes $K + 1$ levels $k = 0, \ldots, K$ in non-overlapping age intervals. Level 0 is the baseline or reference level, representing lack of exposure (or a reference exposure level). The exposure effect for case i is piecewise constant on disjoint intervals $(d_{ir}, d_{ir+1}], r = 0, \ldots, D_i$ with $d_{i0} = a_i$ and $d_{iD_i+1} = b_i$. Generally, the number of intervals D_i will vary between cases: for example, some cases might be exposed more often, or with different exposure levels, than others. The exposure effect is represented by a single age-dependent factor $v_i(t; x_i)$ with

---

* This section may be skipped.

$K + 1$ levels, parameterised by the vector $\boldsymbol{\beta}$ and taking some level k_{ir} on the interval $(d_{ir}, d_{ir+1}]$. The relative incidence function for individual i associated with the exposure is the step function

$$\rho(t|x_i) = \exp\{\boldsymbol{v}_i(t; x_i)^T \boldsymbol{\beta}\} = \exp(\beta_{k_{ir}}) \quad \text{for } t \text{ in } (d_{ir}, d_{ir+1}].$$

Level $k = 0$ being the reference level, we set $\beta_0 = 0$. There are K exposure-related parameters $\beta_1, \ldots, \beta_K$ to be estimated. Parameter β_k represents the log relative incidence associated with exposure level k.

The number of age intervals and exposure levels, and the age and exposure cutpoints, are to be chosen by the investigator, and depend entirely on the application. Some general guidance is provided in Chapter 8.

This simple model may be elaborated in several ways, as described in the applications in this chapter. First, both the age effect and the exposure effect may be modified by time-invariant covariates $\boldsymbol{y}_i$. This is handled by including interactions between the time-varying age factor or the time-varying exposure factor and the $\boldsymbol{y}_i$. Examples were described in Section 4.7.

A further extension of the basic model is to include several distinct exposures, for example different pharmaceutical drugs, whose association with the event is of interest. Distinct exposures may be represented by superscripts $s = 1, \ldots, S$. To each exposure type s, with observation and exposure history x_i^s, corresponds a distinct time-varying factor $\boldsymbol{v}_i^s(t; x_i^s)$. Exposure type s is piecewise constant on intervals $(d_{ir}^s, d_{ir+1}^s]$ for $r = 1, \ldots, D_i^s$, has $K^s + 1$ levels with level 0 as reference, and associated parameter vectors $\boldsymbol{\beta}^s = (\beta_0^s, \beta_1^s, \ldots, \beta_{K^s}^s)^T$ with $\beta_0^s = 0$. Note that the exposure intervals $(d_{ir}^s, d_{ir+1}^s]$ can overlap between different exposures. Examples of SCCS models with more than one exposure type were considered in Section 4.5.

Finally, the age effect may be supplemented by a calendar time effect, such as a seasonal effect. This requires a further individual-specific partition into seasonal components, represented by an additional time-varying factor. Such models were considered in greater detail in Section 4.9.

4.11   Bibliographical notes and further material

The theory of generalised linear models (GLMs) is central to the standard SCCS model, owing to the equivalence between product multinomial models and certain Poisson models. The key reference in this regard is McCullagh and Nelder (1989).

Originally, the SCCS software was developed within GLIM4, a now superseded statistical package for fitting GLMs which had the key advantage of possessing an absorption facility. The R package gnm now also possesses this facility (Turner and Firth, 2015) and is one of several that can be used to fit the models in this chapter. The R package SCCS uses the equivalence between the SCCS model and the conditional logistic regression model described in Section 4.2, implemented with function `clogit` within the R package `survival` (Therneau, 2015). Other software for fitting the standard SCCS model may be found on the SCCS website (see Chapter 1, Section 1.4).

The SCCS model was originally developed for evaluating adverse events potentially associated with vaccination. This remains a major area of application, discussed in Andrews (2002) and reviewed in Weldeselassie et al. (2011). To our knowledge, the first use of the method in non-vaccine pharmacoepidemiology was Hubbard et al. (2003). This has now become a major field of application, notably in conjunction with administrative or clinical databases. Reviews of studies using the SCCS method in pharmacoepidemiology include Nordmann et al. (2012), Gault et al. (2017) and Ghebremichael-Weldeselassie et al. (2018), the latter encompassing other applications in non-vaccine epidemiology.

5

Checking model assumptions

Like all statistical methods, the SCCS method relies on assumptions. In this chapter, we describe some techniques for checking whether the assumptions of the SCCS method are reasonable, in the sense that departure from them is unlikely to produce grossly inaccurate inferences. Assumptions may be grouped in several categories, detailed in the following paragraphs.

First are the assumptions about the nature of the underlying process that generates the data. These include assumptions 1, 2 and 3 described in Chapter 3, Section 3.7. They are: (1) events are uncommon or arise in a nonhomogeneous Poisson process; (2) events do not influence observation periods; and (3) events do not influence subsequent exposures.

Then there are assumptions about how the data were sampled, for example assumption 4 in Chapter 3, Section 3.7 (namely, that exposures do not influence ascertainment of cases). It may also be relevant to know whether the data comprise all or a random sample of events occurring within a defined population.

In addition, modelling assumptions are required in specifying the form of the statistical model for the incidence rate function $\lambda(t|x_i, y_i)$. For example, all SCCS models considered in this book assume that age and exposure effects combine multiplicatively. For the standard SCCS model, modelling assumptions also include the number and placing of age and exposure categories.

Other modelling assumptions relate directly to the subject matter of the specific application, notably the choice of variables to include in the model. Examples include interactions with effect modifiers, seasonal effects, and additional time-varying exposures.

Finally, there are assumptions about the validity of the inferential framework, for example whether asymptotic likelihood theory is reliable in the finite sample at hand.

We will not consider sampling and subject matter assumptions in any detail, as these require application-specific information. Likewise, issues regarding the validity of asymptotic likelihood theory are not specific to the SCCS method, so will only be considered briefly.

Our approach to the other categories of assumptions is guided by two principles. First, given that assumptions are unlikely to be true in any absolute sense, what matters primarily is whether the results obtained are sensitive to departures from these assumptions. Thus, we need to establish whether our model is *useful*, rather than whether it is *right*. Second, investigating the validity of and sensitivity to assumptions should be straightforward, otherwise it will not be done. Thus, we restrict the discussion to methods that are easy to use. We focus on the standard SCCS model, though many of the techniques apply more generally. In Chapter 7 we will consider more complicated extensions of SCCS models which may be appropriate when failure of the key assumptions is likely to have a major impact on the results.

The techniques described in this chapter are not intended as a set of recipes to be applied in all circumstances. As with any other statistical model, which assumptions ought to be checked depends on the specific application, and is a matter of judgement. For example, the Poisson assumption for recurrent events need only be checked when there are substantial numbers of recurrences. Event-dependence of observation periods need only be investigated when the event carries substantial short-term mortality. Long-term event-dependence of exposures requires attention only when there is reason a priori to suspect that it might be an issue.

Although the methods described are simple to use, in a few cases their justification involves a technical argument. This material is in Sections 5.1.2, 5.3.4 and 5.4.5, which are starred and may be skipped.

5.1 Rare disease assumption for non-recurrent events

If the event of interest is non-recurrent, the SCCS method works provided that the event is rare. But how rare is 'rare'? In this section we provide some guidance.

Briefly, this may be summarised as follows: if, in the population from which cases are drawn, the probability of the event occurring during a typical observation period is p, conditional on no event having occurred before that, then the relative bias in the relative incidence is of order $\frac{1}{2}p$. Assessing whether such a relative bias is acceptable then depends on context, notably the degree of uncertainty in the estimates (as indicated by the width of the confidence intervals) and the use to which these estimates are to be put.

For example, if the probability that an event will occur within a typical observation period is about 0.1, then the relative bias in the relative incidence is about 0.05, or 5%. This could mean that a relative incidence of 2 is estimated as 2.1.

Evaluating p cannot be achieved using case series data alone: it requires denominator information. However, for our present purpose only rough orders of magnitude are sufficient, and approximate denominator or rate information is usually not difficult to obtain. Two examples are provided in Section 5.1.1. The relative bias is derived in starred Section 5.1.2.

Summary

- A rare disease assumption is required to apply the SCCS method to non-recurrent events.

- The relative bias in the relative incidence is of order $\frac{1}{2}p$, where p is the probability of an event occurring in a typical observation period.

5.1.1 Evaluation of absolute risks: convulsions and stroke

In this section we provide two examples of evaluations of event probabilities. These evaluations aim only to establish orders of magnitude, rather than precise estimates: only rough estimates are required for our purpose.

MMR vaccine and convulsions
In the first example, we evaluate the absolute risk of a child experiencing a first febrile convulsion in the second year of life. Our purpose in doing so is to assess whether a SCCS analysis of MMR vaccine and first convulsion in this age group is valid. Thus, the population we are primarily interested in includes children eligible for MMR vaccination. We use data from Farrington et al. (1995), a record linkage study undertaken in five Health Districts of England. In this study, 952 first admissions for febrile convulsion were recorded in children who received an MMR vaccine before or after their convulsion. It was estimated that, during the study period, 97 300 doses of MMR vaccine had been given in the study districts. Thus, a rough estimate of the probability of experiencing one or more convulsions during the second year of life is $952/97300 \simeq 0.01$. This in turn suggests that the relative bias in the relative incidence estimate in a SCCS study restricted to first convulsions will be of the order of 0.5% or less. A relative bias of this magnitude is sufficiently small to be of no practical concern.

Antipsychotics and stroke
The second example, in contrast, relates to an elderly population. It is based on a SCCS study undertaken to assess the possible association between antipsychotic drugs and first stroke (Douglas and Smeeth, 2008). The median age at stroke in the cases is 80.7 years, with interquartile range (IQR) 73.0–86.8 years. The observation periods span a median of 6.1 years, IQR 3.1–9.8 years. The study was undertaken in England, with stroke cases ascertained in 1988–2002.

Incidence rates for stroke in England may be obtained from Scarborough et al. (2009), Table 2.1. The annual incidence rates vary between studies. Averaging values for men and women, a lower estimate, for Great Britain in 2004, is 837 per 100 000 per year in the 75+ years age group. A higher estimate, for Oxfordshire in 2005, is 1097 per 100 000 per year in the 75–84 year age group. Applying these rates over a period of observation of 6.1 years gives a probability of stroke in the range 0.05–0.07. Thus, the relative bias in a SCCS study of stroke resulting from the rare disease assumption would be expected to be of the order of about 3% or less. This is not likely to be of major concern.

5.1.2 Quantifying the bias for non-recurrent events*

The relative bias is derived in a simple but extreme scenario, in which there are no age effects. Including age effects in the model would be expected to reduce the bias.

We assume that the baseline event hazard λ is constant. Suppose that each individual has the same observation period $(0, b]$ and experiences a single risk period of fixed duration, defined as $(u, u + d]$ with $0 \leq u \leq b - d$. We investigate the asymptotic (large sample) bias in the relative incidence $\rho = \exp(\beta)$ associated with this risk period in a SCCS analysis that makes no allowance for age.

Let Λ denote the cumulative hazard over the entire observation period $(0, b]$, including the exposure period. Thus,

$$\Lambda = \rho \lambda d + \lambda(b - d).$$

The probability that an event occurs in the risk period $(u, u + d]$, conditional on it occurring in $(0, b]$, is

$$P_1 = P(u < T \leq u + d | T \leq b) = \frac{e^{-\lambda u}(1 - e^{-\rho \lambda d})}{1 - e^{-\Lambda}}.$$

Similarly, the conditional probability that an event does not occur in the risk period is

$$P_0 = P(T \leq u \text{ or } T \geq u + d | T \leq b) = \frac{1 - e^{-\lambda(b-d)-\rho\lambda d} - e^{-\lambda u}(1 - e^{-\rho \lambda d})}{1 - e^{-\Lambda}}.$$

The likelihood for a SCCS model with common observation period $(0, b]$, common risk period $(u, u + d]$ and no age effects is binomial. If N is the total number of cases (and therefore of events, since these are non-recurrent), N_1 is the number of events in the risk period, and N_0 the number of events in the control period, then the maximum likelihood estimator of ρ is

$$\hat{\rho} = \frac{N_1}{N_0} \times \frac{b - d}{d}.$$

Asymptotically as $N \to \infty$,

$$\hat{\rho} \to \bar{\rho} = \frac{P_1}{P_0} \times \frac{b - d}{d} \quad \text{in probability.}$$

---

* This section may be skipped.

We consider the limit in which λ, and hence Λ, are small. Using standard approximations,

$$\bar{\rho} = \frac{e^{-\lambda u}(1 - e^{-\rho\lambda d})}{1 - e^{-\lambda(b-d)-\rho\lambda d} - e^{-\lambda u}(1 - e^{-\rho\lambda d})} \times \frac{b-d}{d}$$

$$\simeq \rho[1 + \frac{1}{2}\Lambda(1 - 2\frac{u}{b-d})],$$

to first order in Λ. Thus, the relative bias is of order $\Lambda/2$ if $u = 0$, $-\Lambda/2$ if $u = b - d$, and 0 if $u = (b - d)/2$. In general, to first order,

$$|\frac{\bar{\rho} - \rho}{\rho}| \leq \frac{1}{2}\Lambda.$$

Thus the relative bias in this setting is at most $\frac{1}{2}\Lambda$ in absolute value.

When Λ is small, the probability of an event occurring in the observation period is $p = 1 - \exp(-\Lambda) \simeq \Lambda$, to first order in Λ. Thus the relative bias is of order $\frac{1}{2}p$ or less in absolute value.

5.2 Poisson assumption for potentially recurrent events

The SCCS likelihood for recurrent events is derived under the assumption that the events arise in Poisson processes modulated within individuals by age and time-varying exposures. In most practical applications, the events of interest are rare, so there are relatively few recurrences. Nevertheless, for applications in which recurrences are more common, it is desirable to check that failure of the Poisson assumption would not substantially bias the estimator of the exposure-related relative incidence.

The Poisson assumption may fail if the event intensity function depends on the event history. This will occur, for example, if the occurrence of an event alters the incidence of subsequent events, as is the case with myocardial infarction since subsequent events are more likely after experiencing a first event. The Poisson assumption may also fail if event ascertainment depends on the event history. For example, if events are ascertained through hospital admissions, and several admissions occur as the result of one event, these will be recorded as several events, even though they are part of the same clinical episode. There is often insufficient information to distinguish between episodes on the basis of clustered event information.

5.2.1 Investigating recurrences

The simplest way to investigate the sensitivity of the SCCS model to the Poisson assumption when first events are rare (see Section 5.1), is to repeat the analysis with only first events, and informally compare the relative incidence associated with exposure in the two models. This will usually suffice.

A more formal test of sensitivity to the inclusion of cases with recurrences in the analysis may be undertaken by carrying out a likelihood ratio test of the interaction between the exposure and the marginal event count n_i, or a grouped version of n_i, for example $n_i = 1$ versus $n_i > 1$. Such a test is acceptable, since the SCCS analysis is conditional on the values n_i. Note, however, that it is not acceptable to include an interaction with the order of each event, namely the variable categorising each event as a first, second, ..., kth event. This is because specifying the order imposes a restriction of the observation period, since the kth event can only occur after the first $k - 1$ events. Restricting the analysis to first events only, on the other hand, is valid provided that these are rare in the sense described in Section 5.1.

If there are large numbers of recurrent events, graphical investigations may be useful. If individual i has n_i events at times $t_{i1}, \ldots, t_{in_i}$, with $n_i > 1$, there are $n_i - 1$ inter-event gap times $w_{ij} = t_{ij+1} - t_{ij}$ between events, starting at the first event, with $j = 1, \ldots, n_i - 1$. To explore recurrences visually, it may be useful to inspect gap times. A histogram of the gap times may reveal unexpected patterns. In a pure Poisson process without censoring, gap times are exponentially distributed, so the histogram would be expected to show an exponential decline.

The histogram of gap times, however, does not allow for differences of follow-up time between individuals. Provided that the case series comprises all cases or was randomly sampled from a cohort, the histogram may be supplemented by a nonparametric estimate of the cumulative hazard function of the gap time distribution for second and subsequent events. As a guide to interpretation, if the gap times are exponentially distributed the cumulative hazard should be a straight line.

The cumulative hazard of gap times for second and subsequent events may be obtained because the case series, conditionally on the occurrence of a first event, comprises full information on such events. The observed gap times w_{ij} described previously are supplemented by censored values $w_{in_i} = b_i - t_{in_i}$, where b_i is the end of observation for individual i. The Nelson–Aalen nonparametric estimator of the cumulative hazard function is

$$\hat{\Lambda}(w) = \sum_{k:w_k^* \leq w} \frac{d_k}{m_k}$$

where the w_k^* are the distinct values among the w_{ij}, $i = 1, \ldots, N$, $j = 1, \ldots, n_i - 1$, d_k is the number of gap times equal to w_k^* and m_k is the number of gap times or censored values greater than or equal to w_k^*. The variance of the Nelson–Aalen estimator is

$$\text{var}\{\hat{\Lambda}(w)\} = \sum_{k:w_k^* \leq w} \frac{d_k}{m_k^2}.$$

For further details of this and other estimators see Cook and Lawless (2007), page 123.

The cumulative hazard plot can be used to investigate whether events tend to be clustered within episodes. This would be revealed by an unexpected preponderance of short gap times, resulting in the cumulative hazard function being concave close to the origin.

Summary

- Recurrent events should arise in a non-homogeneous Poisson process.

- When first events are rare, a simple sensitivity analysis is to refit the model with first events only and compare results.

- More formally, an interaction may be fitted to stratify the exposure effect according to presence or absence of recurrences.

- A histogram or a plot of the cumulative hazard of gap times for second and subsequent events may be used to display recurrent events.

5.2.2 Recurrences for MMR and ITP data

We return to the data on ITP and MMR vaccine introduced in Chapter 4, Section 4.3.1. These data comprise 44 events in 35 individuals. A significantly raised relative incidence was found in the 0–42 day period post-MMR, especially in the two-week period 14–28 days. How sensitive is this finding to the assumption that events arise in a non-homogeneous Poisson process within individuals?

The first step in addressing this question is to describe the recurrences in a little more detail. To this end we use three further variables. Variable `rec` identifies the order of each event within the case, and thus takes the value 1 if the event is the first, 2 if it is the second, and so on. Variable `gap` is the gap time between the event and the next event or, if there is no further event, between the event and the end of observation. Finally, variable `cen` takes the value 1 if `gap` is a gap time between successive events, and 0 if not.

The data are in data frame `itpdat`. As before, age at MMR vaccination is in variable `mmr`; age at ITP is in `itp`. Variables `gap`, `cen` and `rec` can be calculated from variables `case`, `itp` and `end`, but are included in the data frame for simplicity.

We first obtain the distribution of event orders:

```
> table(itpdat$rec)

 1  2  3  4  5
35  6  1  1  1
```

This is just another way of saying that there are 29 individuals with a single event, 5 with two events, and 1 with five. With so few recurrences, we are unlikely to find any strong evidence against (or in favour of) the Poisson assumption.

The Nelson–Aalen estimator of the cumulative hazard may be obtained using functions Surv and survfit from R package survival (Therneau, 2015). The code is as follows:

```
library(survival)
par(mar=c(4.1,4.1,1,1), cex.lab=1.4)
plot(survfit(Surv(itpdat$gap,itpdat$cen)~1,type=
    "fleming-harrington",error="tsiatis"), fun=
    "cumhaz", xlab="gap time (days)",
    ylab="cumulative hazard")
```

This produces the plot shown in Figure 5.1. As expected, the confidence bands

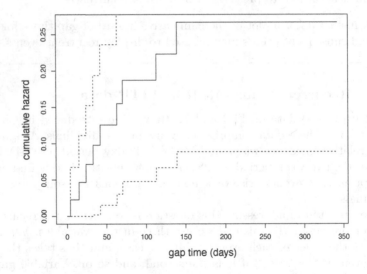

FIGURE 5.1
ITP gap times for second and subsequent events: Nelson–Aalen estimator of the cumulative hazard (full line), with 95% confidence bands (dashed lines).

are very wide. The plot provides little evidence to suggest that gap times are clustered near zero, as the cumulative hazard appears to be linear close to the origin.

Whether or not recurrences satisfy the Poisson assumption remains a moot point. However, what really matters is to what extent the results depend on this assumption. Since ITP is a rare event, we may assess sensitivity to the assumption by repeating the analysis with just the 35 first events. This is achieved using the subset function, as follows.

```
itp.mod7 <- standardsccs(event~mmr+age, indiv=case, astart=
            sta, aend=end, aevent=itp, adrug=mmr, aedrug=
            mmr+42, expogrp=c(0,15,29), agegrp=c(427, 488, 549,
            610, 671), data=subset(itpdat,rec==1))
```

This produces the following results.

```
> itp.mod7
......
      exp(coef) exp(-coef) lower .95 upper .95
mmr1    1.5945     0.6272    0.35544    7.1526
mmr2    7.1921     0.1390    2.91823   17.7251
mmr3    3.2174     0.3108    0.89305   11.5914
```

These results may be contrasted with those obtained in Chapter 4, Section 4.3.1. The relative incidences are a little higher when the analysis is restricted to first events, with the same pattern as observed previously. This is because all recurrences occurred outside risk periods.

The same applies when the three risk periods are combined into one:

```
> itp.mod8 <- standardsccs(event~mmr+age, indiv=case, astart=
              sta, aend=end, aevent=itp, adrug=mmr, aedrug=
              mmr+42, agegrp=c(427,488,549,610,671),
              data=subset(itpdat,rec==1))
> itp.mod8
......
      exp(coef) exp(-coef) lower .95 upper .95
mmr1    3.9415     0.2537    1.78140    8.7209
```

In Chapter 4, Section 4.3.1, the relative incidence in the 0–42 day risk period was found to be 3.23, 95% CI (1.53, 6.79). Thus, neither the results nor their interpretation are substantially altered when recurrences are excluded. We conclude that the analysis is not sensitive to failure of the Poisson assumption.

5.2.3   Recurrent convulsions and MMR vaccine

In the previous example there were rather few recurrences; the present data set is larger and there are more recurrences, enabling a few more analyses to be undertaken. The data comprise the 2435 convulsions in 2201 cases previously described in Chapter 4, Section 4.5.1: thus, there are 234 recurrences.

The data are in data frame `condat`; `mmr` is the age at MMR vaccination and `conv` is the age at convulsion. The data also include variables `gap`, `cen` and `rec` described in Section 5.2.2, and the variable `ngrp` which takes the value 1 if the case has a single event and the value 2 if the case has more than one event. These four variables can be calculated from the others, but are included in the data frame for simplicity.

We begin by describing the recurrences:

```
> table(condat$rec)

    1    2    3    4    5    6    7    8    9
 2201  170   42   13    4    2    1    1    1
```

Thus one case had nine events, one had six, two had five, nine had four, 29 had three, 128 had two and 2031 had one. The gaps between successive events may be represented graphically as follows.

```
par(mar=c(4.1,4.1,1,1), cex.lab=1.4)
hist(ifelse(condat$cen==1,condat$gap,NA), breaks=seq(0,350,10),
     xlab="gap time (days)", main=NULL)
```

This produces the histogram shown in Figure 5.2; note that only uncensored gap times are included. The histogram shows a mode close to zero, as would

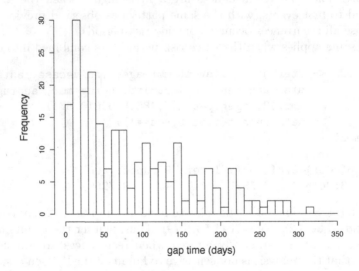

FIGURE 5.2
Histogram of gap times between adjacent recurrences of convulsions.

be expected if the gap times were exponentially distributed – and also if they were clustered in episodes. To get more insight we obtain the Nelson–Aalen estimator of the cumulative hazard; the R code is as follows.

```
library(survival)
par(mar=c(4.1,4.1,1,1), cex.lab=1.4)
plot(survfit(Surv(condat$gap,condat$cen)~1,type=
     "fleming-harrington",error="tsiatis"),
     fun="cumhaz", xlab="gap time (days)",
     ylab="cumulative hazard")
```

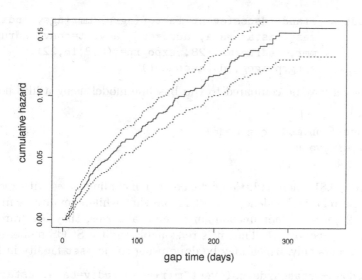

FIGURE 5.3
Gap times for second and subsequent convulsions: Nelson–Aalen estimator of the cumulative hazard (full line), with 95% confidence bands (dashed lines).

The cumulative hazard of the gap times is plotted in Figure 5.3. The estimator displays some concavity close to zero, in the range 0–100 days. This may indicate that short gap times occur too frequently: accordingly, we undertake some further investigations.

First, we fit the baseline model, with 20-day age groups and four weekly risk periods, $[0, 7]$, $[8, 14]$, $[15, 21]$ and $[22, 28]$ days post-MMR.

```
ageg <- seq(387,707,20)
con.mod4 <- standardsccs(event~mmr+age, indiv=case, astart=sta,
            aend=end, aevent=conv, adrug=mmr, aedrug=mmr+28,
            expogrp=c(0,8,15,22), agegrp=ageg, data=condat)
```

This yields the following relative incidence estimates:

```
> con.mod4
......
```

	exp(coef)	exp(-coef)	lower .95	upper .95
mmr1	1.1128	0.8986	0.8600	1.4401
mmr2	2.4669	0.4054	2.0399	2.9832
mmr3	1.1796	0.8477	0.9043	1.5387
mmr4	1.1700	0.8547	0.8950	1.5294

Thus, only in the second week post-MMR is the relative incidence significantly raised, with $RI = 2.47$, 95% CI $(2.04, 2.98)$. We now fit an interaction model, allowing different exposure effects according to the levels of ngrp, as follows.

```
con.mod5 <- standardsccs(event~factor(ngrp)/mmr+age, indiv=
            case, astart=sta, aend=end, aevent=conv, adrug=
            mmr, aedrug=mmr+28, expogrp=c(0,8,15,22),
            agegrp=ageg, data=condat)
```

This model may be compared to the baseline model using a likelihood ratio test:

```
> lrtsccs(con.mod4,con.mod5)
  test df pvalue
  1.58  4 0.8124
```

Since $p = 0.81$, there is little evidence that including cases with recurrences alters the relative incidence. Finally, note that while convulsions in children aged 1–2 years are not uncommon in clinical terms, they are 'rare' by the criterion of Section 5.1. Thus it is reasonable to fit a SCCS model restricted to first events only, which may be done using the subset facility in R:

```
con.mod6 <- standardsccs(event~mmr+age, indiv=case, astart=sta,
            aend=end, aevent=conv, adrug=mmr, aedrug=mmr+28,
            expogrp=c(0,8,15,22), agegrp=ageg,
            data=subset(condat,rec==1))
```

This yields

```
> con.mod6
......
     exp(coef) exp(-coef) lower .95 upper .95
mmr1    1.1127     0.8987    0.8541    1.4496
mmr2    2.5404     0.3936    2.0944    3.0815
mmr3    1.2099     0.8265    0.9228    1.5864
mmr4    1.1857     0.8434    0.9002    1.5619
```

The relative incidence in the second week is only very marginally higher than for the baseline model: RI = 2.54, 95% CI (2.09, 3.08); the RIs for other risk periods are only marginally different as well, and not statistically significant.

We conclude from these analyses that, though there may be some evidence of clustering of events in episodes, as suggested by the slight concavity of the cumulative hazard close to the origin, this has little impact on the results, and hence the baseline SCCS model is sufficiently robust to departures from the Poisson assumption to provide trustworthy estimates.

5.3   Event-dependent observation periods

A key assumption of the SCCS method is that the observation periods are not influenced by the events. This assumption was discussed in Chapter 3,

Section 3.7. The assumption is required to ensure that conditioning on observation periods does not alter the event intensity function, which may in turn bias the relative incidence associated with exposure.

The main scenario in which the assumption may fail is if the event of interest carries high short-term mortality, so that some events are soon followed by an event-induced end of observation. Generally, if there is no (or low) short-term mortality attributable to the event, it is reasonable to regard the assumption as being valid.

If the event is associated with increased short-term mortality, this does not necessarily imply that inferences are biased. When the relative incidence is indeed biased, the bias can be in either direction. If censoring of observation periods primarily affects unexposed or 'control' time, relative incidences associated with exposure will be biased towards zero. If on the other hand the censoring primarily affects exposed or 'at risk' time, the relative incidences will be biased upwards. Generally, bias arises when exposures primarily occur towards one end of the observation period. Event-dependence of observation periods also can wreak havoc with age-related relative incidence estimates, these typically being biased upwards in older age groups.

Note finally that if it is found that failure of the assumption is likely to induce non-ignorable bias, the extension of the SCCS method described in Chapter 7, Section 7.2 may be used.

In the present section we discuss some straightforward methods to investigate the assumption that observation periods are not influenced by events, and the sensitivity of the results to failure of this assumption. We focus entirely on the possibility that observation periods may be curtailed soon after an event. The material in starred Section 5.3.4 is more technical and may be skipped.

5.3.1 Investigating event-dependent observation periods

Suppose that a case i experiences an event at age t_i; if events are recurrent, let t_i be the age at the first event. Let $(a_i, b_i]$ denote the observation period for individual i. If occurrence of an event precipitates the end of observation, one might expect to observe a cluster of short intervals $s_i = b_i - t_i$. Thus, the first step in investigating event-dependence of observation periods ought to be to inspect a histogram of the s_i.

A formal hypothesis test of such clustering may be undertaken by fitting a SCCS model with all the exposures of interest, along with an additional terminal exposure with risk period $(b_i - \tau, b_i]$ where τ is some constant. Then use a likelihood ratio test to test the null hypothesis that the relative incidence associated with this terminal risk period is 1 – that is, test the null hypothesis of no clustering of events close to the end of observation. The likelihood ratio test is preferred to the inspection of parameter estimates from this expanded model, since a degree of confounding between age effects and this terminal exposure period may in certain circumstances affect these estimates. The value

τ is context-dependent. A range of values may be tried; τ must be smaller than the shortest observation period duration $b_i - a_i$.

This test is very limited in scope: it may detect the occurrence of event-dependent observation periods, but does not offer any guide as to whether this influences the estimate of the exposure effect β. As will be shown in Section 5.3.4, it is perfectly possible for event-dependent observation periods not to have any impact on the estimates of β. In order to investigate robustness we need further information – namely whether the observation period has been censored by (possibly event-induced) early termination. To describe this censoring we need to describe the set-up in a little more detail, and introduce some new notation.

In most SCCS studies, observation periods are defined by pre-specified age and calendar time boundaries, which determine the start and end ages of the observation period. In practice, the observation period may stop earlier than the planned value b_i^*, at some age $c_i < b_i^*$. This may be because the individual has died, or for some other reason. If $c_i < b_i^*$, we say the observation period has been censored; if $c_i \geq b_i^*$ the observation period is uncensored. The actual observation period is $(a_i, b_i]$ where b_i is the minimum of c_i and b_i^*.

We define the following censoring indicator:

$$I_i = 1 \text{ if } b_i < b_i^*, \ 0 \text{ if } b_i = b_i^*,$$

and assume that the values of I_i are available in variable `censor`.

To investigate whether censoring of observation periods biases the estimated exposure-related relative incidence, we study the interaction between the exposure of interest and the censoring indicator. Thus, we fit the interaction model with model formula `Censor/Exposure + Age`. As will be shown below, if censoring of observation periods is unrelated to events, then the interaction is zero.

A likelihood ratio test for zero interaction may be undertaken, comparing the interaction model to the standard SCCS model with model formula `Exposure + Age`. Evidence against the null hypothesis of zero interaction suggests that censoring of observation periods may be related to events, and may significantly affect the relative incidence associated with exposure. The interaction with age is not included, as interest focuses on the exposure effects.

In addition, the interaction may be investigated directly, by contrasting the estimated exposure effects in the censored and uncensored groups. Substantial differences in these estimates, even if the interaction is not statistically significant, might indicate that event-dependence of observation periods is likely to affect the results, or their interpretation.

This procedure is only likely to be useful when the numbers of cases with censored observation periods and with uncensored observation periods are both reasonably large. If there are few censored cases, event-dependent censoring of observation periods is unlikely to be a major problem. However, if there are few uncensored cases, then the test may be uninformative. In this situation there is little alternative but to try the extension of the SCCS model to be described in Chapter 7, Section 7.2.

Summary

- Observation periods should not be influenced by events.

- Histograms of the time interval between event and end of observation can help to identify event-induced censoring of observation.

- A simple (but limited) test is to fit a terminal risk period.

- Robustness may be investigated by including an interaction between the exposure and an indicator for early termination of the observation period.

- If the results are not robust to event-dependence of observation periods, an extension from Chapter 7, Section 7.2 may be used.

5.3.2   Planned and actual observation periods: NRT and MI

In Chapter 4, Section 4.8.3, we investigated the association between the initiation of nicotine replacement therapy (NRT) and first myocardial infarction (MI). The start of the observation period was the day NRT began; the planned end of the observation period, in variable **end**, was 365 days after the start of NRT.

In fact, for 39 of the 141 cases, observation ended before the full 365 days had elapsed. For some of these 39, the reason observation ended may have been related to their myocardial infarction: indeed, for 9, observation ended on the day of MI. Thus, a SCCS analysis with the actual observation periods may have biased the estimators, which is why we used the planned observation periods stretching to 365 days after NRT initiation. This was possible in this example because all risk periods were known, by design (because exposure is NRT initiation and all observation periods start at the first NRT prescription).

In the present section, we shall investigate the implications of using the actual observation periods. The data, in data frame **nrtdat**, also contain the actual end of observation for each case in variable **act**. The variable **cen** is equal to 1 if **act** is strictly less than the planned end of observation in variable **end**, and 0 otherwise. As before, **mi** is the age at MI and **nrt** is the age at NRT.

Figure 5.4 shows the histograms of the intervals from MI to the planned (365 days after NRT) and actual ends of observation. The contrast between the two histograms is noticeable: intervals to the actual end of observation display a sharp mode close to zero. This may indicate event-dependence of the actual observation periods.

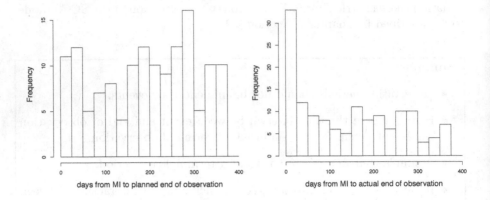

FIGURE 5.4
Intervals between MI and end of observation. Left: planned. Right: actual.

To investigate this further, we first re-fit the SCCS model with the previously used NRT-associated risk periods $[0, 7]$, $[8, 14]$, $[15, 21]$ and $[22, 28]$ days from initiation of NRT, but now using `act` rather than `end` as the end of observation. As before we do not fit an age effect.

```
nrt.mod3 <- standardsccs(event~nrt, indiv=case, astart=nrt,
            aend=act, aevent=mi, adrug=nrt, aedrug=nrt+28,
            expogrp=c(0,8,15,22), agegrp=NULL, data=nrtdat)
```

Now extend the model to include an additional terminal risk period of duration τ; we shall use $\tau = 30$ days. To this end we include the end of observation `act` as an additional exposure, with risk period starting 30 days before that.

```
nrt.mod4 <- standardsccs(event~nrt+act, indiv=case, astart=nrt,
            aend=act, aevent=mi, adrug=list(nrt,act), aedrug=
            list(nrt+28,act), expogrp=list(c(0,8,15,22),-30),
            agegrp=NULL, data=nrtdat)
```

We test the inclusion of the terminal risk period using a likelihood ratio test:

```
> lrtsccs(nrt.mod3,nrt.mod4)
  test df    pvalue
 14.73  1 0.0001241
```

Unsurprisingly, the terminal effect is highly significant, confirming the impression conveyed by the histogram. Finally we fit the SCCS model with an interaction between the exposure and the censoring variable `cen`.

```
nrt.mod5 <- standardsccs(event~factor(cen)/nrt, indiv=case,
            astart=nrt, aend=act, aevent=mi, adrug=nrt,
            aedrug=nrt+28, expogrp=c(0,8,15,22), agegrp=NULL,
            data=nrtdat)
```

We compare this model to the baseline model:

```
> lrtsccs(nrt.mod3,nrt.mod5)
  test df pvalue
 7.073  4 0.1321
```

Since $p = 0.13$, the interaction term is not statistically significant. Thus, there is little evidence that event-dependence of observation periods has a statistically significant impact on the exposure effects. These are as follows, from the baseline model `nrt.mod3`:

```
> nrt.mod3
......
      exp(coef) exp(-coef) lower .95 upper .95
nrt1    0.8863     1.1283    0.3408     2.305
nrt2    1.0129     0.9873    0.3895     2.634
nrt3    0.6753     1.4809    0.2083     2.189
nrt4    0.7366     1.3575    0.2301     2.358
```

None of the relative incidences from this model are statistically significant. This was also the finding in Chapter 4, Section 4.8.3, using the planned observation periods terminating 365 days after initiation of NRT, as obtained from `nrt.mod1` in that section. However, it is instructive to compare informally the results: the relative incidences obtained with the actual observation periods are much lower than those obtained previously. This is because event-dependent censoring shortens the control periods, owing to the fact that risk periods are always at the start of observation. Thus, while the analysis suggest that event-dependent censoring has no statistically significant impact on exposure effects, this may be due to low power of the interaction test. The results obtained using the planned observation periods, rather than the actual ones possibly curtailed by death, are more trustworthy as they are guaranteed to be unaffected by event-dependence.

5.3.3 Heavy censoring: antipsychotics and stroke

In the NRT and MI example of Section 5.3.2, it was possible to use the planned observation periods even if they were curtailed by censoring. This is not generally possible, since exposures after censoring are not usually known (in the NRT application no exposures could occur after censoring, since exposure was NRT initiation, and all observation periods began at the first NRT prescription). In this section we describe such an application. In addition, in this example, the proportions of cases with censored observation periods is high.

The example concerns the potential association between antipsychotics and stroke in patients with and without dementia. The data are simulated, based on Douglas and Smeeth (2008). The data in data frame `apdat` include 2000 cases of first stroke with at least one prescription for an antipsychotic. There are 1500 cases in patients without dementia (`dem = 0`) and 500 cases in

patients with dementia (`dem` = 1). Stroke carries high short-term mortality, so
in this example event-dependent censoring of observation periods is virtually
certain to occur. The issue of primary interest is whether it has any impact
on the estimates of relative incidence for antipsychotics and stroke, and if so,
how much.

Cases can have repeated exposures to antipsychotics. The data are in
the (default) `stack` format, with the exposure endpoints in variables `ap` and
`endap`. Age at stroke is in `stro` and the censoring indicator is in `cen`. The case
identifier is `case`. Figure 5.5 shows the distribution of observation periods for
all 2000 cases.

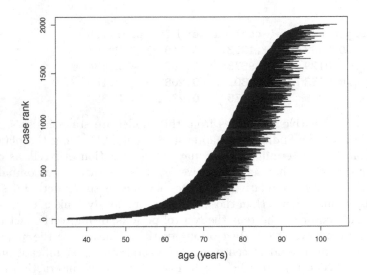

FIGURE 5.5
Observation periods for 2000 stroke cases.

This figure was obtained using the following code.

```
par(mar=c(4.1,4.1,1,1), cex.lab=1.4)
usta <- apdat$sta[duplicated(apdat$case)==0]
uend <- apdat$end[duplicated(apdat$case)==0]
os <- order(usta)
plot(c(min(usta)/365.25, max(uend)/365.25), c(1,length(os)),
     type="n", xlab="age (years)", ylab="case rank")
segments(usta[os]/365.25, 1:length(os),
         uend[os]/365.25, 1:length(os))
```

The observation periods span the age range 35–105 years, each one lasting
up to 15 years. For the dementia cases, the observation periods start later,
from age 60 years (not shown). To assess the potential impact of censoring of

observation periods, we obtain counts of the numbers censored by dementia status.

```
> table(apdat$cen[duplicated(apdat$case)==0],
       apdat$dem[duplicated(apdat$case)==0])
        0    1
  0   394   47
  1  1106  453
```

Thus, of the 1500 cases without dementia, 1106 (74%) are censored; of the 500 cases with dementia, 453 (91%) are censored. For these data, censoring means 'not present in the database at the end of study', so that death due to stroke is not the only cause of censoring; other causes include deaths not associated with stroke. The distributions of intervals from stroke to end of observation in uncensored and censored cases are shown in Figure 5.6.

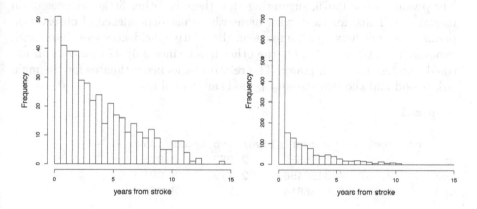

FIGURE 5.6
Intervals between stroke and end of observation. Left: uncensored cases. Right: censored cases.

For the censored cases, the peak in intervals under 6 months is very much more pronounced than for uncensored cases. This is suggestive of event-dependent censoring. In order to throw some light on whether censoring of observation periods is likely to bias the relative incidences associated with antipsychotics, we test the interaction between the exposure and the censoring indicator. We proceed separately for cases with and without dementia.

The risk period is the period on antipsychotics. Douglas and Smeeth (2008) used five 35-day washout periods; we shall use two 91-day washout periods (to save on parameters). As in Douglas and Smeeth (2008) we use 5-year age groups (except at the extremities of the age range where events are sparse).

For cases with dementia, the age range for stroke is 62 to 102 years; the baseline and interaction models are as follows.

```
agedem <- floor(seq(70,95,5)*365.25)
ap.mod1 <- standardsccs(event~ap+age, indiv=case, astart=sta,
          aend=end, aevent=stro, adrug=ap, aedrug=endap,
          washout=c(1,92,182), agegrp=agedem, data=
          subset(apdat,dem==1))
ap.mod2 <- standardsccs(event~factor(cen)/ap+age, indiv=case,
          astart=sta, aend=end, aevent=stro, adrug=ap,
          aedrug=endap, washout=c(1,92,182), agegrp=agedem,
          data=subset(apdat,dem==1))
```

The likelihood ratio test yields:

```
> lrtsccs(ap.mod1,ap.mod2)
   test df  pvalue
  6.875  3 0.07599
```

The p-value is $p = 0.076$, suggesting that there is rather little evidence of an interaction. Thus, for cases with dementia, event-dependence of observation periods may not have much impact on the relative incidences associated with exposure to antipsychotics. On the other hand, since only 47 cases are uncensored, the test may lack power. The relative incidence estimates for the main risk period and the two washout periods are as follows.

```
> ap.mod1
......
      exp(coef) exp(-coef) lower .95 upper .95
ap1      2.963  0.3375332     2.252     3.898
ap2      2.907  0.3439456     2.172     3.891
ap3      1.978  0.5056814     1.278     3.060
```

Thus, in this unadjusted analysis, the relative incidence associated with antipsychotics is 2.96, 95% CI $(2.25, 3.90)$, and declines a little during the washout periods. The relative incidences for censored and uncensored cases obtained from the interaction model are as follows:

```
> ap.mod2
......
                     exp(coef) exp(-coef) lower .95 upper .95
......
factor(cen)0:ap1 3.762e+00  2.658e-01    1.6546     8.555
factor(cen)1:ap1 2.896e+00  3.453e-01    2.1654     3.873
factor(cen)0:ap2 2.223e+00  4.499e-01    0.8196     6.028
factor(cen)1:ap2 2.973e+00  3.363e-01    2.1897     4.037
factor(cen)0:ap3 2.716e-07  3.681e+06    0.0000       Inf
factor(cen)1:ap3 2.211e+00  4.523e-01    1.4185     3.446
```

For example, the relative incidence associated with antipsychotics is 3.76, 95% CI $(1.65, 8.56)$ in the uncensored group, and 2.90, 95% CI $(2.17, 3.87)$

in the censored group. There are no events in the second washout period for uncensored cases. The estimates from the censored and uncensored groups invite similar inferences, further suggesting that event-dependence may not be a serious problem in patients with dementia.

For cases without dementia, the analysis proceeds along similar lines; the age range for stroke is now 36 to 102 years.

```
agenod <- floor(seq(45,95,5)*365.25)
ap.mod3 <- standardsccs(event~ap+age, indiv=case, astart=sta,
          aend=end, aevent=stro, adrug=ap, aedrug=endap,
          washout=c(1,92,182), agegrp=agenod, data=
          subset(apdat,dem==0))
ap.mod4 <- standardsccs(event~factor(cen)/ap+age, indiv=case,
          astart=sta, aend=end, aevent=stro, adrug=ap,
          aedrug=endap, washout=c(1,92,182), agegrp=agenod,
          data=subset(apdat,dem==0))
```

The model without interaction yields the following estimates:

```
> ap.mod3
......
```

	exp(coef)	exp(-coef)	lower .95	upper .95
ap1	1.434	0.6974396	1.2051	1.706
ap2	1.454	0.6876020	1.2047	1.756
ap3	1.140	0.8773626	0.8523	1.524

These suggest that there is a statistically significant effect of antipsychotics on stroke in patients without dementia. However, model `ap.mod4` gives:

```
> ap.mod4
......
```

	exp(coef)	exp(-coef)	lower .95	upper .95
factor(cen)0:ap1	0.9893	1.0108215	0.6907	1.417
factor(cen)1:ap1	1.6198	0.6173424	1.3290	1.974
factor(cen)0:ap2	1.1399	0.8772953	0.7634	1.702
factor(cen)1:ap2	1.5783	0.6336003	1.2756	1.953
factor(cen)0:ap3	0.8620	1.1601524	0.4654	1.597
factor(cen)1:ap3	1.2534	0.7978343	0.9010	1.744

Thus, the relative incidence for antipsychotics exposure is 0.99, 95% CI $(0.69, 1.42)$ in the uncensored group, but 1.62, 95% CI $(1.33, 1.97)$ in the censored group. Similar contrasts may be observed for the washout periods. Though the confidence intervals overlap, the estimates suggest different inferences in the two groups. On the other hand, the likelihood ratio test yields:

```
> lrtsccs(ap.mod3,ap.mod4)
   test df  pvalue
  6.662  3 0.08349
```

Since $p = 0.083$, there is little evidence of an interaction. At this stage, it appears that while the bias from event-dependent censoring of observation periods may not be large in patients without dementia, it might nevertheless affect our conclusions, and thus it warrants further investigation. In Chapter 7, Section 7.2.4 we describe an adjusted SCCS analysis of the full data set.

In these data, information was available on censoring. What if it had not been? In this case we might have tried fitting a terminal risk period of duration $\kappa = 183$ days, to reflect the large number of intervals of under 6 months between stroke and end of observation. The models, for cases with and without dementia, respectively, are:

```
ap.mod5 <- standardsccs(event~ap+end+age, indiv=case,
        astart=sta, aend=end, aevent=stro, adrug=
        list(ap,end),aedrug=list(endap,end),
        expogrp=list(0,-183),washout=list(c(1,92,182),0),
        agegrp=agedem, data=subset(apdat,dem==1))
ap.mod6 <- standardsccs(event~ap+end+age, indiv=case,
        astart=sta, aend=end, aevent=stro, adrug=
        list(ap,end), aedrug=list(endap,end),
        expogrp=list(0,-183), washout=list(c(1,92,182),0),
        agegrp=agenod, data=subset(apdat,dem==0))
```

The terminal risk periods produce highly significant effects. For cases with dementia,

```
> ap.mod5
......
      exp(coef) exp(-coef) lower .95 upper .95
ap1      2.645    0.378039    2.016     3.471
ap2      2.460    0.406481    1.837     3.294
ap3      1.574    0.635519    1.011     2.450
end1     3.908    0.255910    3.150     4.847
```

Thus, in this group, the relative incidence parameter associated with the terminal risk period is 3.91, 95% CI $(3.15, 4.85)$. The relative incidence associated with antipsychotics remains high, at 2.65, 95% CI $(2.02, 3.47)$, though slightly lower than the value 2.96 from model ap.mod1.

For cases without dementia, we obtain:

```
> ap.mod6
......
      exp(coef) exp(-coef) lower .95 upper .95
ap1     1.1945    0.83717   1.0044     1.421
ap2     1.1963    0.83588   0.9885     1.448
ap3     0.9676    1.03352   0.7209     1.299
end1    2.8370    0.35248   2.4717     3.256
```

The relative incidence associated with the terminal risk period is 2.84, 95% CI (2.47, 3.26). The relative incidence associated with antipsychotics is 1.19, 95% CI (1.00, 1.42). This is closer to the value obtained in the uncensored group from model `ap.mod4`. Thus, fitting a suitably chosen terminal risk period, in this case, may help to reduce the bias.

Finally, note that event-dependence of observation periods is likely to have a big effect on the estimated age effects, especially at older ages, since observation time in these age groups is censored. Typically, age-related relative incidences are inflated in older age groups. Age effects, however, are seldom the focus of inference in SCCS studies.

5.3.4   Censoring of observation periods*

In this section we provide the rationale for the interaction test suggested in Section 5.3.1. Related material is also provided in Chapter 7, Section 7.2.

We modify the SCCS likelihood to incorporate censoring that may lead to the observation period being curtailed. We assume that censoring arises with hazard $\mu_i(s|h_i^s)$ for individual i, where h_i^s is the event history to age s. When there is no event history, that is $h_i^s = \emptyset$, which occurs when no event has occurred by age s, then $\mu_i(s|h_i^s) \equiv \mu_i(s)$. The censoring hazard may depend on the exposure history and time-invariant covariates, though such dependence is not made explicit to simplify the notation. Let $S_i(t|h_i^t)$ denote the survivor function of the censoring event for individual i, that is, the probability that no censoring has occurred by age t given the event history:

$$S_i(t|h_i^t) = \exp\left(-\int_0^t \mu_i(s|h_i^s)ds\right).$$

We now obtain the SCCS likelihood contributions for cases with uncensored and censored observation periods, that is, cases for whom $c_i \geq b_i^*$ (uncensored) or $c_i < b_i^*$ (censored). Because the hazards $\mu_i(s|h_i^s)$ are left unspecified, it is convenient to use the general SCCS likelihood formulation of Chapter 3, Section 3.5. Suppose that case i has events at ages $t_{i1}, \ldots, t_{in_i}$, with $t_{i1} < t_{i2} < \cdots < t_{in_i}$. At b_i, the event history for case i is thus

$$h_i^{b_i} = \{t_{i1}, \ldots, t_{in_i}\}.$$

Suppose first that case i is uncensored, so $I_i = 0$ (I_i is defined in Section 5.3.1). The SCCS likelihood contribution then becomes:

$$L_i = \frac{\prod_{j=1}^{n_i} \lambda_i(t_{ij}|x_i, y_i) S_i(b_i|t_{i1}, \ldots, t_{in_i})}{\int_{a_i}^{b_i} \cdots \int_{s_{n_i-1}}^{b_i} \prod_{j=1}^{n_i} \lambda_i(s_j|x_i, y_i) S_i(b_i|s_1, \ldots, s_{n_i}) ds_{n_i} \ldots ds_1},$$

$$(5.1)$$

---

* This section may be skipped.

with $s_0 = a_i$ if $n_i = 1$. Now suppose that case i is censored, so $I_i = 1$. The SCCS likelihood contribution L_i is now:

$$\frac{\prod_{j=1}^{n_i} \lambda_i(t_{ij}|x_i, y_i)\mu_i(b_i|t_{i1}, \ldots, t_{in_i})S_i(b_i|t_{i1}, \ldots, t_{in_i})}{\int_{a_i}^{b_i} \cdots \int_{s_{n_i-1}}^{b_i} \prod_{j=1}^{n_i} \lambda_i(s_j|x_i, y_i)\mu_i(b_i|s_1, \ldots, s_{n_i})S_i(b_i|s_1, \ldots, s_{n_i})ds_{n_i} \cdots ds_1}.$$

$$(5.2)$$

Suppose that the censoring hazard does not depend on the event history, so that $\mu_i(s|h_i^s) \equiv \mu_i(s)$, and therefore $S_i(t|h_i^t) \equiv S_i(t)$. Then the terms involving $\mu_i(b_i)$ and $S_i(b_i)$ in these likelihood contributions cancel out, leaving just

$$
\begin{aligned}
L_i &= \frac{\prod_{j=1}^{n_i} \lambda_i(t_{ij}|x_i, y_i)}{\int_{a_i}^{b_i} \cdots \int_{s_{n_i-1}}^{b_i} \prod_{j=1}^{n_i} \lambda_i(s_j|x_i, y_i)ds_{n_i} \cdots ds_1} \\
&= n_i! \times \frac{\prod_{j=1}^{n_i} \lambda_i(t_{ij}|x_i, y_i)}{\left(\int_{a_i}^{b_i} \lambda_i(s|x_i, y_i)ds\right)^{n_i}}.
\end{aligned}
$$

This last expression follows from the fact that there are $n_i!$ different orderings of the n_i event times; it may be proved by induction on n_i. Thus, when the censoring hazard does not depend on the event history, we retrieve the SCCS likelihood from Chapter 3, Equation 3.5.

The key point, for our purpose, is that event-dependent observation periods introduce extra terms in the SCCS likelihood contributions, which differ according to whether observation periods are censored or not. This is what motivates the test based on including an interaction term with the censoring variable. Under the null hypothesis that observation periods are not event-dependent, this interaction is zero. Because we are primarily interested in the possible bias induced by event-dependent observation periods in the exposure-related relative incidences, we implement this test by expanding the SCCS model to include the interaction between the censoring variable and the exposure effect, but not the interaction with age.

We have several times stated that event-dependent censoring of observation periods does not imply that the estimated exposure parameter of interest, β, is biased. Thus, the results need not be sensitive to failure of this assumption. We now demonstrate this in a special case. Suppose that

$$\mu_i(t|h_i^t) = \mu_i(t) + \|h_i^t\|\theta,$$

where $\|h_i^t\|$ is the number of events for individual i that have occurred prior to t in $(a_i, b_i]$. Thus, for case i, the censoring hazard is $\mu_i(t)$ before the first event, and $\mu_i(t) + k\theta$ between the kth and $(k+1)$th events. It follows that

$$
\begin{aligned}
\mu_i(b_i|s_1, \ldots, s_{n_i}) &= \mu_i(b_i) + n_i\theta, \\
S_i(b_i|s_1, \ldots, s_{n_i}) &= e^{-n_ib_i\theta} \times \prod_{j=1}^{n_i} e^{\theta s_j} \times \exp\left(-\int_{a_i}^{b_i} \mu_i(s)ds\right).
\end{aligned}
$$

Inserting these expressions in Equations 5.1 and 5.2, the adjusted SCCS likelihood contribution for case i turns out to be identical whether the case is censored or uncensored. It may be written

$$L_i = \text{constant} \times \frac{\prod_{j=1}^{n_i} \lambda_i^*(t_{ij}|x_i, \boldsymbol{y}_i)}{\left(\int_{a_i}^{b_i} \lambda_i^*(s|x_i, \boldsymbol{y}_i)ds \right)^{n_i}},$$

where $\lambda_i^*(t|x_i, \boldsymbol{y}_i) = \lambda_i(t|x_i, \boldsymbol{y}_i)\exp(\theta t)$. The term $\exp(\theta t)$ is incorporated into the age effect of the proportional incidence model (see Chapter 4, Expression 4.1), which becomes $\psi^*(t) = \psi(t)\exp(\theta t)$, leaving the exposure effect unchanged.

Note that L_i is a standard SCCS likelihood contribution. The likelihood will yield unbiased estimates of β, though the estimate of the age effect is likely to be seriously upwardly biased (if $\theta > 0$), especially at older ages.

5.4 Event-dependent exposures

The third key assumption of the SCCS method is that events do not influence subsequent exposures. Specifically, exposures are required to be external, or exogenous, in the sense described in Chapter 3, Section 3.7. This assumption is required to ensure that conditioning on exposure histories over the observation period does not alter the intensity function of the event; this in turn is needed to ensure that the relative incidence associated with exposure is not biased.

There are two specific scenarios in which the assumption may fail, which invite different adjustments. The first, more benign, scenario arises when occurrence of an event affects the exposure process for a fixed, and usually short, period. This typically occurs with routine childhood vaccinations, which are generally only administered to well individuals: if an event occurs, administration of the vaccine in the days following the event may be delayed until the child has recovered. The second, more challenging, scenario arises when occurrence of an event permanently alters the subsequent exposure process. This may occur, for example, if the event is a contra-indication to treatment with the drug of interest.

Event-dependent exposures will usually bias the estimators of relative incidence associated with exposure (though the bias may be small). On the other hand, the direction of bias is often predictable: if occurrence of an event delays or reduces the probability of subsequent exposures, then the relative incidence associated with exposure will be biased upwards. If, on the other hand, the occurrence of an event precipitates subsequent exposures, or increases their probability, then the relative incidence will be biased downwards, towards zero.

If the impact of an event on subsequent exposures is short-lived, as is most often the case, then a simple adjustment to the standard SCCS model can be applied. If, on the other hand, events affect the subsequent exposure process over the long term, then the extension of the SCCS model described in Chapter 7, Section 7.1 may be used.

In Section 5.4.1, some straightforward methods are described to investigate the assumption that exposures are not influenced by events. These are followed by some examples. Starred Section 5.4.5 is a little more technical and may be skipped.

5.4.1 Investigating event-dependent exposures

We assume that events do not influence observation periods, and investigate whether events might influence exposures. Suppose first that the event of interest is non-recurrent, and that each case experiences at most one exposure. Suppose that case i has an event at age t_i and a point exposure, or start of exposure, at age u_i. Suppose now that occurrence of an event reduces the chance of an exposure occurring (or starting) during the subsequent time interval of duration τ. This would result in a dearth of exposures in the post-event period $(t_i, t_i + \tau]$. Conversely, if occurrence of an event increases the chance of an exposure occurring during the subsequent time interval τ, this would result in an excess of exposures in this post-event period.

To identify any unusual patterns of exposures in relation to the timing of events, a histogram of the time intervals $t_i - u_i$ may be useful. We call this the centred event plot. Cases with no exposed time in their observation period are not included in the centred event plot. If a case has several events, or several exposures of the same type, we superimpose the data for each event-exposure combination.

More formally, suppose that case i, $i = 1, \ldots, N$, has events at ages t_{ij}, $j = 1, \ldots, n_i$, and point exposures, or exposure starts, at ages u_{ik}, $k = 1, \ldots, m_i$, with $n_i \geq 1$ and $m_i \geq 0$. The centred event plot includes all $\sum_{i=1}^{N} n_i \times m_i$ values $t_{ij} - u_{ik}$, with $j = 1, \ldots, n_i$ and $k = 1, \ldots, m_i$; if $m_i = 0$, the intervals are undefined and case i is left out. If there are different exposure types, separate centred event plots for each exposure type can be obtained.

In the SCCS model, event times are random, while exposures are treated as fixed, and are conditioned upon. Thus, for a case i with observation period $(a_1, b_i]$ and an exposure at age u_{ik}, the values of $t_{ij} - u_{ik}$ in the centred event plot are limited to the interval $(a_i - u_{ik}, b_i - u_{ik}]$. This is because t_{ij} could in principle take any value in $(a_i, b_i]$, since under the Poisson assumption the ordering of event times within individuals is immaterial.

The distribution of the ranges $(a_i - u_{ik}, b_i - u_{ik}]$ may affect the appearance of the plot. It may be useful, therefore, to supplement the centred event plot with a second centred plot, showing the maximum possible number of events, given the constraints imposed by the observation periods, numbers of events per case, and exposure histories. We call this the centred observation plot. It is obtained by plotting $E(t)$ against t, where

$$E(t) = \sum_{i=1}^{N} \sum_{k=1}^{m_i} n_i \times I_{ik}(t).$$

Here $I_{ik}(t)$ is the indicator function for the interval $(a_i - u_{ik}, b_i - u_{ik}]$, taking the value 1 if $t \in (a_i - u_{ik}, b_i - u_{ik}]$ and 0 otherwise. Again, if $m_i = 0$ then the interval is undefined and case i is left out. $E(t)$ is the number of events in exposed cases whose observation periods include the time interval t from exposure; we call this the number under observation. In particular, $E(0)$ is the number of events in exposed cases.

In centred event plots, interest focuses on the shape of the histogram in pre-exposure intervals $[-\tau, 0)$ for relevant positive values of τ. For example, a dearth of events in $[-\tau, 0)$ may indicate that exposures are postponed after an event until an interval τ has elapsed. A cluster of events at positive values, on the other had, may reflect the association of primary interest – but this is not our present focus. This aspect of centred event plots will be discussed in Section 5.5.

Observing a dearth or an excess of events in an interval of duration τ prior to exposure is exactly equivalent to observing a dearth or an excess of exposures in an interval of duration τ after an event. This suggests a simple test for short-term event-dependence of exposures: expand the standard SCCS model to include the pre-exposure risk period $[-\tau, 0)$ prior to each point exposure or prior to the start of each extended exposure. Note, however, that this pre-exposure interval is not actually associated with any exposure-induced risk. Under the null hypothesis that there is no short-term event-dependence of exposures of duration τ, the relative incidence parameter corresponding to this pre-exposure risk period is $\exp(\xi) = 1$. This null hypothesis can be tested using a likelihood ratio test; it is also important to know whether inclusion of a pre-exposure risk period alters the relative incidences associated with exposure.

Several potentially useful graphical representations can be based on this test. For example, the parameter estimate $\exp(\hat{\xi})$ can be plotted against τ, for a range of values τ. This plot, with confidence limits on the estimates, helps to indicate the duration of exposure-related event-dependence. In addition, the robustness of a relative incidence parameter of primary interest, β, to event-dependent exposures, may be visualised by plotting the estimated values $\exp(\hat{\beta})$ obtained with pre-exposure risk periods of different durations τ.

As previously remarked, the relative incidence parameter $\exp(\xi)$ associated with a pre-exposure risk period is not an exposure-related quantity. However, in certain conditions (for example, when τ is small or repeat events are uncommon) it approximates the relative incidence of exposures after events. For example, if $\exp(\xi) = 0.5$, this signifies that an exposure is half as likely to occur in an interval τ after an event than it would have had no event occurred.

This interpretation is explored further in starred Section 5.4.5, which may be skipped.

However, some caution is required in the interpretation of the pre-exposure risk period parameter when there are overlaps between the pre-exposure risk period and the exposure risk periods. Such overlaps may occur when cases experience several exposure episodes. Then it is advisable to include an interaction term between pre-exposure and post-exposure risk periods, to provide greater flexibility in modelling the relative event rate on the overlaps.

Summary

- Exposures should not be influenced by events. For example, the event should not be a contra-indication to the exposure of interest.

- A histogram of the time interval between the start of exposure and the event can help to identify event-dependence of exposures.

- A simple test for short-term event-dependence of exposures is to expand the model to include a pre-exposure risk period.

- Robustness may be investigated graphically by varying the duration of pre-exposure risk periods and plotting the results.

- If the results are not robust to event-dependence of exposures, the extension of Chapter 7, Section 7.1 may be used.

5.4.2 Event-dependence of exposures: ITP and MMR

We return to the data on ITP and MMR vaccine previously considered in Section 5.2.2 of the present chapter, and in Chapter 4, Section 4.3.1. A priori, it is likely that, in the event of a child being admitted to hospital for ITP, vaccination would be postponed for a short period until the child had recovered. However, it is unlikely that vaccination would be affected long after the event. We examine the data to throw light on the matter; we shall use the data frame `itpdat` previously described.

Recall that the observation period is $[366, 730]$ days, and that the post-MMR risk period of interest is 0–42 days. Thus only MMR vaccinations in the age range $[324, 730]$ days of age are relevant. The centred event and observation plots are obtained as follows.

```
par(mfrow=c(1,2), mar=c(4.1,4.1,1,1), cex.lab=1.4)
mmrx <- ifelse(itpdat$mmr<366-42|itpdat$mmr>730, NA, itpdat$mmr)
timint <- itpdat$itp - mmrx
hist(timint, breaks=seq(-350,350,25), xlab="days since MMR",
     ylab="number of events", main=NULL)
xtime <- seq(min(itpdat$sta-mmrx,na.rm=T),
```

```
          max(itpdat$end-mmrx,na.rm=T), 1)
ytime <- NULL
for (i in 1:length(xtime)){
ytime[i] <- sum((itpdat$sta-mmrx<=xtime[i])*
          (xtime[i]<=itpdat$end-mmrx), na.rm=T)
}
plot(xtime, ytime, type="s", xlab="days since MMR",
     ylab="number under observation")
abline(v=2, lty=2)
```

The two centred plots are in Figure 5.7. The panel on the left shows the event

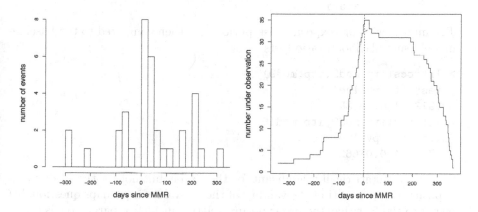

FIGURE 5.7
Centred plots for ITP data. Left: event plot. Right: observation plot.

plot. The cluster of events at short positive intervals reflects the association between MMR and ITP. There are no events at short negative intervals (the first such event is at -46 days). Indeed, there are only 9 events at negative intervals – however, this is likely to reflect the lack of observation time shown in the panel on the right, itself due to the fact that most primary MMR vaccines are administered early in the second year of life. (The number under observation at t, plotted in the observation plot, is the number of events in exposed cases, whose observation periods include the interval t from exposure.) The absence of events at short negative intervals may be a chance effect, or it may be due to delay in vaccination following an event.

We investigate further the potential impact of delayed vaccination on the relative incidence estimates. To keep matters simple, we use the relative incidence for the $[0, 42]$ day post-MMR risk period. The baseline model `itp.mod2` (with no pre-exposure risk period), and models with pre-exposure risk periods of $\tau = 14$ days (model `itp.mod9`) and $\tau = 28$ days (model `itp.mod10`) are specified as follows; model `itp.mod2` was originally fitted in Section 4.3.1, and is re-fitted here for completeness.

```
itp.mod2 <- standardsccs(event~mmr+age, indiv=case, astart=sta,
             aend=end, aevent=itp, adrug=mmr, aedrug=mmr+42,
             expogrp=0, agegrp=c(427,488,549,610,671),
             data=itpdat)
itp.mod9 <- standardsccs(event~mmr+age, indiv=case, astart=sta,
             aend=end, aevent=itp, adrug=mmr, aedrug=mmr+42,
             expogrp=c(-14,0), agegrp=c(427,488,549,610,671),
             data=itpdat)
itp.mod10 <- standardsccs(event~mmr+age, indiv=case, astart=sta,
              aend=end, aevent=itp, adrug=mmr, aedrug=mmr+42,
              expogrp=c(-28,0), agegrp=c(427,488,549,610,671),
              data=itpdat)
```

The models with pre-exposure risk periods are then compared to the baseline model using likelihood ratio tests.

```
> lrtsccs(itp.mod2,itp.mod9)
  test df  pvalue
 2.979  1 0.08435
> lrtsccs(itp.mod2,itp.mod10)
  test df  pvalue
 5.736  1 0.01662
```

The effect is statistically significant for the 28-day but not for the 14-day pre-exposure risk period (but the validity of these p-values is perhaps questionable owing to the fact that the pre-exposure relative incidence parameter is 0 and hence lies on the boundary of the parameter space). The key issue, however, is whether including a pre-exposure risk period substantially alters the relative incidence associated with MMR. To evaluate this, we try a sequence of values of τ, and loop through them as follows.

```
tau <- seq(14,84,14)
pre.ri <- pre.lo <- pre.hi <- NULL
ri <- lo <- hi <- NULL
for (i in 1:length(tau)){
d <- -tau[i]
mod <- standardsccs(event~mmr+age, indiv=case, astart=sta,
        aend=end, aevent=itp, adrug=mmr, aedrug=mmr+42,
        expogrp=c(d,0), agegrp=c(427,488,549,610,671),
        data=itpdat)
pre.ri[i] <- mod$conf.int[1,1]
pre.lo[i] <- mod$conf.int[1,3]
pre.hi[i] <- mod$conf.int[1,4]
ri[i] <- mod$conf.int[2,1]
lo[i] <- mod$conf.int[2,3]
hi[i] <- mod$conf.int[2,4]
}
```

These parameter values may then be plotted, as follows.

```
par(mfrow=c(1,2), mar=c(4.1,4.1,1,1), cex.lab=1.4)
plot(tau, pre.ri, type="p", pch=16, xlim=c(0,100),
    ylim=c(0,2.5), xlab="pre-exposure interval (days)",
    ylab="relative incidence")
abline(1, 0, lty=2)
segments(tau, pre.lo, tau, pre.hi)
plot(tau, ri, type="p", pch=16, xlim=c(0,100), ylim=c(0,7),
    xlab="pre-exposure interval (days)", ylab=
    "relative incidence")
segments(tau, lo, tau, hi)
abline(itp.mod2$conf.int[1,1], 0, lty=2)
points(0, itp.mod2$conf.int[1,1], pch=16)
segments(0, itp.mod2$conf.int[1,3], 0, itp.mod2$conf.int[1,4])
```

These plots are displayed in Figure 5.8. The plot on the left shows the esti-

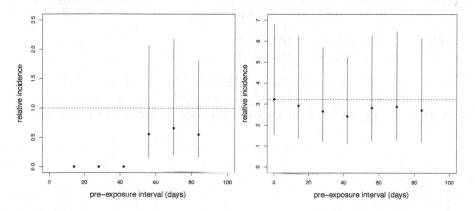

FIGURE 5.8
Relative incidences and 95% CIs, by duration of pre-exposure risk period. Left: relative incidence associated with the pre-exposure interval. Right: relative incidence associated with MMR vaccine.

mated relative incidences $\exp(\hat{\xi})$ associated with the pre-exposure risk period. The estimates for $\tau = 14, 28, 42$ days are presented without confidence intervals, as these cannot be calculated using asymptotic methods, because there are no events in these intervals (profile likelihood confidence limits could be used instead). For other values of τ, the confidence intervals include 1. The plot on the right shows the estimated relative incidences associated with MMR vaccine with a 0–42 day risk period. The baseline model with no pre-exposure risk period yields $RI = 3.23$, 95% $(1.53, 6.79)$. With a pre-exposure risk period of $\tau = 42$ days, $RI = 2.41$, 95% CI $(1.11, 5.26)$; other values of τ yield estimates closer to that of the baseline model. We conclude that while there is some evidence that MMR vaccination may be delayed after a hospital admission for ITP, and that this inflates the estimated relative incidence, the conclusion that ITP is associated with MMR vaccination is robust to such a departure from the assumption that events do not influence subsequent exposures.

5.4.3   Event-dependence with multiple exposures: NSAIDs, antidepressants and GI bleeds

In Chapter 4, Sections 4.5.2 and 4.7.2 we considered analyses of simulated data on gastro-intestinal (GI) bleeds, non-steroidal anti-inflammatory drugs (NSAIDs) and antidepressants (ADs). Might occurrence of a GI bleed delay subsequent administration of NSAIDs or ADs? We consider the evidence. The data are in data frame `addat` and are arranged in format `stack`, with repeat exposures and events in separate rows. Thus the intervals between GI bleeds and the start of NSAID and AD exposures, for all within-case combinations of events and exposures, are simple to obtain:

```
nsint <- addat$bleed - addat$ns
adint <- addat$bleed - addat$ad
```

In this case the range of the GI to NSAID or GI to AD intervals is wide, so we shall focus on intervals of about a year on either side of the exposures. The centred event plots, for NSAIDs and ADs respectively, are in Figure 5.9.

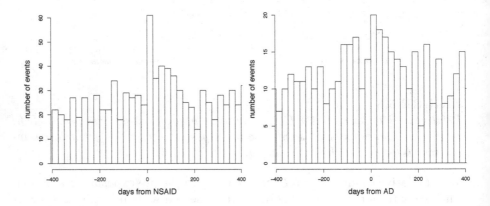

FIGURE 5.9
Centred event plots for GI bleed data. Left: days from start of NSAID prescription. Right: days from start of AD prescription.

Interval zero corresponds to the start of the prescription. Both plots show a clustering of events at short positive intervals, more pronounced for NSAIDs, corresponding to the association between these exposures and occurrence of GI bleeds. There is no clear evidence of an unusually pronounced peak or trough at short negative intervals, suggesting that events do not appear to impact substantially upon exposures.

We investigate this further by including pre-exposure risk periods for both NSAIDs and ADs. Normally we would use a short interval such as $\tau = 14$ days, as any effect is likely to be short-lived. However, to illustrate how to handle overlaps between pre-exposure and post-exposure risk periods we shall use $\tau = 60$ days (there are no overlaps with $\tau = 14$ days). We first refit the baseline model ad.mod5; to keep matters simple we use the model without interaction, without changing the reference age group.

```
ageq <- floor(quantile(addat$bleed[duplicated(addat$case)==0],
        seq(0.025,0.975,0.025), names=F))
ad.mod5 <- standardsccs(event~ns+ad+age,
            indiv=case, astart=sta, aend=end, aevent=bleed,
            adrug=cbind(ns,ad), aedrug=cbind(endns,
            endad), agegrp=ageq, data=addat)
ad.mod6 <- standardsccs(event~ns+ad+age,
            indiv=case, astart=sta, aend=end, aevent=bleed,
            adrug=cbind(ns,ad), aedrug=cbind(endns,
            endad), expogrp=list(c(-60,0),c(-60,0)),
            agegrp=ageq, data=addat)
```

The likelihood ratio test yields:

```
> lrtsccs(ad.mod5,ad.mod6)
   test df pvalue
  2.508  2 0.2854
```

The p-value is $p = 0.29$, which suggests there is little evidence of event-dependence in a 60-day period. More important, however, is to assess the robustness of the baseline model. The estimated relative incidences for model ad.mod6 are:

```
> ad.mod6
. . . . . .
```

	exp(coef)	exp(-coef)	lower .95	upper .95
ns1	1.231	0.812648	0.9351	1.619
ns2	2.075	0.481884	1.6792	2.565
ad1	1.065	0.938760	0.7257	1.564
ad2	1.281	0.780734	0.9585	1.712

Thus, the estimated pre-exposure relative incidences are 1.23 for the 60-day period prior to NSAIDs, and 1.07 for the 60-day period prior to ADs – both are close to 1 and not statistically significant. The relative incidences associated with NSAIDs and ADs are 2.08 and 1.28, respectively. In Chapter 4,

Section 4.7.2, the estimated values without a pre-exposure risk period were 1.99 and 1.28, respectively: including a 60-day pre-exposure risk period has little impact on these estimates.

However, this analysis ignores possible overlaps between pre-exposure and post-exposure risk periods, which may arise since each case can experience several exposure episodes. In such circumstances it is advisable to fit a model including the interaction between pre- and post-exposure risk periods. To do so, it is necessary to redefine the pre-exposure risk periods as relating to distinct exposures. Thus, define new variables nspre and adpre as follows:

```
nspre <- addat$ns-60
adpre <- addat$ad-60
```

The main effects model (without interactions) may then be fitted as follows:

```
ad.mod7 <- standardsccs(event~ns+nspre+ad+adpre+age,
          indiv=case, astart=sta, aend=end, aevent=bleed,
          adrug=cbind(ns,ad,nspre,adpre), aedrug=cbind(endns,
          endad,ns-1,ad-1), agegrp=ageq, data=addat)
```

This relative incidence estimates for model ad.mod7 are as follows.

```
> ad.mod7
......
```

	exp(coef)	exp(-coef)	lower .95	upper .95
ns1	2.016	0.496028	1.6380	2.481
nspre1	1.141	0.876758	0.8706	1.494
ad1	1.284	0.778986	0.9656	1.707
adpre1	1.043	0.958460	0.7143	1.524

The estimated relative incidences for the pre-exposure periods are 1.14 for NSAIDs and 1.04 for ADs. These differ (slightly) from those obtained using model ad.mod6. The discrepancies are due to the different conventions used to handle overlaps. In model ad.mod6, precedence is given to the most recent exposure, whereas in model ad.mod7 overlaps are modelled by combining parameters for the two intervals involved. These conventions are discussed in detail in Chapter 4, Section 4.5.4.

The interactions between pre and post-exposure risk periods for each exposure may be included as follows in the model (again, for simplicity, we have not included interactions between the two exposures).

```
ad.mod8 <- standardsccs(event~ns*nspre+ad*adpre+age,
          indiv=case, astart=sta, aend=end, aevent=bleed,
          adrug=cbind(ns,ad,nspre,adpre), aedrug=cbind(endns,
          endad,ns-1,ad-1), agegrp=ageq, data=addat)
```

The relative incidence estimates and the interactions for model ad.mod8 are as follows.

```
> ad.mod8
......
```

	exp(coef)	exp(-coef)	lower .95	upper .95
ns1	2.0775	0.481338	1.6808	2.568
nspre1	1.2190	0.820349	0.9184	1.618
ad1	1.2838	0.778953	0.9605	1.716
adpre1	1.0440	0.957848	0.7006	1.556

```
......
```

	exp(coef)	exp(-coef)	lower .95	upper .95
ns1:nspre1	0.5501	1.817807	0.2148	1.409
ad1:adpre1	1.0022	0.997767	0.2927	3.432

Neither interaction term is statistically significant. The relative incidences for the pre-exposure risk periods are 1.22 for NSAIDs and 1.04 for ADs. The exposure-related relative incidences are 2.08 for NSAIDs and 1.28 for ADs. These results differ only marginally from those obtained from models ad.mod6 and ad.mod7. We conclude that, in these data, overlaps between pre-exposure and post-exposure risk periods have little impact on the results.

Finally, the likelihood ratio test to compare models ad.mod5 (without pre-exposure risk periods) and ad.mod8 (with pre-exposure risk periods, including interactions) is as follows.

```
> lrtsccs(ad.mod5,ad.mod8)
   test df pvalue
  2.752   4 0.6001
```

As before, the p-value $p = 0.60$ suggests there is little evidence of event-dependence of exposures in a 60-day period.

Our substantive conclusion from this analysis is that the assumption that events do not exert a short-term influence on subsequent exposures is reasonable in this application.

5.4.4 Long-term dependence: influenza vaccine and GBS

Our final example is one in which the SCCS model is *not* robust to failure of the assumption that events do not influence subsequent exposures.

In Chapter 4, Section 4.9.1, we discussed a possible association between influenza vaccine and Guillain–Barré syndrome (GBS). Administration of the seasonal influenza vaccine may not be appropriate for patients with a history of GBS. This is likely to introduce long-term dependence of exposures on events: patients who have had GBS are less likely subsequently to receive the influenza vaccine.

The centred event and observation plots are shown in Figure 5.10. The event plot, on the left, shows that, of the 52 GBS cases with an influenza vaccination, only one had an event before the vaccine. On the other hand, the observation plot, on the right, shows a sharp increase in the number under observation before 0. (The number under observation at t is the number

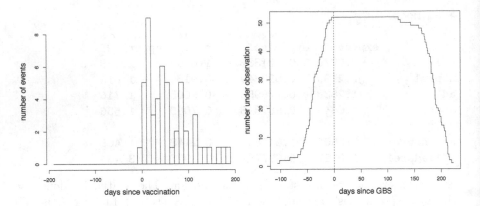

FIGURE 5.10
Centred event and observation plots for GBS and influenza vaccination.

of events in exposed cases whose observation period includes the interval t from exposure.) Thus, the vaccinated cases had less opportunity for GBS to arise before vaccination – largely due to the fact that influenza vaccination is encouraged early in the influenza season.

Figure 5.10 is obtained with the following code.

```
gint <- gbsdat$gbs - gbsdat$flu
par(mfrow=c(1,2), mar=c(4.1,4.1,1,1), cex.lab=1.4)
gcuts <- seq(-190,190,10)
hist(gint, breaks=gcuts, xlab="days since vaccination",
     ylab="number of events", main=NULL)
xtime <- seq(min(gbsdat$sta-gbsdat$flu, na.rm=T),
        max(gbsdat$end-gbsdat$flu,na.rm=T), 1)
ytime <- NULL
for (i in 1:length(xtime)){
ytime[i] <- sum((gbsdat$sta-gbsdat$flu <= xtime[i])*
        (xtime[i] <= gbsdat$end-gbsdat$flu), na.rm=T)
}
plot(xtime, ytime, type="s", xlab="days since GBS",
     ylab="number under observation")
abline(v=0, lty=2)
```

A priori, we must assume that there is strong event-dependence of exposures, and thus the standard SCCS model is unlikely to be appropriate. Consequently, these data will be reanalysed using the extension of the SCCS model to be described in Chapter 7, Section 7.1. Nevertheless, it is instructive to examine the impact of including a pre-exposure risk period in the standard SCCS model.

We begin by fitting a SCCS model with a pre-exposure risk interval of duration $\tau = 120$ days, and monthly season groups as in Chapter 4, Section 4.9.1:

```
seas   <- cumsum(c(31,30,31,31,28,31))
gbs.mod4 <- standardsccs(event~flu+age, indiv=case, astart=
            sta, aend=end, aevent=gbs, adrug=flu, aedrug=flu+42,
            expogrp=c(-120,0), agegrp=seas, data=gbsdat)
```

This produces the following estimates.

```
> gbs.mod4
......
      exp(coef) exp(-coef) lower .95 upper .95
flu1    0.09418    10.6180   0.01215    0.7298
flu2    1.82738     0.5472   0.96901    3.4461
```

The pre-exposure effect is statistically significant, with $RI = 0.094$, 95% CI $(0.012, 0.73)$. The relative incidence associated with influenza vaccination is now marginally statistically non-significant: $RI = 1.83$, 95% CI $(0.97, 3.45)$. Other values of τ confirm these results, as shown in Figure 5.11, for values $\tau = 20(20)120$. The R code is omitted, as it is similar to that of Section 5.4.2.

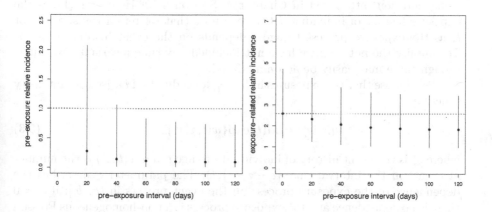

FIGURE 5.11
Relative incidences and 95% CIs, by duration of pre-exposure risk period. Left: relative incidence associated with the pre-exposure interval; the dashed line is at $RI = 1$. Right: relative incidence associated with influenza vaccine; the dashed line is at $RI = 2.58$.

The plot on the left shows the relative incidences associated with the pre-exposure risk interval. For the larger values of τ, the effects are statistically significant, in that the 95% confidence interval is entirely located below 1, suggesting that there is indeed a significant dearth of GBS events prior to influenza vaccination. The impact this has on the relative incidences associated with influenza vaccination are shown in the plot on the right.

When no pre-exposure risk period is included, $RI = 2.58$, 95% $(1.42, 4.71)$. When a pre-exposure risk period is included, the relative incidence is reduced to such an extent that it may become marginally statistically non-significant. We conclude that, in this application, the results are sensitive to the assumption that exposures are not event-dependent.

5.4.5   Interpretation of pre-exposure risk period*

In this section we explore a little further the idea of including a pre-exposure risk period in a standard SCCS model in order to identify short-term dependence of exposures on events. We need to consider both the event and the exposure processes simultaneously. We suppose that exposures are point events, such as vaccinations; more general formulations in which the point exposure marks the start of a treatment period could also be considered.

Suppose that events, which may be recurrent for an individual i, arise in a process with intensity function

$$\lambda_i(t|x_i^t) = \phi_i \psi_i(t) \exp\{v_i(t, x_i^t)^T \beta\},$$

using notation introduced in Chapter 4, Section 4.10. Here x_i^t includes the exposure history of individual i to age t; note that we retain the superscript t, as the exposure process to age t depends on the event history to age t. To simplify the notation we have not included any time-invariant covariates, though these may easily be accommodated.

We suppose that the exposures in $(a_i, b_i]$ for individual i arise with intensity function

$$\mu_i(t|z_i^t) = \mu_i(t) \exp\{w(t, z_i^t)\xi\}, \tag{5.3}$$

where z_i^t is the event history of individual i to age t and $w(t, z_i^t)$ is the number of events in the interval $(\max\{t - \tau, a_i\}, t)$. The parameter ξ describes the dependence of the exposure process on the event process in $(a_i, b_i]$: if $\xi = 0$ there is no dependence and the exposure process is a non-homogeneous Poisson process with intensity $\mu_i(t)$. If $\xi > 0$, events precipitate exposures within an age interval τ, and if $\xi < 0$ then events inhibit exposures within this interval. Dependence on the event process prior to age a_i is assumed to be incorporated into $\mu_i(t)$.

We consider the joint density of event and exposure times for one individual i over an age interval $(a_i, b_i]$. For greater clarity we shall suppress the individual identifier i, and write $v_i(t, x_i^t)$ as $v(t)$ and $w(t, z_i^t)$ as $w(t)$. Suppose the individual has n events at ages $t = \{t_1, \ldots, t_n\}$ and m exposures at ages $u = \{u_1, \ldots, u_m\}$, where $a < t_1 < \cdots < t_n \le b$ and $a < u_1 < \cdots < u_m \le b$.

---

* This section may be skipped.

Given the exposure and event histories to age a, the joint density of the n event times and m exposure times is

$$f(n, m, \boldsymbol{t}, \boldsymbol{u}) = \phi^n \prod_{j=1}^{n} \psi(t_j) \exp\{\boldsymbol{v}(t_j)^T \boldsymbol{\beta}\} \exp\left(-\int_a^b \phi\psi(s) \exp\{\boldsymbol{v}(s)^T \boldsymbol{\beta}\} ds\right)$$

$$\times \prod_{k=1}^{m} \mu(u_k) \exp\{w(u_k)\xi\} \exp\left(-\int_a^b \mu(s) \exp\{w(s)\xi\} ds\right).$$

$$(5.4)$$

Let $I_A(t)$ denote the indicator function for a time interval A, taking the value 1 when t lies in A and the value 0 otherwise. Define

$$r(t) = \sum_{k=1}^{m} I_{(u_k - \tau, u_k)}(t).$$

We then have

$$\sum_{k=1}^{m} w(u_k) = \sum_{j=1}^{n} r(t_j). \tag{5.5}$$

Note also that if $n \geq 2$ and $t_j - t_{j-1} > \tau$ for all $j = 2, \ldots, n$, then

$$\int_a^b \mu(s) \exp\{w(s)\xi\} ds$$

$$= \sum_{j=1}^{n} \int_a^b \mu(s) \exp\{I_{(t_j, t_j+\tau)}(s)\xi\} ds - (n-1) \int_a^b \mu(s) ds. \tag{5.6}$$

If the condition $t_j - t_{j-1} > \tau$ is not satisfied for some $j \geq 2$, then identity 5.6 holds only approximately: there is an additional term of order $O(\tau)$ corresponding to the overlaps between the intervals $(t_j - \tau, t_j)$.

Substituting Expressions 5.5 and 5.6 in Equation 5.4, and rearranging, yields:

$$f(n, m, \boldsymbol{t}, \boldsymbol{u}) \simeq \left[\prod_{j=1}^{n} \psi^*(t_j) \exp\{\boldsymbol{v}(t_j)^T \boldsymbol{\beta} + r(t_j)\xi\}\right]$$

$$\times \phi^n \prod_{k=1}^{m} \mu(u_k) \exp\left(-\int_a^b \phi\psi(s) \exp\{\boldsymbol{v}(s)^T \boldsymbol{\beta}\} ds\right)$$

$$\times \exp\left((n-1) \int_a^b \mu(s) ds\right), \tag{5.7}$$

where

$$\psi^*(t) = \psi(t) \exp\left(-\int_a^b \mu(s) \exp\{I_{(t, t+\tau)}(s)\} ds\right).$$

Equation 5.7 is exact when $n = 1$ or when $t_j - t_{j-1} > \tau$ for $j = 2, \ldots, n$. Note that only the expression in square brackets in Equation 5.7 involves the event times $t_1 < \cdots < t_n$. Now, as previously seen in Section 5.3.4,

$$\int_a^b \int_{t_1}^b \cdots \int_{t_{n-1}}^b \prod_{j=1}^n \psi^*(t_j) \exp\{v(t_j)^T \beta + r(t_j)\xi\} dt_n \ldots dt_2 dt_1$$

$$= \frac{1}{n!} \left[\int_a^b \psi^*(s) \exp\{v(s)^T \beta + r(s)\xi\} ds \right]^n.$$

Thus, integrating out the event times in Equation 5.7 yields the following approximate expression for the marginal density:

$$\begin{aligned}
f(n, m, u) \quad &\simeq \quad \frac{1}{n!} \left[\int_a^b \psi^*(s) \exp\{v(s)^T \beta + r(s)\xi\} ds \right]^n \\
&\times \quad \phi^n \prod_{k=1}^m \mu(u_k) \exp\left(- \int_a^b \phi\psi(s) \exp\{v(s)^T \beta\} ds \right) \\
&\times \quad \exp\left((n-1) \int_a^b \mu(s) ds \right).
\end{aligned} \tag{5.8}$$

We now reinstate the individual identifiers i. The conditional likelihood contribution of case i with event times $t_{i1}, \ldots, t_{in_i}$, given that n_i events occurred, and given the observed exposures over $(a_i, b_i]$, is obtained by dividing Equation 5.7 by Equation 5.8. Thus it is

$$L_i \simeq n_i! \times \frac{\prod_{j=1}^{n_i} \psi_i^*(t_{ij}) \exp\{v_i(t_{ij})^T \beta + r_i(t_{ij})\xi\}}{\left[\int_{a_i}^{b_i} \psi_i^*(s) \exp\{v_i(s)^T \beta + r_i(s)\xi\} ds \right]^{n_i}}.$$

This has the form of a SCCS likelihood contribution, with baseline age effect $\psi_i^*(t)$, exposure-related parameter vector β, and an additional time-varying covariate $r_i(t)$, which is the number of exposures experienced by case i in $(t, t + \tau)$ within $(a_i, b_i]$, with associated parameter ξ.

Thus, when events are rare (so that $n_i = 1$ for most cases i, for which the likelihood contributions L_i are then exact) or τ is small, we retrieve a SCCS likelihood. For small values τ, or when each case experiences at most one exposure, the number of exposures in any interval $(t, t + \tau)$ is 0 or 1. In this case, including the covariate $r_i(t)$ is the same as defining a pre-exposure risk period of duration τ. From its definition in Equation 5.3, the exponentiated parameter value $\exp(\xi)$ represents the relative incidence of exposure during an interval of duration τ after an event.

5.5   Modelling assumptions

By modelling assumptions, we specifically refer to the specification of the model for the incidence function $\lambda_i(t|x_i, y_i)$. In the case of the standard SCCS model, this includes the appropriateness of the choice of risk periods and age groups, and the age homogeneity of the exposure effect. In this section we briefly discuss how to evaluate these aspects of the SCCS model.

5.5.1   Checking the model

We do not propose any formal, data-driven methods for choosing risk periods: indeed we do not recommend using such techniques, other than in the very specific situation where a SCCS study is undertaken solely as a hypothesis-generating exercise. The reason is that, when used with the analysis methods described in this book, data-driven choices of risk periods may produce spurious inferences about the association between the exposure and event of interest (this is explored further in Chapter 8, Section 8.1.2). On the other hand, it can be useful to represent the data in such a way as to display temporal associations or their absence. This is achieved by the centred event plot described in Section 5.4.1, possibly supplemented by the centred observation plot also described there.

In contrast to risk periods, it does make sense to check that the age groups used in the standard SCCS model are appropriate. The key issue is not usually to obtain a valid estimate of the age effect (though in some applications this may also be required), but to ensure that the estimate of the exposure effect is not biased owing to an inappropriate choice of age categories. A simple way to check this is to refit the model with a finer age categorisation, and informally compare the estimates of β. If there is little practical difference, the original choice of age groups is likely to be adequate.

Finally, the proportional incidence model implies that the relative incidence associated with exposure is constant at different ages, in other words, that the exposure effect is homogeneous. This can be explored by including an `Age * Exposure` interaction term. A likelihood ratio test can be used to check whether including the interaction improves the model fit, though it may be more useful to supplement this by an informal assessment of whether the estimates of β vary with age in practically important ways. To avoid sparse or empty categories and a profusion of parameters, the interaction may best be explored with grouped versions of the original age and exposure levels. If the interaction is found to be statistically significant, this may indicate heterogeneity of the exposure effect, or may call into question the multiplicative effect assumption upon which the proportional incidence model is based. The relative incidence estimated from the standard SCCS model without the interaction should then be interpreted as an average effect.

Summary

- Modelling assumptions include the specification of risk periods and age categories.

- While a data-driven choice of risk periods is generally to be avoided, a centred event plot of the time interval between the start of exposure and the event can help visualise temporal associations.

- Robustness to the choice of age groups may be investigated by using a finer age categorisation.

- Homogeneity of the exposure effect may be investigated by including a (possibly grouped) age by exposure interaction.

5.5.2   Risk periods and age groups: MMR and convulsions

In Section 5.2.3 we explored recurrences of convulsions in data on MMR vaccination. The data, which are in data frame `condat`, were originally analysed in Chapter 4, Section 4.5.1. In this analysis, age was grouped in 20-day periods, and four 1-week risk periods were used: $[0, 7]$, $[8, 14]$, $[15, 21]$ and $[22, 28]$ days post-MMR. A significantly raised relative incidence was found for the $[8, 14]$-day period after MMR, but not for the other risk periods.

To investigate the appropriateness of these preselected risk intervals we construct the centred event and observation plots, restricting attention to MMR vaccines given in the age range $366 - 42 = 324$ to 730 days.

```
par(mfrow=c(1,2), mar=c(4.1,4.1,1,1), cex.lab=1.4)
mmrx <- ifelse(condat$mmr<366-42|condat$mmr>730, NA, condat$mmr)
timint <- condat$conv - mmrx
timhis <- hist(timint, breaks=seq(-400,400,5), xlab=
          "days since MMR", ylab="number of events",
          main=NULL)
xtime <- seq(min(condat$sta-mmrx,na.rm=T), max(condat$end-mmrx,
          na.rm=T), 1)
ytime <- NULL
for (i in 1:length(xtime)){
ytime[i] <- sum((condat$sta-mmrx<=xtime[i])*
          (xtime[i]<=condat$end-mmrx), na.rm=T)
}
plot(xtime, ytime, type="s", xlim=c(-400,400),
     xlab="days since MMR", ylab="number under observation")
abline(v=0, lty=2)
```

This produces the graphs shown in Figure 5.12. The centred event plot reveals a very striking pattern close to zero; this aside it broadly mirrors the overall

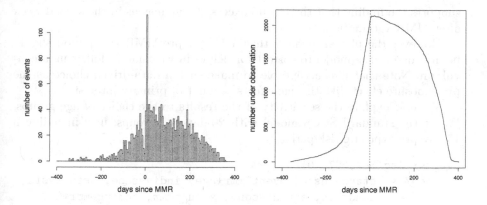

FIGURE 5.12
Centred plots for convulsions. Left: event plot. Right: observation plot.

shape of the centred observation plot. Figure 5.13 zooms in on the neighbourhood of zero; the bin size used is 5 days. The plot shows a large peak in the

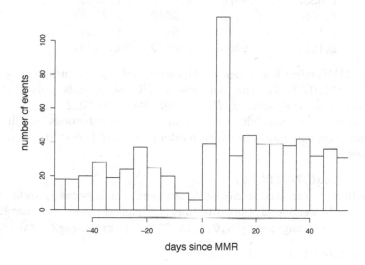

FIGURE 5.13
Detail of centred event plot for MMR and convulsions.

6–10 day period post-MMR, and a marked trough in the period 15–1 days prior to MMR vaccine. Thus, it appears that the choice of MMR-associated risk periods (weeks one to four post-MMR) is adequate: the plot certainly supports the finding that there is an excess of convulsions in the second week after MMR vaccination.

However the plot also shows that a 15-day pre-MMR risk period should be included in the model to correct for delays in vaccination following a convulsion. Note that it is acceptable to make such a data-driven choice as the pre-exposure effect, like the age effects, are not of primary interest.

We now explore the sensitivity of the results to the choice of age groups. We fit the standard SCCS model with 20-day age groups, now including a 15-day pre-exposure risk period.

```
ageg <- seq(387,707,20)
con.mod7 <- standardsccs(event~mmr+age, indiv=case, astart=sta,
            aend=end, aevent=conv, adrug=mmr, aedrug=mmr+28,
            expogrp=c(-15,0,8,15,22), agegrp=ageg, data=condat)
```

The exposure effects are as follows:

```
> con.mod7
......
      exp(coef) exp(-coef) lower .95 upper .95
mmr1    0.3717    2.6900    0.2683    0.5152
mmr2    1.0332    0.9679    0.7977    1.3383
mmr3    2.3014    0.4345    1.9010    2.7863
mmr4    1.1058    0.9043    0.8472    1.4435
mmr5    1.1028    0.9068    0.8432    1.4423
```

The pre-MMR effect is significant, the associated relative incidence being 0.37, 95% CI $(0.27, 0.52)$. For the four post-MMR risk periods, only the effect in the second week is significant, $RI = 2.30$, 95% CI $(1.90, 2.79)$.

To investigate sensitivity to the choice of age categories, we fit a model with more age categories, in which model con.mod7 is nested. We use 10-day age categories:

```
ageg2 <- seq(377,717,10)
con.mod8 <- standardsccs(event~mmr+age, indiv=case, astart=sta,
            aend=end, aevent=conv, adrug=mmr, aedrug=mmr+28,
            expogrp=c(-15,0,8,15,22), agegrp=ageg2, data=condat)
```

The exposure effects for this model are:

```
> con.mod8
......
      exp(coef) exp(-coef) lower .95 upper .95
mmr1    0.3705    2.6992    0.2673    0.5134
mmr2    1.0318    0.9691    0.7965    1.3367
mmr3    2.2903    0.4366    1.8908    2.7741
mmr4    1.1043    0.9056    0.8459    1.4417
mmr5    1.1053    0.9047    0.8451    1.4457
```

The estimates of the exposure effect are very similar to those obtained from model con.mod7. Specifically, the estimate for the second week post-MMR is $RI = 2.29$ rather than 2.30. Thus, the original choice of age categories was adequate.

5.5.3   Homogeneity of effect: MMR and convulsions

We now turn to verifying the homogeneity of the exposure effect. Since only the pre-MMR risk period and the $[8, 14]$ day risk period are associated with convulsions, it makes sense to limit the exposure effects to these two periods. Since they are not adjacent, they cannot be specified using expogrp. Instead we define a new exposure variable pre containing the values mmr-15. We also coarsen the age groups, in order to avoid empty categories when fitting interactions. The reduced model is defined as follows.

```
pre <- condat$mmr-15
ageg3 <- c(427,487,547,607,667)
con.mod9 <- standardsccs(event~mmr+pre+age, indiv=case,
              astart=sta, aend=end, aevent=conv, adrug=
              list(mmr,pre), aedrug=list(mmr+14,pre+14),
              expogrp=list(8,0), agegrp=ageg3, data=condat)
```

The estimated exposure effects are then:

```
> con.mod9
......
```

	exp(coef)	exp(-coef)	lower .95	upper .95
mmr1	2.2822	0.4382	1.8898	2.7562
pre1	0.3666	2.7277	0.2649	0.5073

Parameter pre1 corresponds to the pre-MMR risk period and parameter mmr1 to the 8–14 days post-MMR risk period; the estimates are close to those obtained with model con.mod7 in Section 5.5.2 which included three additional risk periods and three times as many age categories.

We now investigate a possible interaction between the post-MMR exposure effect and age.

```
con.mod10 <- standardsccs(event~age/mmr+pre, indiv=case,
              astart=sta, aend=end, aevent=conv, adrug=
              list(mmr,pre), aedrug=list(mmr+14,pre+14),
              expogrp=list(8,0), agegrp=ageg3, data=condat)
```

```
> lrtsccs(con.mod9,con.mod10)
   test df    pvalue
  18.31  5 0.002582
```

The interaction is highly statistically significant ($p = 0.003$) suggesting that the MMR effect may vary with age, and in this sense is not homogeneous. To

examine this further, we obtain two graphs: first, the relative age effect from
model `con.mod9`, and second, the age by exposure interaction from model
`con.mod10`. The code for these graphs is as follows.

```
par(mfrow=c(1,2), mar=c(4.1,4.1,1,1), cex.lab=1.4)
ar <- c(1,con.mod9$conf.int[3:7,1],con.mod9$conf.int[7,1])
as <- c(366,ageg3,730)/30.5
plot(as, ar, type="s", xlim=c(12,24), ylim=c(0.6,1.1),
     xlab="age (months)", ylab="relative incidence")
ri <- con.mod10$conf.int[7:12,1]
lo <- con.mod10$conf.int[7:12,3]
hi <- con.mod10$conf.int[7:12,4]
ag <- 0.5*(c(ageg3,730)+c(366,ageg3))/30.5
plot(ag, ri, pch=16, xlim=c(12,24), ylim=c(0,16), xlab=
     "age group midpoint (months)", ylab="relative incidence")
segments(ag,lo,ag,hi)
abline(h=con.mod9$conf.int[1,1], lty=2)
```

The graphs are shown in Figure 5.14. The estimated age effect decreases mono-

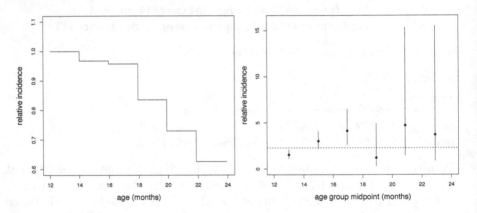

FIGURE 5.14
*Left: relative age effect for convulsions data. Right: relative incidence associ-
ated with MMR, by age group. The horizontal dashed line indicates the relative
incidence without interaction.*

tonically. The MMR-associated relative incidences from the interaction model
are not monotone, though perhaps consistent with an increase. Taken together, these plots might indicate that the exposure and age effects combine
additively rather than multiplicatively. Though the interaction is statistically
significant, the relative incidence estimate from model `con.mod9`, represented
as the dashed line in the right panel of Figure 5.14, nevertheless provides a
useful summary of the association between MMR vaccination and convulsions,
and may be interpreted as an average effect over this age range.

5.6   Asymptotic assumptions

The maximum likelihood inference framework relies on asymptotic arguments, which may or may not be valid in small samples, especially when few events occur in the risk period of interest. In such circumstances it might be possible to combine risk periods to reduce such sparseness problems. Alternatively, an analysis method other than the asymptotic likelihood ratio test may be used.

We shall describe one such alternative: a permutation test; for more detail on such tests see Davison and Hinkley (1997) and Manly (1997). Suppose that N cases are available with observation periods $(a_i, b_i]$, $i = 1, \ldots, N$, and furthermore assume that these observation periods are not determined by the exposure histories. Suppose also that exposure histories are obtained over an age interval $(a, b]$ that includes all the $(a_i, b_i]$, and that case i experiences n_i events. Thus there are $M = \sum_{i=1}^{N} n_i$ events. Each event is assigned the exposure history of the corresponding case; if $n_i > 1$ the exposure history of case i is replicated n_i times. Under the null hypothesis of no association between exposures and events, the exposure histories associated with the M events may be permuted without altering the distribution of the test statistic.

Asymptotically as N grows large, the null distribution of the likelihood ratio test statistic LRT comparing the model Exposure + Age with the model Age is chi-squared on k degrees of freedom, k being the number of exposure parameters. The permutation test, instead, uses the null distribution of LRT obtained by permuting the exposure histories associated with the M events.

Often, the distinct permutations are too numerous to explore them exhaustively, in which case a randomly selected subset of permutations is chosen. Let T_0 denote the observed likelihood ratio test statistic, and $T_1, \ldots, T_R$ the likelihood ratio test statistics obtained from R randomly chosen permutations of the exposure histories. The empirical p-value is then

$$ p = \frac{1 + \|\{T_r : T_r \geq T_0, r = 1, \ldots, R\}\|}{1 + R} $$

where $\|A\|$ denotes the size of set A. The Monte Carlo standard error associated with p is of order $\sqrt{p * (1 - p)/R}$. Calculating the Monte Carlo standard error can help in the choice of R and in the interpretation of discrepancies between asymptotic and empirical p-values.

Summary

- The validity of asymptotic assumptions may be questionable in small samples.

- In some circumstances, a permutation test may be undertaken to supplement the likelihood ratio test.

5.6.1   Permutation test for the aseptic meningitis data

We return to the data on MMR vaccine and aseptic meningitis described in Chapter 3, Sections 3.4 and 3.6. There were just 10 cases, each with a single event, all with observation period 366 to 730 days, and nine of whom received MMR vaccine. We used two age groups: [366, 456] days and [457, 730] days, and the risk period was 15 to 35 days post-MMR. The data are in data frame amdat. First, we obtain the asymptotic likelihood ratio test statistic, and store it in t0.

```
am.mod1 <- standardsccs(event~age, indiv=case, astart=sta,
               aend=end, aevent=am, adrug=mmr, aedrug=mmr+35,
               expogrp=15, agegrp=457, data=amdat)
am.mod2 <- standardsccs(event~mmr+age, indiv=case, astart=sta,
               aend=end, aevent=am, adrug=mmr, aedrug=mmr+35,
               expogrp=15, agegrp=457, data=amdat)
t0 <- lrtsccs(am.mod1,am.mod2)$test
```

The exposure effect estimated in model am.mod2, and the likelihood ratio test, are as follows.

```
> am.mod2
......
     exp(coef) exp(-coef) lower .95 upper .95
mmr1    17.8004    0.05618    4.6476    68.175
......
> lrtsccs(am.mod1,am.mod2)
   test df     pvalue
  14.91  1 0.0001128
```

The relative incidence is 17.8 with 95% CI (4.6, 68.2). The significance of the exposure effect is confirmed by the likelihood ratio test, for which the test statistic is 14.91 on 1 degree of freedom, $p = 0.00011$.

However, the very small sample size (10 events) means that the relevance of asymptotic theory is at the very least questionable. The asymptotic null distribution for the likelihood ratio test is $\chi^2(1)$, the chi-squared distribution on 1 degree of freedom. We explore its validity in the present context by undertaking a permutation test. There are $10! = 3\,628\,800$ permutations of the 10 exposure histories, too many to calculate exhaustively. Instead we randomly sample $R = 999$ permutations, and for each of these obtain the likelihood ratio test statistic. These are stored in vector test. The following code is appropriate for data in which each line corresponds to a separate event, as is the case here.

```
set.seed(54321)
R <- 999
perm <- amdat
test <- NULL
```

```
for (i in 1:R){
perm$expo <- sample(perm$mmr, replace=F)
mod2 <- standardsccs(event~expo+age, indiv=case, astart=sta,
        aend=end, aevent=am, adrug=expo, aedrug=expo+35,
        expogrp=15, agegrp=457, data=perm)
mod1 <- standardsccs(event~age, indiv=case, astart=sta,
        aend=end, aevent=am, adrug=expo, aedrug=expo+35,
        expogrp=15, agegrp=457, data=perm)
test[i] <- lrtsccs(mod1,mod2)$test
}
```

The permutation test p-value is as follows.

```
> (1+sum(test>=t0)))/(1+R)
[1] 0.004
```

The p-value is 0.004: some way from the asymptotic value 0.00011, but still highly statistically significant; the Monte Carlo standard error is 0.002. The null distribution estimated from these 999 permutations, together with the asymptotic $\chi^2(1)$ distribution, may be represented graphically as follows.

```
par(mar=c(4.1,4.1,1,1), cex.lab=1.4)
xval <- seq(0, ceiling(max(test)), 0.1)
hist(test, freq=F, xlab="test statistic", ylab="density",
     breaks=seq(0,ceiling(max(test)),0.25), main=NULL)
abline(v=t0, lty=2)
lines(xval, dchisq(xval,df=1))
```

The resulting plot is in Figure 5.15. The estimated null distribution is distinctly discontinuous, here supported on just six points. (The last support point is indicated by the small bar at 14.91 on Figure 5.15.) These correspond, from left to right on Figure 5.15, to permutations in which 1, 0, 2, 3, 4, 5 events lie within the risk period, respectively. More support points may appear with different permutations. For example, with $R = 9999$ in the code above there are seven, and the p-value is 0.0037 (Monte Carlo standard error 0.0006). Thus, in this example, asymptotic theory is clearly not applicable, but the conclusions are not materially affected by this failure of asymptotic assumptions.

5.6.2 Permutation test for the ITP data

In Section 5.2.2 we investigated the Poisson assumption for the ITP and MMR data. We return to these data, which are in data frame itpdat, to study the validity of asymptotic assumptions. There are 44 events in 35 individuals.

We consider first the model with three risk periods, $[0, 14]$, $[15, 28]$ and $[29, 42]$ days post-MMR. To obtain the likelihood ratio test statistic, we refit models itp.mod1 and itp.mod3 previously explored in Chapter 4, Section 4.6.1. The likelihood ratio test statistic is stored in t0 as follows.

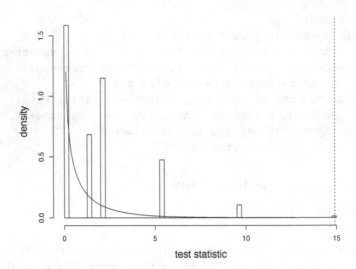

FIGURE 5.15
Estimated probability mass function of the permutation distribution (histogram) and asymptotic $\chi^2(1)$ density. The vertical dashed line indicates the observed value of the test statistic, 14.91.

```
itp.mod1 <- standardsccs(event~mmr+age, indiv=case, astart=sta,
            aend=end, aevent=itp, adrug=mmr, aedrug=mmr+42,
            expogrp=c(0,15,29), agegrp=c(427,488,549,610,671),
            data=itpdat)
itp.mod3 <- standardsccs(event~age, indiv=case, astart=sta,
            aend=end, aevent=itp, adrug=mmr, aedrug=mmr+42,
            expogrp=c(0,15,29), agegrp=c(427,488,549,610,671),
            data=itpdat)
t0 <- lrtsccs(itp.mod1,itp.mod3)$test
```

The likelihood ratio test statistic, and the p-value based on the asymptotic $\chi^2(3)$ distribution, are:

```
> lrtsccs(itp.mod1,itp.mod3)
   test df    pvalue
  13.43  3 0.003793
```

Thus, the exposure effect is highly statistically significant, with asymptotic p-value 0.0038. We investigate the reliability of this value using a permutation test. This is possible because, for these data, exposure histories are available over the age range 366 to 730 days (and beyond), which contains all 35 observation periods.

The data comprise one line per event. The permutation test is implemented as follows, with $R = 999$ permutations of the exposures.

```
set.seed(54321)
R <- 999
perm <- itpdat
test <- NULL
for (i in 1:R){
perm$expo <- sample(perm$mmr, replace=F)
mod2 <- standardsccs(event~expo+age, indiv=case, astart=sta,
        aend=end, aevent=itp, adrug=expo, aedrug=expo+42,
        expogrp=c(0,15,29), agegrp=c(427,488,549,610,671),
        data=perm)
mod1 <- standardsccs(event~age, indiv=case, astart=sta,
        aend=end, aevent=itp, adrug=expo, aedrug=expo+42,
        expogrp=c(0,15,29), agegrp=c(427,488,549,610,671),
        data=perm)
test[i] <- lrtsccs(mod1,mod2)$test
}
```

The p-value is estimated as

```
> (1+sum(test>=t0))/(1+R)
[1] 0.008
```

which is about twice the value obtained using the asymptotic $\chi^2(3)$ distribution. The Monte Carlo standard error is of the order of 0.003. The asymptotic and permutation null distributions of the likelihood ratio test statistic are plotted as follows.

```
par(mar=c(4.1,4.1,1,1), cex.lab=1.4)
xval <- seq(0, ceiling(max(test)), 0.1)
hist(test, freq=F, xlab="test statistic", ylab="density",
        breaks=seq(0,ceiling(max(test)),0.5), main=NULL)
abline(v=t0, lty=2)
lines(xval, dchisq(xval,df=3))
```

The resulting plot is shown in the left panel of Figure 5.16. The asymptotic $\chi^2(3)$ distribution has a single mode; in contrast the permutation null distribution has an additional mode at around 5. It is apparent that the asymptotic distribution differs substantially from its permutation-based counterpart. Nevertheless, the conclusions are unaffected: there is a highly statistically significant exposure effect.

The additional mode at 5 corresponds to those permutations in which one or more of the three risk periods contain zero events. It is instructive to repeat the analysis using the combined $[0, 42]$-day risk period. The R code is similar to that previously given and is not shown. In this case, the asymptotic test statistic is 8.57 on 1 degree of freedom, $p = 0.0034$. The p-value using the permutation test (with $R = 999$ samples) is 0.007. But now the asymptotic distribution, which is $\chi^2(1)$, much more closely matches the permutation-based null distribution. These are shown in the right-hand panel of Figure 5.16.

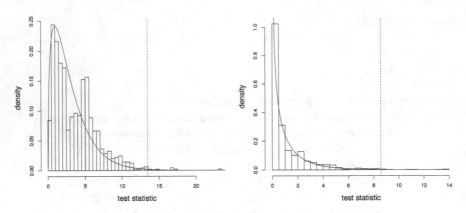

FIGURE 5.16

*Estimated probability mass functions of the permutation distributions (his-
tograms) and asymptotic densities. Left: model with three risk periods. Right:
model with a single 0–42 day risk period. The vertical dotted lines indicate the
observed values.*

Thus, combining risk periods to avoid sparseness improves the validity of
asymptotic approximations.

5.7   Bibliographical notes and further material

Several of the methods described in this chapter were originally suggested
in Farrington (1995) and Farrington and Whitaker (2006). The rare events
assumption discussed in Section 5.1 is studied in Whitaker et al. (2018b).
More detailed empirical investigations of the tests described in Sections 5.3
and 5.4 may be found in Whitaker et al. (2018a). Andrews (2002) describes a
range of sensitivity analyses to investigate the robustness of the SCCS model.

Within-individual dependence of recurrent events is discussed further in
Farrington and Hocine (2010). Simpson (2013) proposed an extension of the
SCCS model to cater for positive dependence between successive events.

The small-sample performance of the standard SCCS method is studied
in Musonda et al. (2008b). In this paper, the small-sample bias in the relative
incidence is quantified. Zeng et al. (2013), on the other hand, discuss the
application of bias correction methods to the SCCS model.

Mohammed et al. (2012) developed an extension of the SCCS model to
correct for measurement error in risk period endpoints, which may bias the
relative incidence. The impact of such measurement errors on hypothesis tests
is studied in Mohammed et al. (2013b). Misclassification of events, and its

impact on estimates derived using the SCCS method, is discussed in Quantin et al. (2013).

In this chapter we have not recommended using data-driven choices of risk periods, owing to their likely impact on the validity of the inferences drawn from the models we have described. In exploratory investigations of a hypothesis-generating, rather than hypothesis-testing, character, however, data-driven choices of risk periods can be justified. Methods to this effect have been proposed by Xu et al. (2011) and Xu et al. (2013).

6

Further SCCS models

The standard SCCS models considered so far share the following characteristics: the age effect is assumed to be constant on pre-defined age groups; the exposure effect is also assumed to be piecewise constant on pre-defined risk periods; events are of a single type; and exposures are discrete. In the present chapter, we relax the constraints imposed by these characteristics, and introduce a wider range of models. The likelihood for these models is still of the general SCCS form specified in Chapter 3, Section 3.5, and the primary focus for inference remains the estimation of exposure effects.

We begin, in Section 6.1, with a semiparametric SCCS model, in which the age effects need not be pre-specified by the user. This model is only of practical use for datasets of moderate size (typically, up to a few hundred cases), so in Section 6.2 we consider SCCS models in which the age effects are represented by spline functions. These models are extended in Section 6.3 so that exposure effects are also modelled by spline functions. Throughout the sections on semiparametric and spline-based SCCS models, we assume age is the time line of primary interest, but it could just as well be calendar time.

In Section 6.4 we consider SCCS models for events of several different types. In Section 6.5 we present a SCCS model for quantitative exposures. Finally, in Section 6.6 we discuss SCCS models for environmental exposures, and their relationship with other Poisson models. Bibliographical details, and brief mention of some other SCCS models not considered here, are given in Section 6.7. As in other chapters, material of a more technical nature has been confined to separate starred sections which may be skipped: these include Sections 6.1.4, 6.2.5, 6.3.6 and 6.4.4.

6.1 Semiparametric SCCS model

In the standard SCCS model described in Chapter 4, the relative age effect is piecewise constant on user-specified age groups. However, an inappropriate choice of age groups could, in principle, bias the estimator of the exposure effect, so it can be advantageous to avoid such choices. This is the idea of the semiparametric SCCS model: while the exposure effect of primary interest remains user-defined (this is the parametric half of the model), the age effect is determined solely by the data (and is estimated nonparametrically).

In the semiparametric SCCS model, the age effect is left completely unspecified, other than it being non-negative and bounded. It turns out that the maximum likelihood estimator of the cumulative relative age effect is a non-decreasing step function, taking steps only at event times. Details of the model, and of its properties and limitations, are given in Section 6.1.1, which is followed by some examples. The derivation of the semiparametric model, and some further properties, are described in starred Section 6.1.4, which may be skipped.

6.1.1   Formulation of the semiparametric model

Recall from Chapter 4, Equation 4.1, that the rate kernel for a case i observed over the age interval $(a_i, b_i]$ is defined as follows:

$$\nu(t|x_i) = \psi(t)\rho(t|x_i).$$

Time-invariant covariates y_i have been omitted to keep the notation simple; they may be introduced into the semiparametric SCCS model in the same way as for the standard model. The function $\psi(t)$ is the relative age effect, to be estimated nonparametrically.

We define the cumulative relative age effect from age a to be

$$\Psi(t) = \int_a^t \psi(s)ds.$$

Suppose that there are N cases, observed over the intervals $(a_i, b_i]$, $i = 1, \ldots, N$. We set $a = \min\{a_i : i = 1, \ldots, N\}$. Let $n_i \geq 1$ be the number of events experienced by case i, at ages $t_{i1}, \ldots, t_{in_i}$, $i = 1, \ldots, N$. Define $\mathfrak{S}$ to be the set of distinct event ages t_{ij} across all N cases. Suppose that there are $M + 1$ such distinct event ages, listed in increasing order as $s_0, \ldots, s_M$.

We assume only that the relative age effect $\psi(t)$ is non-negative and bounded. The nonparametric maximum likelihood estimator of the cumulative relative age effect $\Psi(t)$ is a non-decreasing step function, taking steps only at ages in $\mathfrak{S} = \{s_0, \ldots, s_M\}$; why this is so is explained in Section 6.1.4. Suppose that the step at age s_r is of size $\exp(\alpha_r)$, for $r = 0, \ldots, M$. The reference level is at the earliest event at age s_0, so we set $\alpha_0 = 0$. The maximum likelihood estimate of $\Psi(t)$ may thus be written

$$\hat{\Psi}(t) = \sum \{\exp(\hat{\alpha}_r) : s_r \leq t\}.$$

The maximum likelihood estimator of $\psi(t)$ consists of a series of spikes at the ages in $\mathfrak{S}$, and is zero elsewhere.

At this point, one might query why a supposedly nonparametric estimator of $\Psi(t)$ should be expressed in terms of parameters α_r. The key point is that this parameterisation is not pre-specified, but is entirely determined by the data – specifically, by the distinct event times in $\mathfrak{S}$.

In contrast, the exposure effect $\rho(t|x_i)$ in the rate kernel is explicitly specified as piecewise constant on $K \geq 1$ risk groups, as for the standard SCCS model.

There are $M + K$ parameters to be estimated: the M parameters $\alpha_1, \ldots, \alpha_M$ corresponding to the steps in the cumulative relative age effect function $\Psi(t)$, and the K exposure parameters $\beta_1, \ldots, \beta_K$. Like the standard SCCS model, the semiparametric likelihood is product multinomial, and may be fitted using similar algorithms to those used for the standard model. Further details are in Section 6.1.4.

One important feature to note, however, is that the age effect parameter α is high-dimensional, involving M elements. Typically, M is of the same order as the number of cases, N. This has two consequences. First, and most problematically, fitting the semiparametric SCCS model can be computationally demanding owing to the large number of age-related parameters. This limits the practical usefulness of the model for large data sets, comprising more than a few hundred cases. For large data sets, the standard SCCS model with a large number of age categories, or the spline model described in Section 6.2, may be used instead. Second, because the number of parameters increases with the sample size, some special asymptotic theory is required. This is discussed further in Section 6.1.4. It turns out that treating α as if it were of fixed dimension is reasonable, so fitting algorithms based on standard asymptotic likelihood theory will yield valid estimates and standard errors.

We end this section with one further remark concerning temporal effects. Suppose that the baseline incidence of events depends on calendar time u as well as the individual's age t through a calendar time effect $\eta(u)$. A simple multiplicative model for the event incidence is:

$$\lambda_i(t, u|x_i) = \phi_i \psi(t) \eta(u) \rho(t|x_i).$$

Now suppose that the temporal effect $\eta(u)$ is exponential, with $\eta(u) = \exp(u\delta)$. Let u_i denote the time of birth of an individual i, so that $u = t + u_i$, t denoting the age of this individual. The terms ϕ_i and $\exp(u_i\delta)$ are time-invariant and so drop out of the likelihood, leaving the rate kernel

$$\nu(t|x_i) = \psi^*(t) \rho(t|x_i),$$

with $\psi^*(t) = \psi(t) \exp(t\delta)$. Thus, the calendar time effect is absorbed into the relative age effect. In the semiparametric SCCS model, we estimate age effect parameters $\log\{\psi^*(s_r)\} = \alpha_r^* = \alpha_r + s_r\delta$. In other words, the estimated age effect includes the contribution of any exponential time trends present.

The benefit of this feature is that the semiparametric SCCS model adjusts implicitly for exponential time trends in the baseline incidence. Other SCCS models – notably the standard SCCS model – may be expected to be robust to monotone calendar time effects. The downside is that care is required in interpreting the estimates of $\psi(t)$ and $\Psi(t)$, which incorporate exponential calendar time as well as age components.

This property has been described when age is the time line of primary interest. If the analysis is undertaken with calendar time as the primary time line, a similar argument applies to monotone age effects: the semiparametric SCCS model then adjusts implicitly for exponential age trends in the baseline incidence. Thus, the estimated temporal effect incorporates the contribution of any exponential age trends.

In the R package SCCS, the semiparametric model is fitted using function semisccs. The syntax is similar to that of function standardsccs. For the reasons given above, however, the function can only handle data sets up to a moderate size (a few hundred cases). The next sections provide examples of its application.

Summary

- In the semiparametric SCCS model, the exposure effect is piecewise-constant as in the standard SCCS model, but the age effect is estimated nonparametrically.

- The estimated cumulative relative age effect is a step function with jumps only at the distinct event times.

- The semiparametric SCCS model avoids the need to specify age categories. However, estimation is computationally demanding, and this restricts the applicability of the method.

- The semiparametric SCCS model automatically adjusts for exponential calendar time trends.

6.1.2   Semiparametric model for the MMR and ITP data

We illustrate the semiparametric SCCS model with the ITP and MMR data introduced in Chapter 4, Section 4.3.1, with the three risk periods $[0, 14]$, $[15, 28]$ and $[29, 42]$ days after MMR vaccination. The semiparametric SCCS model is fitted as follows:

```
itp.mod12 <- semisccs(event~mmr, indiv=case, astart=sta,
              aend=end, aevent=itp, adrug=mmr, aedrug=mmr+42,
              expogrp=c(0,15,29), data=itpdat)
```

The main difference with the standard SCCS model is that the model formula is specified by

$$event{\sim}mmr$$

rather than

$$event{\sim}mmr{+}age.$$

The age effect in the semiparametric model is included automatically. The argument `agegrp` is no longer used. In other respects – for example, handling of data formats `stack` and `multi`, and inclusion of several exposure types – the function is identical to `standardsccs`. The parameter estimates are:

```
> itp.mod12
.....
          exp(coef) exp(-coef) lower .95 upper .95
mmr1         1.4620     0.6840   0.32378     6.601
mmr2         5.4460     0.1836   2.17091    13.662
mmr3         2.0435     0.4893   0.55674     7.501
```

These values may be compared to those obtained in Chapter 4, Section 4.3.1 – the differences are not materially important. The estimated cumulative relative age effect $\hat{\Psi}(t)$ is a step function with jumps at the distinct event times. These may be obtained as follows:

```
> devt <- sort(unique(itpdat$itp))
> devt
 [1] 374 381 389 396 402 403 406 407 409 411 412 414 418
[14] 419 425 429 438 440 442 443 452 463 473 477 480 484
[27] 494 522 543 553 564 598 609 612 615 623 633 666 676
[40] 691 705 708 722
```

There are 43 distinct event times, so there are 43 steps, the first being (arbitrarily) of size 1 at 374 days. The estimated cumulative relative age effect over the maximum observation period [366, 730] days is shown in Figure 6.1.

The cumulative relative age effect at age t represents the cumulative age-specific incidence in the age interval [366, t] days, relative to the reference age. If the age-specific incidence were constant, the cumulative relative age effect would be a straight line. The bulge between 400 and 500 days of age in Figure 6.1 represents clustering of ITP in this age range. This figure was obtained using the following code:

```
par(mar=c(4.1,4.1,1,1), cex.lab=1.4)
psi <- cumsum(c(1,itp.mod12$coefficients[4:45,2]))
plot(c(366,devt,730), c(0,psi,max(psi)), type="s", xlab=
    "age (days)", ylab="cumulative relative age effect")
```

Interactions with the exposure effect may be fitted in the same way as with the standard SCCS model. For example, whether sex is an effect modifier may be investigated as follows:

```
itp.mod13 <- semisccs(event~factor(sex)*mmr, indiv=case,
              astart=sta, aend=end, aevent=itp, adrug=mmr,
              aedrug=mmr+42, expogrp=c(0,15,29), data=itpdat)
```

and tested using the likelihood ratio test:

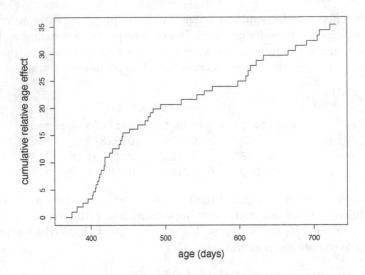

FIGURE 6.1
Estimated cumulative relative age effect for the ITP data.

```
> lrtsccs(itp.mod12,itp.mod13)
    test df pvalue
  0.8648  3 0.8339
```

which, as in Chapter 4, Section 4.7.1, yields a statistically non-significant result ($p = 0.83$).

6.1.3 Semiparametric model for the MMR and autism data

The semiparametric model may be used with indefinite risk periods in the same circumstances as the standard SCCS model, as described in Chapter 4, Section 4.8. We illustrate such an application with the autism and MMR vaccine data of Chapter 4, Section 4.8.2.

Suppose first that we use a single indefinite risk period stretching from age at MMR vaccination to end of observation. The semiparametric model is specified as follows; the argument `expogrp=0` is the default and is included only for emphasis.

```
aut.mod4 <- semisccs(event~mmr, indiv=case, astart=sta,
              aend=end, aevent=diag, adrug=mmr, aedrug=end,
              expogrp=0, data=autdat)
```

This model may take some time to run, depending on your computer: there are 319 distinct event ages, and hence 318 age-related parameters to estimate.

The relative incidence associated with MMR vaccine obtained with this model is as follows:

```
> aut.mod4
. . . . .
                 exp(coef) exp(-coef) lower .95 upper .95
mmr1               0.8002    1.24966   0.36712      1.744
```

The relative incidence is 0.80, 95% CI $(0.37, 1.74)$ and is therefore statistically non-significant. The relative incidence obtained with the standard SCCS model was 1.05, 95% CI $(0.52, 2.13)$. As in the standard SCCS model, we can study how the exposure effect varies with time since vaccination. Using the same time intervals as in Chapter 4, Section 4.8.2, the semiparametric SCCS model is specified as follows.

```
exint <- c(0,731,1461,2191)
aut.mod5 <- semisccs(event~mmr, indiv=case, astart=sta,
            aend=end, aevent=diag, adrug=mmr, aedrug=end,
            expogrp=exint, data=autdat)
```

This yields the following results.

```
> aut.mod5
. . . . .
                 exp(coef) exp(-coef) lower .95 upper .95
mmr1               0.7928    1.26143   0.36123      1.740
mmr2               0.6967    1.43536   0.28713      1.690
mmr3               0.5956    1.67912   0.18683      1.898
mmr4               0.9886    1.01158   0.26204      3.729
```

The cumulative relative age effect from model `aut.mod5` is shown in Figure 6.2. The steep rise in the plot between 2 and 5 years of age indicates that most autism diagnoses occur within this age range. The code for producing Figure 6.2 is as follows.

```
devt <- sort(unique(autdat$diag))
par(mar=c(4.1,4.1,1,1), cex.lab=1.4)
psi <- cumsum(c(1,aut.mod5$coefficients[5:322,2]))
plot(c(min(autdat$sta),devt,max(autdat$end))/365.25,
    c(0,psi,max(psi)), type="s", xlab="age (years)",
    ylab="cumulative relative age effect")
```

6.1.4   Further details of the semiparametric model*

This section provides some further material about three aspects of the semiparametric SCCS model. First, we explain informally why the maximum likelihood estimator of the cumulative relative age effect $\Psi(t)$ is a step function with jumps at the event times. Second, we provide more detail on the product multinomial representation of the semiparametric SCCS model. And finally,

---

* This section may be skipped.

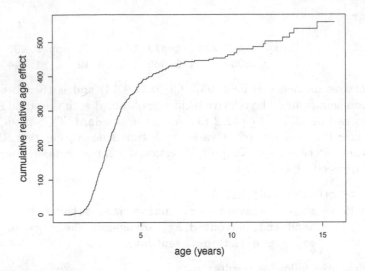

FIGURE 6.2
Estimated cumulative relative age effect for the autism data.

we briefly discuss asymptotics.

Maximum likelihood estimator
Let $\{\hat{\psi}(t), \hat{\boldsymbol{\beta}}\}$ denote the semiparametric maximum likelihood estimator. We show, informally, that $\hat{\psi}(t)$ takes positive values only at event times in $\mathfrak{S}$, and is zero elsewhere – or equivalently, that $\hat{\Psi}(t)$, the maximum likelihood estimator of the cumulative relative age effect, is a step function with jumps at the event times.

To handle these jumpy estimators, it is convenient to rewrite the likelihood in a form that can accommodate such jumps. In the notation of Chapter 4, Section 4.10,

$$\rho(t|x_i) = \exp\{\boldsymbol{v}_i(t; x_i)^T \boldsymbol{\beta}\}.$$

The SCCS likelihood contribution of a case i with n_i events at ages $t_{i1}, \ldots, t_{in_i}$ may be written

$$L_i = \text{constant} \times \frac{\prod_{j=1}^{n_i} \psi(t_{ij}) \exp\{\boldsymbol{v}_i(t_{ij}; x_i)^T \boldsymbol{\beta}\}}{\left[\int_{a_i}^{b_i} \exp\{\boldsymbol{v}_i(t; x_i)^T \boldsymbol{\beta}\} d\Psi(t)\right]^{n_i}}. \tag{6.1}$$

The only change is that the integral in the denominator has been written in a form that accommodates point masses.

We argue by contradiction: suppose that $\hat{\psi}(t)$ is not zero outside $\mathfrak{S}$. Thus, there are ages t outside $\mathfrak{S}$ where $\hat{\psi}(t) > 0$. Let $\tilde{\psi}(t)$ be equal to $\hat{\psi}(t)$ on $\mathfrak{S}$, but zero elsewhere. Then, for all event times t_{ij}, $\tilde{\psi}(t_{ij}) = \hat{\psi}(t_{ij})$, and $\hat{\psi}(t) \geq \tilde{\psi}(t)$ at all t. For all cases i we have

$$\int_{a_i}^{b_i} \exp\{v_i(t; x_i)^T \hat{\beta}\} d\tilde{\Psi}(t) \leq \int_{a_i}^{b_i} \exp\{v_i(t; x_i)^T \hat{\beta}\} d\hat{\Psi}(t),$$

and there is at least one case i for which the inequality is strict, since $\hat{\psi}(t) > 0$ at some values t outside $\mathfrak{S}$ (such a case i includes some or all of these values in its observation period). Let $\hat{L}_i$ and $\tilde{L}_i$ denote L_i with $\psi(t_{ij}), \Psi(t), \beta$ replaced, respectively, with $\hat{\psi}(t_{ij}), \hat{\Psi}(t), \hat{\beta}$ and $\tilde{\psi}(t_{ij}), \tilde{\Psi}(t), \hat{\beta}$. From Equation 6.1, $\tilde{L}_i \geq \hat{L}_i$ for all i, and $\tilde{L}_i > \hat{L}_i$ for at least one i. It follows that, since the overall likelihood is greater with $\tilde{\psi}(t)$, $\hat{\psi}(t)$ cannot be the maximum likelihood estimator. Our original supposition must therefore be wrong, and $\hat{\psi}(t)$ must be zero outside $\mathfrak{S}$. Thus, $\hat{\psi}(t)$ consists of a series of spikes at the event times, and $\hat{\Psi}(t)$ is a step function, with jumps only at event times.

Semiparametric likelihood and product multinomial model
Let $r(i, j)$ denote the value r such that $s_r = t_{ij}$, and let $w_{ir} = I_{(a_i, b_i]}(s_r)$. Thus, w_{ir} is equal to 1 if s_r is in $(a_i, b_i]$, and is 0 otherwise. The contribution of a case i to the semiparametric SCCS likelihood is then:

$$L_i = \text{constant} \times \frac{\prod_{j=1}^{n_i} \exp\{\alpha_{r(i,j)} + v_i(t_{ij}; x_i)^T \beta\}}{\left[\sum_{r=0}^{M} w_{ir} \exp\{\alpha_r + v_i(s_r; x_i)^T \beta\}\right]^{n_i}}. \tag{6.2}$$

Note that the semiparametric SCCS likelihood depends on the ages s_r only through their ranks and through the covariate values $v_i(s_r; x_i)$.

We consider the semiparametric SCCS model with no interactions and a single exposure type. For a case i with observation period $(a_i, b_i]$, let $\mathfrak{S}_i$ denote the set $\mathfrak{S}_i = \mathfrak{S} \cap (a_i, b_i]$ of all distinct event times in $(a_i, b_i]$. The rate kernel for case i is defined for ages s_r in $\mathfrak{S}_i$:

$$\nu_{ir} = \nu(s_r | x_i) = \exp\{\alpha_r + v(s_r; x_i)^T \beta\}.$$

Suppose that case i experiences n_{ir} events at age s_r, and let n_i denote the vector of counts $\{n_{ir} : s_r \in \mathfrak{S}_i\}$. The semiparametric SCCS model is then

$$n_i \sim \text{Multinomial}(n_i, p_i)$$

where the probability vector p_i has elements

$$p_{ir} = \frac{\nu_{ir}}{\sum_{s_k \in \mathfrak{S}_i} \nu_{ik}}.$$

This formulation matches the likelihood contribution in Equation 6.2 because $\sum_{s_k \in \mathfrak{S}_i} \nu_{ik} = \sum_{k=0}^{M} w_{ik} \nu_{ik}$.

Asymptotics

A central feature of standard parametric asymptotic theory is that the parameter to be estimated is finite-dimensional. This helps to ensure that, as the sample size N increases, the amount of information available on each parameter increases at the same rate $O(N)$. In the semiparametric SCCS model, on the other hand, as the number of cases N increases, the size of $\mathfrak{S}$ and hence the number M of age-related parameters to be estimated also increases: $\Psi(t)$ is an infinite-dimensional parameter. For this reason, standard parametric asymptotic theory cannot be assumed to work. However, the more generally applicable methods of empirical process theory may be invoked (Van der Vaart and Wellner, 1996). Applied with suitable regularity conditions, these methods may be used to show that the maximum likelihood estimators $\hat{\beta}$ and $\hat{\Psi}(t)$ are consistent, that $\hat{\beta}$ is asymptotically normally distributed with efficient variance, and that the profile log-likelihood for β is asymptotically χ^2 on K degrees of freedom under the null hypothesis $\beta = \beta_0$. These results are reported in Farrington and Whitaker (2006).

Since the profile log-likelihood for β is the same whether the model parameters are regarded as finite or infinite-dimensional, the variance of the parameter $\hat{\beta}$ may be approximated as if the model parameters were finite dimensional – that is, as if the model were parameterised with pre-specified age effect parameters α of fixed, finite dimension M.

Note finally that these complications are primarily conceptual. In practice, event ages are only ever measured to some pre-determined accuracy – usually days – and so the size of the set $\mathfrak{S}$ is bounded. However, the number of parameters α_r can be large. Whatever theoretical point of view is adopted, the relevance of asymptotic results to finite samples must be verified empirically through simulations. For the semiparametric SCCS model, simulation evidence in Farrington and Whitaker (2006) suggests that the approximations are acceptable even in samples of small to moderate size.

6.2 SCCS model with spline-based age effect

The semiparametric SCCS model sidesteps the need to specify the age effect, but there is a cost, both computationally and in terms of efficiency, because the age effect is replaced by a high-dimensional parameter. In most practical applications, the relative age effect can reasonably be assumed to vary smoothly, with few turning points. In SCCS models with spline-based age effect, the relative age effect is represented by a smooth function obtained by splicing together polynomials of low dimension.

An advantage of splines is that, being smooth functions, they provide a more realistic representation of the age effect than the step functions used in the standard SCCS model. From a more technical point of view, an advantage of spline models is that the flexibility of the semiparametric SCCS model is retained, but without some of its computational and efficiency limitations. In addition, spline models can help mitigate confounding between age and exposure effects.

In this section the SCCS model with spline-based age effect is described and illustrated with practical examples. In Section 6.2.4 we compare the estimates obtained with different SCCS models. More technical material on the spline-based model is included in starred Section 6.2.5. This material is also relevant to the models described in Section 6.3, in which splines are used to represent the exposure effect.

6.2.1 Splines for the relative age effect

Our starting point, as in Section 6.1.1, is the rate kernel for a case i observed over an age interval $(a_i, b_i]$, namely:

$$\nu(t|x_i) = \psi(t)\rho(t|x_i).$$

Time-invariant covariates y_i have been omitted for simplicity. As for the standard and semiparametric SCCS models, the exposure effect $\rho(t|x_i)$ will be assumed to be piecewise constant on pre-defined risk periods, with exposure-related parameter β.

The relative age effect $\psi(t)$, on the other hand, is to be represented by a linear combination of cubic M-splines. This is constructed as follows. Suppose that there are N cases, and let $a = \min\{a_i, i = 1, \ldots, N\}$ and $b = \max\{b_i, i = 1, \ldots, N\}$, so that $(a, b]$ includes all the observation periods $(a_i, b_i]$. The cubic M-spline is a linear combination of specially defined cubic polynomials constituting an M-spline basis (this is described in Section 6.2.5). These basis functions are defined piecewise at fixed points in $[a, b]$ called knots, including the endpoints a and b. We choose K knots $\tau_k, k = 1, \ldots, K$ with $a = \tau_1 < \tau_2 < \cdots < \tau_K = b$. Then $\psi(t)$ is a linear combination of $S = K + 2$ non-negative M-splines or piecewise cubic polynomials $M_s(t)$:

$$\psi(t) = \sum_{s=1}^{S} \alpha_s^2 M_s(t).$$

The constants α_s, which are squared to ensure that $\psi(t)$ is non-negative, are parameters to be estimated. The component polynomials $M_s(t)$ are the M-spline basis functions. Varying the number of knots K and the parameters α_s provides a suitably rich family of flexible parametric forms; the greater the number of knots, the more flexible the spline function is.

M-splines have the property that the basis elements $M_s(t)$ integrate to 1 over $(a, b]$. We shall also use integrated splines or I-splines, whose basis functions $I_s(t)$ are obtained from the M-spline basis functions by integration:

$$I_s(t) = \int_a^t M_s(u)du.$$

The $I_s(t)$ are non-decreasing polynomials of order 4, with $I_s(a) = 0$ and $I_s(b) = 1$. They provide a convenient representation of integrals of spline functions. This feature is particularly useful for the SCCS model, since the SCCS likelihood involves integrals in its denominator. For example, suppose that case i experiences a single event at age t_i, and has a single risk period $(d_{i1}, d_{i2}]$. Let $x_i(t)$ be 1 if t is in $(d_{i1}, d_{i2}]$ and 0 otherwise. The SCCS likelihood contribution for this case is then

$$
\begin{aligned}
L_i &= \frac{\psi(t_i) \exp\{x_i(t_i)\beta\}}{\int_{a_i}^{b_i} \psi(s) \exp\{x_i(s)\beta\}ds} \\
&= \frac{\{\sum_{s=1}^{S} \alpha_s^2 M_s(t_i)\} \exp\{x_i(t_i)\beta\}}{\Psi(b_i) - \Psi(a_i) + \{\exp(\beta) - 1\}\{\Psi(d_{i2}) - \Psi(d_{i1})\}},
\end{aligned}
$$

where

$$
\Psi(t) = \int_a^t \psi(u)du = \sum_{s=1}^{S} \alpha_s^2 I_s(t).
$$

Cases with multiple risk periods are dealt with in a similar manner. In the standard SCCS model, $\psi(t)$ was set to be 1 in a particular age group chosen as reference level; such a constraint is necessary as $\psi(t)$ is the relative, not the absolute age effect. In the absence of discrete age groups, other constraints are required. The constraint used here is to rescale the α_s so that $\psi(a) = 1$. Alternatively, we can set $\int_a^b \psi(t)dt = 1$, which is achieved by requiring $\sum_{s=1}^{S} \alpha_s^2 = 1$.

Further details of the construction of M-splines and I-splines for the purposes of SCCS models is provided in Section 6.2.5. Figure 6.3 shows the $S = 7$ basis functions when $a = 0$, $b = 4$ with $K = 5$ internal knots at $\tau_1 = 0$, $\tau_2 = 1$, $\tau_3 = 2$, $\tau_4 = 3$ and $\tau_5 = 4$.

Approximating $\psi(t)$ with splines requires choosing and placing a suitable number K of knots. If K is too low, the spline will not approximate $\psi(t)$ correctly. On the other hand, if K is too high, the spline will follow the data too closely, producing a function that is too variable because it reproduces random fluctuations.

The fitting technique we use is called penalised likelihood estimation. A relatively large number K of knots is chosen in advance to ensure that the spline is sufficiently flexible, and the smoothness of the estimate of $\psi(t)$ is controlled by penalising choices of the parameter $\alpha = (\alpha_1, \ldots, \alpha_S)$ that produce very wiggly estimates.

Penalised likelihood estimation involves maximising the quantity

$$
PL(\alpha, \beta) = \sum_{i=1}^{N} \log L_i(\alpha, \beta) - 2\lambda \int \left(\sum_{s=1}^{S} \alpha_s^2 M_s^{''}(u) \right)^2 du
$$

where $L_i(\alpha, \beta)$ is the SCCS likelihood contribution of case i and $M_s^{''}(t)$ is the second derivative of $M_s(t)$. The second term in the penalised log likelihood

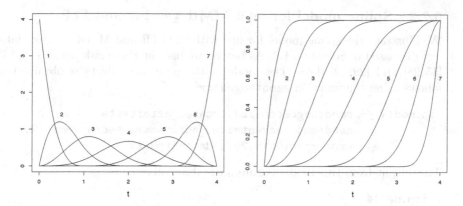

FIGURE 6.3

Cubic spline basis functions on $[0,4]$ with knots at 0,1,2,3 and 4. Left: M-spline basis functions $M_s(t)$. Right: corresponding I-spline basis functions $I_s(t)$. The integer labels are the values of $s = 1, \ldots, 7$.

function $PL(\alpha, \beta)$ is a measure of the smoothness of the estimate of $\psi(t)$, known as the penalty. The non-negative parameter λ is a smoothing parameter: the larger the value of λ, the smoother the estimated relative age effect $\hat{\psi}(t)$ will be. The parameter λ may be chosen automatically, using the method of cross-validation, or an approximation to it. Further details of this and other aspects of the fitting procedure are provided in Section 6.2.5.

In the R package SCCS, the SCCS model with spline-based relative age effect is fitted using the function smoothagesccs. The function may be used when there is a single exposure, with one or more contiguous risk or washout periods.

Summary

- For the SCCS model with spline-based relative age effect, the exposure effect is piecewise constant as in the standard SCCS model. The relative age effect is represented by a cubic M-spline function.

- This allows a flexible yet parsimonious representation of the relative age effect. However, the method requires the selection of a parameter that controls the smoothness of the estimated relative age effect.

- The smoothing parameter may be chosen automatically using the method of cross-validation. The model is then fitted by penalised likelihood estimation.

6.2.2   Spline model for age: MMR vaccine and ITP

We illustrate the spline model for age with the ITP and MMR vaccine data, last discussed in Section 6.1.2. As before, we use the three risk periods $[0, 14]$, $[15, 28]$ and $[29, 42]$ days. The model with spline age effects is obtained as follows using the function smoothagesccs.

```
itp.mod14 <- smoothagesccs(indiv=case, astart=sta,
            aend=end, aevent=itp, adrug=mmr, aedrug=mmr+42,
            expogrp=c(0,15,29), data=itpdat)
```

The output from this model is summarised as follows.

```
> itp.mod14
......
      exp(coef) exp(-coef) lower .95 upper .95
mmr1    1.358     0.7364    0.3081     5.985
mmr2    6.273     0.1594    2.6600    14.794
mmr3    2.605     0.3838    0.7470     9.087


spline based age relative incidence function:
 Smoothing parameter = 2.8e+04
 Cross validation score = 252.98
```

The parameters quoted are the relative incidences associated with the exposure. Thus, the relative incidence in the $[0, 14]$ day risk period is 1.36, 95% CI $(0.31, 5.99)$. In the $[15, 28]$ day risk period, $RI = 6.27$, 95% CI $(2.66, 14.8)$. And in the $[29, 42]$ day risk period, it is 2.61, 95% CI $(0.75, 9.09)$. These values differ only slightly from those obtained with the standard SCCS model in Chapter 4, Section 4.3.1. Nor do they differ substantially from those obtained with the semiparametric model in Section 6.1.2.

The output also gives the value of the smoothing parameter and the corresponding cross-validation score: 2.8e+04 and 252.98, respectively. The smoothing parameter is obtained automatically, so as to minimise the approximate cross-validation score for the number of knots used, which by default is 12, placed at equal intervals.

A plot of the estimated relative age effect is shown in Figure 6.4. The plotted value at each age t is the age-specific relative incidence at t; the plot is scaled so that the relative incidence at the lowest age is 1. This plot was obtained as follows.

```
> par(mar=c(4.1,4.1,1,1), cex.lab=1.4)
> plot(itp.mod14)
```

The smoothness of the estimated age effect can be controlled by the user. There are two ways to do this: the first is to vary the number of knots kn (though at least 5 knots must be used). The second, more direct, way is to vary the smoothing parameter sp. The automatic selection procedure yielded

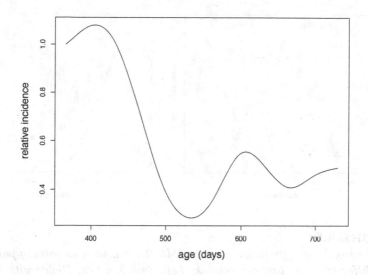

FIGURE 6.4
Fitted smooth age effect for ITP and MMR data, using default settings.

the optimal value of the smoothing parameter, sp = 2.8e+04. Suppose we halve this value:

```
itp.mod15 <- smoothagesccs(sp=1.4e+04, indiv=case, astart=sta,
                aend=end, aevent=itp, adrug=mmr, aedrug=mmr+42,
                expogrp=c(0,15,29), data=itpdat)
```

This produces the following results.

```
> itp.mod15
......
      exp(coef) exp(-coef) lower .95 upper .95
mmr1    1.380     0.7246    0.3133     6.080
mmr2    6.136     0.1630    2.5892    14.542
mmr3    2.481     0.4030    0.7062     8.719

spline based age relative incidence function:
 Smoothing parameter = 1.4e+04
 Cross validation score = 253.67
```

The exposure-related relative incidences are similar to those obtained with the optimal smoothing parameter. As expected, since we have reduced the smoothing parameter, the estimated smooth age effect, shown in the left panel of Figure 6.5, is rather more wavy than in Figure 6.4. Now try doubling the optimal value of the smoothing parameter:

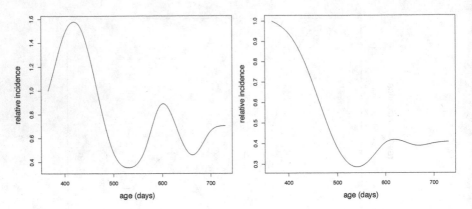

FIGURE 6.5
Fitted smooth age effects for ITP and MMR data, with smoothing parameters
that differ from the optimal value λ. Left: with λ × 1/2. Right: with λ × 2.

```
itp.mod16 <- smoothagesccs(sp=5.6e+04, indiv=case, astart=sta,
                  aend=end, aevent=itp, adrug=mmr, aedrug=mmr+42,
                  expogrp=c(0,15,29), data=itpdat)
```

This yields the following results.

```
> itp.mod16
. . . . . .
      exp(coef) exp(-coef) lower .95 upper .95
mmr1    1.343     0.7444     0.3066     5.886
mmr2    6.332     0.1579     2.6924    14.893
mmr3    2.678     0.3735     0.7715     9.293


spline based age relative incidence function:
 Smoothing parameter = 5.6e+04
 Cross validation score = 253.62
```

Again, these values differ little from those obtained with automatic selection
of the smoothing parameter. As expected, since the smoothness parameter
has been increased, the estimated smooth age effect, shown in the right panel
of Figure 6.5, is less wavy than with the automatically chosen smoothing
parameter. This figure was obtained using the following code.

```
par(mfrow=c(1,2), mar=c(4.1,4.1,1,1), cex.lab=1.4)
plot(itp.mod15)
plot(itp.mod16)
```

Automatic selection of the smoothing parameter is convenient, and frees
the user from having to make arbitrary choices. However, it need not always

produce entirely compelling results. For example, the estimated age effect in
Figure 6.4 is perhaps a little too wavy at higher ages, suggesting a degree of
undersmoothing; the curve in the right panel of Figure 6.5 is perhaps more realistic. However, the estimated exposure effects, which are of primary interest,
are not substantially affected. It is a good idea to check that the exposure-
related relative incidences are not overly sensitive to the choice of smoothing
parameter.

6.2.3   Spline model for age: antidepressants and hip fracture

In Chapter 4, Section 4.3.3, we used the standard SCCS model to investigate
the association between antidepressants and hip fractures in the elderly. The
data, in data frame `hipdat`, comprise 1000 cases. Particular interest focuses
on the initiation of treatment. Thus, we defined three risk periods: $[0, 14]$
days and $[15, 42]$ days after the start of treatment, and the rest of time on
antidepressants. We also used two 91-day washout periods.

The analysis with the standard SCCS model included 20 age groups defined
by the quantiles of age at hip fracture. An alternative is to model the age effect
using splines. The model is specified as follows.

```
hip.mod2 <- smoothagesccs(indiv=case, astart=sta,
                aend=end, aevent=frac, adrug=ad, aedrug=endad,
                expogrp=c(0,15,43), washout=c(1,92,182),
                data=hipdat)
```

This yields the following output.

```
> hip.mod2
......
          exp(coef) exp(-coef) lower .95 upper .95
ad1         2.150     0.4651     1.2609    3.666
ad2         1.855     0.5390     1.2069    2.852
ad3         1.506     0.6639     1.2497    1.816
washout1    1.267     0.7895     0.9370    1.712
washout2    1.029     0.9719     0.7382    1.434

spline based age relative incidence function:
  Smoothing parameter = 1.5e+08
  Cross validation score = 7535.5
```

The results are very similar to those obtained with the standard SCCS
model: there is a strong association between antidepressants and hip fracture,
particularly at the initiation of therapy. Thus, in the $[0, 14]$ day risk period,
$RI = 2.15$ with 95% CI $(1.26, 3.67)$. The smooth age effect estimated from
this model is shown in Figure 6.6, obtained as follows:

```
par(mar=c(4.1,4.1,1,1), cex.lab=1.4)
plot(hip.mod2)
```

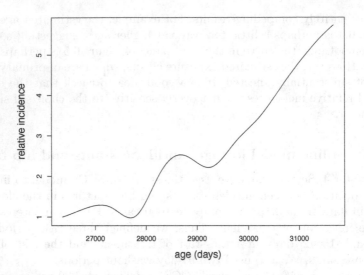

FIGURE 6.6
*Fitted smooth age effect for antidepressants and hip fracture data, obtained
with default settings.*

The sensitivity of the results to the choice of smoothing parameter may
be assessed by refitting the model with different values. The optimal value
obtained by automatic selection was $\lambda = 1.5e+08$. First we reduce this tenfold:

```
hip.mod3 <- smoothagesccs(sp=1.5e+07, indiv=case, astart=sta,
            aend=end, aevent=frac, adrug=ad, aedrug=endad,
            expogrp=c(0,15,43), washout=c(1,92,182),
            data=hipdat)
```

which yields the following:

```
> hip.mod3
......
         exp(coef) exp(-coef) lower .95 upper .95
ad1        2.145     0.4662    1.2580    3.658
ad2        1.852     0.5401    1.2044    2.847
ad3        1.504     0.6648    1.2480    1.813
washout1   1.266     0.7902    0.9362    1.711
washout2   1.028     0.9731    0.7372    1.432

spline based age relative incidence function:
 Smoothing parameter = 1.5e+07
 Cross validation score = 7538.5
```

Next, we increase the smoothing parameter tenfold:

```
hip.mod4 <- smoothagesccs(sp=1.5e+09, indiv=case, astart=sta,
               aend=end, aevent=frac, adrug=ad, aedrug=endad,
               expogrp=c(0,15,43), washout=c(1,92,182),
               data=hipdat)
```

which gives:

```
> hip.mod4
......

          exp(coef) exp(-coef) lower .95 upper .95
ad1           2.154     0.4643    1.2632     3.672
ad2           1.860     0.5376    1.2101     2.859
ad3           1.511     0.6618    1.2538     1.821
washout1      1.268     0.7884    0.9384     1.714
washout2      1.033     0.9683    0.7410     1.439


spline based age relative incidence function:
 Smoothing parameter = 1.5e+09
 Cross validation score = 7536.23
```

The results are insensitive to the choice of smoothing parameter. The estimated smooth age effects obtained with hip.mod3 and hip.mod4 are shown in Figure 6.7. As expected, the plot on the left is slightly more wavy than in

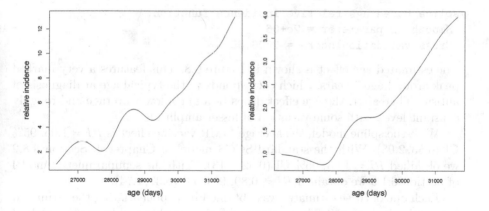

FIGURE 6.7
Fitted smooth age effect for antidepressants and hip fracture data with user-defined smoothing parameter values. Left: $\lambda=1.5e+07$; right: $\lambda = 1.5e+09$.

Figure 6.6; the plot on the right is slightly smoother. The ranges plotted on the vertical axes are also very different. This is due to the different shapes of the estimated age effects at low ages, where the data are sparse, both graphs being scaled to take the value 1 at the lowest age.

The values of the cross-validation score are only marginally affected by these large changes in the smoothing parameter: clearly, the cross-validation score is a very flat function of the smoothing parameter.

6.2.4   Precision of estimators: MMR and autism

In Chapter 4, Section 4.8.2 we fitted the standard SCCS model to data on MMR vaccine and autism; in Section 6.1.3 of the present chapter we fitted the semiparametric model. In the present example, we fit the spline model for age, and compare the precisions (that is, the reciprocals of the variances) of the estimators from the three models. We also comment on the use of spline models when the exposure and age effects are confounded.

The model with spline-based age effect is specified as follows:

```
aut.mod6 <- smoothagesccs(indiv=case, astart=sta, aend=end,
             aevent=diag, adrug=mmr, aedrug=end, data=autdat)
```

This yields the following estimate:

```
> aut.mod6
......
      exp(coef) exp(-coef) lower .95 upper .95
mmr1     1.047     0.9549    0.5266     2.082


spline based age relative incidence function:
 Smoothing parameter = 2e+06
 Cross validation score = 2606.65
```

The estimated age effect is shown in Figure 6.8. This features a very marked peak around age 3 years, which corresponds to the typical age at diagnosis of autism. Thereafter, the age effect drops to a much lower average and roughly constant level, with some variation of lesser amplitude.

With the spline model, the average MMR vaccine effect is $RI = 1.05$, 95% CI $(0.53, 2.08)$. With the standard SCCS model of Chapter 4, Section 4.8.2 we obtained $RI = 1.05$, 95% CI $(0.52, 2.13)$. With the semiparametric model of Section 6.1.3 we obtained $RI = 0.80$, 95% CI $(0.37, 1.74)$.

Each one of these estimates was obtained by exponentiating the estimated log relative incidence $\hat{\beta}$. The variance of $\hat{\beta}$ may be obtained from the standard errors listed in the output of each model. It may also be calculated directly from the 95% confidence limits (preferably, before rounding), as follows:

$$\mathrm{var}(\hat{\beta}) = \left(\frac{\log(RI^+) - \log(RI^-)}{2 \times 1.96} \right)^2,$$

where RI^+, RI^- are the upper and lower 95% confidence limits for $RI = \exp(\beta)$, respectively.

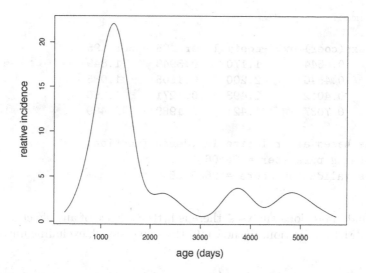

FIGURE 6.8
Fitted smooth age effect for the MMR vaccine and autism data.

Using this expression, we obtain $\text{var}(\hat{\beta}) = 0.123$ for the spline model, 0.130 for the standard SCCS model, and 0.158 for the semiparametric SCCS model. The estimate obtained with the spline model is the most precise, as $\text{var}(\hat{\beta})$ is lowest for this model. The semiparametric model (which makes the fewest assumptions about the shape of the age effect) gives the least precise estimate for these data, because it requires the largest number of parameters to model the age effect. This example illustrates how the spline model provides both great flexibility and good efficiency.

A further advantage of spline models is that they can provide more stable estimates than the standard SCCS model when there is substantial confounding between age and exposure effects. This may occur, for example, when there is little variation in age at exposure, and few unexposed cases.

Recall that in Chapter 4, Section 4.8.2, we fitted the standard SCCS model to the autism data with unvaccinated cases removed, and observed that the parameter estimates for the vaccine effect in successive time intervals after vaccination were inflated, with very wide confidence limits. We repeat these analyses with the SCCS spline model for age, starting with the whole data.

```
exint <- c(0,731,1461,2191)
aut.mod7 <- smoothagesccs(indiv=case, astart=sta, aend=end,
            aevent=diag, adrug=mmr, aedrug=end,
            expogrp=exint, data=autdat)
```

This yields the following estimates for the effect of MMR vaccine at different times from vaccination:

```
> aut.mod7
......
      exp(coef) exp(-coef) lower .95 upper .95
mmr1    0.8544     1.170     0.3948    1.849
mmr2    0.4546     2.200     0.1905    1.085
mmr3    0.4012     2.493     0.1271    1.266
mmr4    0.7037     1.421     0.1989    2.489


spline based age relative incidence function:
 Smoothing parameter = 2e+06
 Cross validation score = 2606.65
```

As found in previous analyses, there is little evidence of any effect at any time since MMR vaccination. We now refit the spline model, excluding unvaccinated cases:

```
aut.mod8 <- smoothagesccs(indiv=case, astart=sta, aend=end,
            aevent=diag, adrug=mmr, aedrug=end,
            expogrp=exint, data=subset(autdat,mmr>0))
```

This yields the following results:

```
> aut.mod8
......
      exp(coef) exp(-coef) lower .95 upper .95
mmr1    0.9203     1.0866    0.3648    2.322
mmr2    0.4741     2.1092    0.1679    1.338
mmr3    0.5924     1.6880    0.1372    2.558
mmr4    1.5757     0.6346    0.3213    7.728


spline based age relative incidence function:
 Smoothing parameter = 2.9e+05
 Cross validation score = 2099.39
```

Other than in the last time period, these estimates are not strikingly different from those obtained with model `aut.mod7` using the whole data. Certainly, the parameters are not as seriously inflated as they were when the analyses were undertaken with the standard SCCS model; see models `aut.mod2` and `aut.mod3` in Chapter 4, Section 4.8.2.

This example illustrates how using a spline model can mitigate the estimation problems resulting from confounding of age and exposure effects. However, spline models cannot be expected to resolve such problems entirely: including unexposed cases in such circumstances is strongly recommended.

6.2.5 Modelling with M-splines*

In this section, some further material is provided on M-spline basis functions, the selection of the smoothing parameter λ, and the estimation procedure. More details on M-splines may be found in Ramsay (1988). The approach used to fit the SCCS model with spline-based relative age effect is similar to that used by Joly et al. (1998).

M-spline basis functions

The K knots $a = \tau_1 < \tau_2 < \cdots < \tau_K = b$ are supplemented by six further dummy knots, three at a and three at b. The knots are relabelled k_1 to k_{K+6}, with $\tau_r = k_{r+3}$ for $r = 1, \ldots, K$. Define functions $M_s(t|q)$ on $(a, b]$ for $q = 1, 2, \ldots$ and $s = 1, \ldots, K + 2 = S$ recursively on q as follows.

For $q = 1$,

$$M_s(t|1) = \begin{cases} \frac{1}{(k_{s+1}-k_s)} & k_s \leq t < k_{s+1}, \\ 0 & \text{elsewhere on } (a, b]. \end{cases}$$

Note that $M_s(t|1)$ is identically zero for $s = 1, 2, 3$, since for these values $k_s = k_{s+1} = a$. Then for $q \geq 2$ define in turn:

$$M_s(t|q) = \begin{cases} \frac{q\{(t-k_s)M_s(t|q-1)+(k_{s+q}-t)M_{s+1}(t|q-1)\}}{(q-1)(k_{s+q}-k_s)} & k_s \leq t < k_{s+q}, \\ 0 & \text{elsewhere on } (a, b]. \end{cases}$$

Finally, set $M_s(t) = M_s(t|4)$. This function is a positive cubic polynomial on $(\tau_{\max\{1,s-3\}}, \tau_{\min\{S-2,s+1\}})$, $s = 1, \ldots, S$, is zero elsewhere on (a, b), and is twice differentiable on (a, b). The set of functions $M_s(t), s = 1, \ldots, S$ is the M-spline basis.

The I-spline basis functions $I_s(t)$ are obtained by integrating the M-spline basis functions $M_s(t)$. They can also be defined recursively in terms of M-spline basis functions. See Ramsay (1988) for details.

Smoothing parameter selection

The smoothing parameter λ is chosen by maximising an approximation to the cross-validation score obtained when the exposure effect parameter $\beta = 0$. The method closely follows that of Joly et al. (1998). The cross-validation score is defined as

$$V(\lambda) = \sum_{i=1}^{N} \log L_i(\hat{\boldsymbol{\alpha}}_{-i}),$$

where $L_i(\boldsymbol{\alpha})$ is the contribution of case i to the SCCS likelihood and $\hat{\boldsymbol{\alpha}}_{-i}$ is the maximum penalised likelihood estimate obtained when case i is removed, both with $\beta = 0$. The cross-validation score printed by R function `smoothagesccs`

---

* This section may be skipped.

is actually $-V(\lambda)$, which is positive. In the estimation, we use the constraint $\alpha_r = 1$ for $r = [(S+1)/2]$, rounded up when S is even.

Following O'Sullivan (1988), the leave-one-out estimator $\hat{\boldsymbol{\alpha}}_{-i}$ is replaced by its 1-step Newton–Raphson approximation $\bar{\boldsymbol{\alpha}}_{-i}$:

$$\bar{\boldsymbol{\alpha}}_{-i} = \hat{\boldsymbol{\alpha}} - \mathbf{W}^{-1}\hat{\mathbf{d}}_{-i},$$

where $\mathbf{W}$ is the $(S-1) \times (S-1)$ Hessian of $PL(\boldsymbol{\alpha})$ and $\mathbf{d}_{-i}$ is the gradient of the penalised log likelihood function with case i removed; both are evaluated at the maximum penalised likelihood estimator $\hat{\boldsymbol{\alpha}}$ of $\boldsymbol{\alpha}$. The second term is $O_p(N^{-1})$. Since the gradient of $PL(\boldsymbol{\alpha})$ is zero at $\hat{\boldsymbol{\alpha}}$,

$$
\begin{aligned}
\hat{\mathbf{d}}_{-i} &= \frac{\partial\{PL(\boldsymbol{\alpha}) - \log L_i(\boldsymbol{\alpha})\}}{\partial \boldsymbol{\alpha}}\Big|_{\hat{\alpha}} \\
&= -\frac{\partial \log L_i(\boldsymbol{\alpha})}{\partial \boldsymbol{\alpha}}\Big|_{\hat{\alpha}} \\
&= -\hat{\mathbf{d}}_i
\end{aligned}
$$

where $\mathbf{d}_i$ is the gradient of $\log L_i(\boldsymbol{\alpha})$. Substituting this expression in $\log L_i(\hat{\boldsymbol{\alpha}}_{-i})$ and expanding around $\hat{\boldsymbol{\alpha}}$, we obtain

$$\log L_i(\hat{\boldsymbol{\alpha}}_{-i}) \simeq \log L_i(\hat{\boldsymbol{\alpha}}) + \hat{\mathbf{d}}_i^T \hat{\mathbf{W}}^{-1} \hat{\mathbf{d}}_i.$$

Let $\mathbf{H}$ denote the Hessian of the SCCS log likelihood function $\sum_{i=1}^{N} \log L_i(\boldsymbol{\alpha})$ with $\beta = 0$ and the constraint $\alpha_r = 1$. Write $\mathbf{W} = \mathbf{H} - 2\lambda\mathbf{P}$, the second term representing the Hessian of the penalty. Using the approximation

$$\hat{\mathbf{H}} \simeq -\sum_{i=1}^{N} \hat{\mathbf{d}}_i \hat{\mathbf{d}}_i^T,$$

derived from the second Bartlett identity $E(l'^2) = -E(l'')$ for a log likelihood function l, and summing over i,

$$
\begin{aligned}
V(\lambda) &\simeq \sum_{i=1}^{N} \log L_i(\hat{\boldsymbol{\alpha}}) + \sum_{i=1}^{N} \hat{\mathbf{d}}_i^T \hat{\mathbf{W}}^{-1} \hat{\mathbf{d}}_i \\
&\simeq \sum_{i=1}^{N} \log L_i(\hat{\boldsymbol{\alpha}}) - \text{trace}([\hat{\mathbf{H}} - 2\lambda\hat{\mathbf{P}}]^{-1}\hat{\mathbf{H}}).
\end{aligned}
$$

Finally, we obtain an explicit expression for $\hat{\mathbf{P}}$, which depends on $\boldsymbol{\alpha}$. Let $\mathbf{A}$ denote the symmetric matrix with entries

$$A_{jk} = \int_a^b M_j''(u)M_k''(u)du.$$

Then

$$\int_a^b \left(\sum_{s=1}^{S} \alpha_s^2 M_s''(u)\right)^2 du = \boldsymbol{\alpha}^{2T}\mathbf{A}\boldsymbol{\alpha}^2,$$

α^2 denoting the vector with elements α_s^2. Let

$$\mathbf{P}^+ = 4\{\mathbf{A} \circ (\boldsymbol{\alpha}\boldsymbol{\alpha}^T)\} + 2\{\mathrm{diag}(\mathbf{A}\boldsymbol{\alpha}^2)\},$$

where $\circ$ denotes the element-wise matrix product. Finally, let $\mathbf{P}$ equal $\mathbf{P}^+$ with row r and column r removed. The optimal value of the smoothing parameter λ is selected to maximise this approximation to $V(\lambda)$.

Estimation procedure
In most applications, we would not expect the age-related effect to have many turning or inflexion points. Typically, between 8 and 15 knots should suffice; the default number in R function smoothagesccs is 12, and we require at least 5. The knots are equally spaced in $[a, b]$. The optimal value of the smoothing parameter λ is selected with the exposure effect β set to zero, as described above. This value λ is then fixed, and the estimates $\hat{\alpha}$ and $\hat{\beta}$ are the values that maximise the penalised log likelihood function $PL(\alpha, \beta)$ with the constraint $\alpha_r = 1$, for $r = [(S+1)/2]$, rounded up if S is even. The constant trace$([\hat{\mathbf{H}} - 2\lambda\hat{\mathbf{P}}]^{-1}\hat{\mathbf{H}})$ may be interpreted as the model degrees of freedom associated with the relative age effect.

We follow Rondeau and Gonzalez (2005) and use the inverse of minus the Hessian of the maximised penalised log likelihood $PL(\hat{\alpha}, \hat{\beta})$ as an approximation to the covariance matrix for the parameters. From this, approximate confidence intervals for the exposure effect parameters β may be derived. Finally, the parameters α_s are scaled to meet our preferred constraint, namely $\psi(a) = 1$.

6.3 SCCS models with spline-based exposure effect

In Section 6.2 we described a spline-based SCCS model in which the relative age effect is represented by cubic M-splines. In the present section, cubic M-splines are used to represent the exposure effect. We describe two SCCS models. In the first, only the exposure effect is spline-based: the age effect is piecewise constant on pre-defined age groups. In the second, both exposure and age effects are represented by cubic M-splines.

When the risk period of primary interest is very short – a few days or weeks, say – then a SCCS model with piecewise constant exposure effect, such as the standard, semiparametric, or spline model for age, is recommended. However, when the risk period is long, and there is interest in describing the risk profile associated with exposure, then a spline model may provide a more realistic representation of the exposure effect. This can also be used to verify the validity of parametric representations.

Representing the exposure effect with a spline function means that it is no longer assumed to take a set of discrete values, but is a relative incidence function that varies smoothly with time since the start of exposure. Such a representation is useful especially in an exploratory rather than hypothesis testing context, when the shape of the exposure-associated risk profile is of interest, or the timing of the exposure effect in relation to the start of exposure is uncertain.

In Section 6.3.1 we describe the models. In subsequent sections we provide practical examples of their application. Some technical material relating to both models is included in starred Section 6.3.6, which may be skipped.

6.3.1   Splines for exposure effects

In Section 6.2, we described a model for the rate kernel in which the exposure effect is taken to be piecewise constant and the relative age effect is represented by a spline function. We now describe SCCS models in which the exposure effect is represented by a spline function. To keep matters simple, we assume that each case i experiences one period of exposure within the observation period $(a_i, b_i]$, starting at age d_{i1} and ending at age d_{i2}. For example, age d_{i1} might represent the age at vaccination, while d_{i2} represents an age at which the vaccination may be assumed to have no further impact. Alternatively, d_{i1} may represent age at the start of treatment, while d_{i2} is the age at the end of treatment (or some time after that). If the risk period associated with exposure is indefinite, then $d_{i2} = b_i$.

We now set

$$d = \max\{d_{i2} - d_{i1} : i = 1, \ldots, N\}.$$

The interval $(0, d]$ is the nominal risk period from the start of exposure, over which the spline function describing the exposure effect will be defined. It is called nominal because it may be longer than the actual risk period. The interval $(0, d]$ includes all intervals $(0, d_{i2} - d_{i1}]$, $i = 1, \ldots, N$. Note that times within the interval $(0, d]$ are not ages, but times since the start of exposure.

The effect of exposure is described by a spline-based relative incidence function $\rho(u)$, defined on the nominal risk period $(0, d]$. We choose $K \geq 5$ knots $\tau_k, k = 1, \ldots, K$ with $0 = \tau_1 < \tau_2 < \cdots < \tau_K = d$. The exposure-related relative incidence function $\rho(u)$ is a linear combination of $S = K + 2$ M-spline basis functions $M_s(u)$ defined for values u in $(0, d]$:

$$\rho(u) = \sum_{s=1}^{S} \beta_s^2 M_s(u). \tag{6.3}$$

The M-spline basis functions are the same as those described in Section 6.2, and are defined in Section 6.2.5. The constants β_s are parameters to be estimated, and are squared to ensure that $\rho(t)$ is non-negative. No constraint is placed on the parameters $\beta_1, \ldots, \beta_S$.

For a case i with exposure history in x_i determined by the risk period

$(d_{i1}, d_{i2}]$, the exposure effect at age t is:

$$\rho(t|x_i) = \begin{cases} \sum_{s=1}^{S} \beta_s^2 M_s(t - d_{i1}) & \text{for } t \text{ in } (d_{i1}, d_{i2}], \\ 1 & \text{elsewhere on } (a_i, b_i]. \end{cases}$$

To avoid a proliferation of symbols we use ρ to describe both $\rho(u)$ and $\rho(t|x_i)$. The relative incidence function $\rho(u)$ is a function of duration of exposure, whereas the exposure effect $\rho(t|x_i)$ is a function of age, given the exposure history in x_i.

The relative age effect $\psi(t)$ is represented in one of two ways, which we consider in turn. The first option is to assume the relative age effect is constant on pre-defined age groups, as for the standard SCCS model. Thus, the exposure effect is represented by a spline function, but the age effect is piecewise constant with parameter vector α; level 0 is the reference level, for which $\alpha_0 = 0$. The reference level is usually the earliest age group.

Estimating the parameters of the model involves striking a compromise between correctly representing genuine variation in the exposure-related relative incidence function $\rho(u)$ in Equation 6.3, without producing an unduly wiggly estimate. We use the penalised likelihood technique described in Section 6.2 to control the smoothness of the estimate of $\rho(u)$. This is determined by a single smoothing parameter λ. The penalised likelihood function is

$$PL(\alpha, \beta) = \sum_{i=1}^{N} \log L_i(\alpha, \beta) - 2\lambda \int \left(\sum_{s=1}^{S} \beta_s^2 M_s^{''}(u) \right)^2 du,$$

where $L_i(\alpha, \beta)$ is the SCCS likelihood contribution of case i and $M_s^{''}(u)$ is the second derivative of $M_s(u)$. The smoothing parameter λ may be chosen by the method of cross-validation, or an approximation to it. The penalised likelihood estimates of α and β are the values that maximise $PL(\alpha, \beta)$ for this optimal value of λ. Approximate confidence bands for the exposure-related relative incidence function $\rho(t)$ may be obtained by inverting the Hessian of the penalised likelihood function.

The second option is to represent the relative age effect by a separate spline function. In this model, both the exposure effect and the relative age effect are represented by M-splines. Insofar as spline-based models may be regarded as nonparametric, this SCCS model is then fully nonparametric. The spline function for the relative age effect involves K_1 knots and $S_1 = K_1 + 2$ parameters α_s, $s = 1, \ldots, S_1$, with $\alpha^T \alpha = 1$ or $\psi(a) = 1$, as described in Section 6.2. The spline function for the exposure effect uses K_2 knots and $S_2 = K_2 + 2$ parameters, as described earlier in the present section. Thus, for case i with observation period $(a_i, b_i]$ and exposure history in x_i determined by the single exposure period $(d_{i1}, d_{i2}]$, the rate kernel $\nu_i(t|x_i) = \psi(t)\rho(t|x_i)$

is represented by the product of the following two spline functions:

$$\psi(t) \;=\; \sum_{s=1}^{S_1} \alpha_s^2 M_{1s}(t) \quad \text{for } t \text{ in } (a_i, b_i], \text{ and}$$

$$\rho(t|x_i) \;=\; \sum_{s=1}^{S_2} \beta_s^2 M_{2s}(t - d_{i1}) \quad \text{for } t \text{ in } (d_{i1}, d_{i2}] \text{ and 1 otherwise.}$$

The functions $M_{1s}(t)$, $s = 1, \ldots, S_1$, denote the cubic M-spline basis functions for the relative age effect, defined as in Section 6.2 on the age interval $(a, b]$, and the functions $M_{2s}(t)$, $s = 1, \ldots, S_2$, are the S_2 basis functions for the exposure effect, defined at times in $(0, d]$ after the start of exposure. The penalised likelihood now involves two penalty terms with two distinct smoothing parameters, λ_1 controlling the smoothness of the age effect and λ_2 controlling the smoothness of the exposure effect:

$$PL(\boldsymbol{\alpha}, \boldsymbol{\beta}) = \sum_{i=1}^{N} \log L_i(\boldsymbol{\alpha}, \boldsymbol{\beta}) \;-\; 2\lambda_1 \int \Big(\sum_{s=1}^{S_1} \alpha_s^2 M_{1s}^{''}(u) \Big)^2 du$$

$$-\; 2\lambda_2 \int \Big(\sum_{s=1}^{S_2} \beta_s^2 M_{2s}^{''}(u) \Big)^2 du.$$

As before, optimal values of λ_1 and λ_2 are selected by a cross-validation method. The penalised likelihood is then maximised to obtain estimates of the parameters $\boldsymbol{\alpha}$ and $\boldsymbol{\beta}$.

So far we have assumed that each case has at most one risk period $(d_{i1}, d_{i2}]$. Multiple non-overlapping risk periods may also, in principle, be accommodated in much the same way. Brief details may be found in Ghebremichael-Weldeselassie et al. (2017b).

For both these SCCS models with spline-based exposure effects, further details of the SCCS likelihood contributions, the choice of smoothing parameters and the calculation of approximate confidence bands for the exposure-related relative incidence function $\rho(u)$ are provided in Section 6.3.6.

In the R package SCCS, the SCCS model with spline-based exposure effect and piecewise constant relative age effect is fitted using the function smoothexposccs. The default number of knots is kn=12 and the smoothing parameter sp can be specified explicitly, or optimised automatically (the default).

The nonparametric SCCS model with spline-based age and exposure effects is fitted using the function nonparasccs. The numbers of knots are kn1 and kn2 for the age and exposure effects, respectively. The smoothing parameters are sp1 and sp2, and are automatically optimised by default.

Both these functions may be used when each case experiences at most one exposure period. Both models may take some time to run. Fitting problems may arise when events are sparse at some ages, or at some times since exposure, in which case another SCCS model should be fitted instead.

These R functions also produce pointwise 95% confidence bands for the exposure effect. These confidence bands are generally wider than the 95% confidence intervals for the exposure effects in pre-defined risk periods, obtained from the standard SCCS model. This is because the pointwise confidence bands quantify the uncertainty of the exposure-related relative incidence at each time point since the start of exposure, rather than the uncertainty of the average relative incidence over each risk period.

Summary

- Rather than representing the exposure effect by a step function, it may be described by a smooth exposure-related relative incidence function. M-splines may be used to represent this function.

- In one version of this model, the age effect is assumed to be constant on pre-defined age groups. There is a single smoothing parameter determining the smoothness of the exposure effect.

- In a second version, splines are used to represent both the age effect and the exposure effect. There are then two smoothing parameters, controlling the smoothness of the age and exposure effects, respectively. This model may be regarded as nonparametric.

- The models are fitted using cross-validation and penalised likelihood methods similar to those used for the SCCS model with spline-based age effect.

6.3.2 Spline model for exposure: MMR and autism

In Section 6.2.4 we fitted the spline model for age to the data on MMR vaccine and autism. In this application, the risk periods stretch from age at primary MMR vaccination to the end of observation: thus, the risk periods can be very long. With the models we have fitted so far, we obtained estimates of the average MMR-related relative incidence. In Chapter 4, Section 4.8.2 and in Section 6.1.3 we also fitted models with time since MMR vaccine grouped in 4 categories (1, 2, 3, and 4 or more years).

The spline model for the exposure effect allows for a more detailed assessment of the risk profile by time since MMR vaccination. Using the same age groups as for the standard SCCS model, the spline model for exposure is specified as follows using R function smoothexposccs:

```
ageq <- quantile(autdat$diag, seq(0.025,0.975,0.025), names=F)
aut.mod9 <- smoothexposccs(indiv=case, astart=sta, aend=end,
            aevent=diag, adrug=mmr, aedrug=end, agegrp=ageq,
            data=autdat)
```

This yields the following results (all but the first and last of the age parameters have been omitted):

```
> aut.mod9
......
       exp(coef) exp(-coef) lower .95 upper .95
age2     6.774    0.14762    2.5599    17.927
......
age40    2.171    0.46070    0.6642     7.093


Spline based exposure relative incidence function:
 Smoothing parameter =  5.9e+00
 Cross validation score =  2404.15
```

Our main interest lies in the plot of the estimated exposure-related relative incidence function, shown in Figure 6.9.

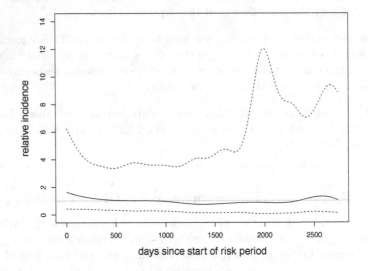

FIGURE 6.9

Fitted smooth exposure effect for MMR vaccine and autism (full line), with pointwise 95% confidence bands (dashed lines). The horizontal dotted line is at RI = 1.

This figure is obtained using the following code:

```
par(mar=c(4.1,4.1,1,1), cex.lab=1.4)
plot(aut.mod9)
abline(h=1, lty=3)
```

The estimated exposure-related relative incidence function remains close to

1 throughout the post-MMR risk period. Figure 6.9 thus supports the use of the model in which the MMR-related relative incidence is represented by a single constant value, as in Section 6.2.4. In that model, $RI = 1.05$, with 95% CI $(0.53, 2.08)$.

Note that the pointwise 95% confidence bands in Figure 6.9 are much wider than this confidence interval. This is because they represent the uncertainty in different quantities. The pointwise 95% confidence bands represent the uncertainty in the relative incidence at each time since MMR vaccination. The confidence interval for the average RI represents the uncertainty in the estimated average RI over all times post-MMR. Figure 6.9 shows that such an average is a reasonable summary measure, and so can validly be used as the target for inference.

6.3.3 Spline model for exposure: antidiabetics and fracture

In Chapter 4, Section 4.8.1 we used the standard SCCS model to analyse data on antidiabetics and fracture. The model identified a significantly increased risk over the risk period, which extended from the age at the first antidiabetic prescription to end of observation. A further analysis, with time at risk grouped into 7 categories, suggested that the risk increased up to 4–5 years after the start of treatment, and then declined.

The risk profile can also be investigated using the spline model for the exposure effect. Using the same age groups as previously, the model is specified as follows.

```
ageq <- quantile(adidat$frac, seq(0.025,0.975,0.025), names=F)
adi.mod3 <- smoothexposccs(indiv=case, astart=sta, aend=end,
            aevent=frac, adrug=adi, aedrug=end, agegrp=ageq,
            data=adidat)
```

This yields the following output (only the first and last of the 39 age parameters are displayed):

```
> adi.mod3
......
       exp(coef) exp(-coef) lower .95 upper .95
age2      0.8483    1.1788    0.5650    1.274
......
age40     3.7148    0.2692    1.2548   10.998

Spline based exposure relative incidence function:
  Smoothing parameter =   3.9e+02
  Cross validation score =   16547.31
```

The main interest resides in the plot of the exposure effect in Figure 6.10. This shows that the relative incidence increases to about 2.5, reaching this peak about 1500 days (4.1 years) after the start of treatment, then declines to

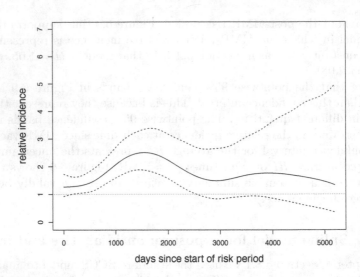

FIGURE 6.10

Fitted smooth exposure effect for antidiabetics and fracture (full line), with pointwise 95% confidence limits (dashed lines). The horizontal dotted line is at RI = 1.

a value a little in excess of 1.5 at around 2500 days (6.8 years) after the start of treatment, thereafter remaining roughly constant.

The main advantage of the spline model for the exposure effect is that it provides a more flexible estimate of the risk profile over the whole risk period than is available from parametric or semiparametric models. Note that, above about 6.5 years (2374 days), the risk profile is roughly constant. Thus it is appropriate to summarise it with a constant average value.

In Chapter 4, Section 4.8.1, the estimated relative incidence from model `adi.mod2` for the period 6+ years (about 2200+ days) after the start of treatment was 1.60, 95% CI $(1.16, 2.21)$. This confidence interval is much narrower than the confidence bands for this age range displayed in Figure 6.10, which relate to the uncertainty at individual time points.

For the purpose of inference about defined time periods after the start of exposure, we can also use the spline model for age. Using the same groupings of time since exposure as in Chapter 4, Section 4.8.1, the model is specified as follows.

```
exint <- c(0,366,731,1096,1461,1826,2191)
adi.mod4 <- smoothagesccs(indiv=case, astart=sta, aend=end,
            aevent=frac, adrug=adi, aedrug=end, expogrp=exint,
            data=adidat)
```

This gives the following estimates.

```
> adi.mod4
......

        exp(coef) exp(-coef) lower .95 upper .95
adi1      1.279     0.7816     1.069     1.532
adi2      1.421     0.7037     1.155     1.748
adi3      1.908     0.5242     1.531     2.377
adi4      2.565     0.3899     2.025     3.249
adi5      2.681     0.3731     2.048     3.508
adi6      2.243     0.4459     1.629     3.086
adi7      1.551     0.6446     1.118     2.152


spline based age relative incidence function:
 Smoothing parameter = 1.5e+08
 Cross validation score = 16581.88
```

The final parameter represents the relative incidence 6+ years after the start of treatment. This is $RI = 1.55$, with 95% CI $(1.12, 2.15)$, similar to the estimate obtained with the standard SCCS model. The smooth age effect is shown in Figure 6.11.

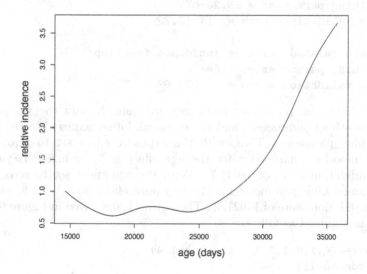

FIGURE 6.11
Fitted smooth age effect for antidiabetics and fracture.

6.3.4 Nonparametric model: MMR and convulsions

In Chapter 4, Section 4.5.1 and also in Chapter 5, Section 5.2.3 we discussed data on MMR vaccine (and other vaccines) and convulsions in children aged

1–2 years. Standard SCCS analyses were undertaken with a range of different risk periods; a significant association was identified in the second week after MMR vaccination, but not at other times.

In the present section we undertake a nonparametric analysis of the association between MMR vaccine and convulsions. That is, we shall represent both the age effect and the exposure effect using spline functions. We shall use the 8-week nominal risk period $[0, 56]$ days. Such an analysis provides a broader picture of the risk profile of the vaccine over this time scale.

The model is specified as follows, using the R function `nonparasccs`. Neither the arguments `expogrp` or `agegrp` are required.

```
con.mod11 <- nonparasccs(indiv=case, astart=sta, aend=end,
          aevent=conv, adrug=mmr, aedrug=mmr+56,
          data=condat)
```

This produces the following output.

```
> con.mod11
Non parametric self controlled case series
Age related relative incidence function:
 Smoothing parameter =   6.2e+07
 Cross validation score =   14042.72

Exposure related relative incidence function:
 Smoothing parameter =   1.5e+00
 Cross validation score =   14021.99
```

Note that no parameter estimates are quoted: only the values of the two smoothing parameters, and the cross-validation scores obtained for each smoothing parameter. Thus, with the exposure effect set to zero, the optimal smoothing parameter for the age effect is $\lambda_1 = 6.2\text{e}+07$, yielding a cross-validation score of 14042.72. With the age effect set to zero, the optimal smoothing parameter for the exposure effect is $\lambda_2 = 1.5$, yielding a cross-validation score of 14021.99. The output is displayed in Figure 6.12; this figure is obtained as follows.

```
par(mar=c(4.1,4.1,1,1), cex.lab=1.4)
plot(con.mod11)
abline(h=1, lty=3)
```

The estimated smooth age effect, shown in the left panel of Figure 6.12, is monotone decreasing from 1 to about 0.5 over the second year of life. The estimated MMR-related exposure effect shows a clear peak rising to about $RI = 2.3$ in the period 4–12 days after MMR vaccine. There is a less pronounced second bump at 18–25 days post MMR, rising to about $RI = 1.4$.

While the confidence bands unequivocally identify the first peak (at 4–12 days post MMR) as statistically significant, the status of the second peak (at

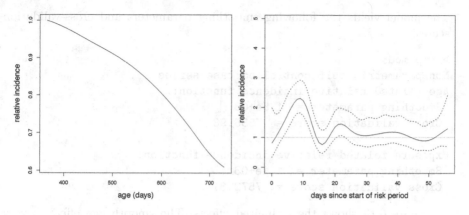

FIGURE 6.12
Nonparametric SCCS model for MMR vaccine and convulsions. Left: age effect. Right: exposure effect (full line) with 95% pointwise confidence bands (dashed lines). The horizontal dotted line is at $RI = 1$.

8–25 days post MMR) is not so clear. This analysis could be used to generate a hypothesis about the presence of a second peak, to be tested in further studies. At other times in the 8-week nominal risk window, there is little evidence of an effect associated with MMR, the relative incidence remaining close to 1.

6.3.5 Nonparametric model: acute risk of hip fracture

In Section 6.2.3 we fitted a spline SCCS model for age to the hip fracture and antidepressants data, first analysed using the standard SCCS model in Chapter 4, Section 4.3.3. These models used 5 risk periods: two initial risk periods $[0, 14]$ and $[15, 42]$ days after the initiation of treatment with antidepressants, followed by the rest of the time on the drug, and two washout periods. The overall risk periods can be very long indeed.

Long risk periods present a challenge for the nonparametric SCCS model, which may fail to converge. In such circumstances it may be necessary to use shorter risk periods, provided these are appropriate in the context of the application.

For the hip fracture data, the model does not converge if we specify `aedrug=endad`. However, interest focuses primarily on the acute risk immediately following initiation of treatment with antidepressants. Accordingly, we restrict the nominal risk period to include only the first year of exposure. This model is specified as follows:

```
hip.mod5 <- nonparasccs(indiv=case, astart=sta,
            aend=end, aevent=frac, adrug=ad,
            aedrug=pmin(endad,ad+365), data=hipdat)
```

The model yields the following smoothing parameters and cross-validation scores.

```
> hip.mod5
Non parametric self controlled case series
Age related relative incidence function:
 Smoothing parameter =  1.5e+08
 Cross validation score =   7535.98

Exposure related relative incidence function:
 Smoothing parameter =  1.1e+03
 Cross validation score =   7572.31
```

Figure 6.13 shows the estimated effects. The smooth age effect is very similar to that obtained in Section 6.2.3 with the spline model for age. The

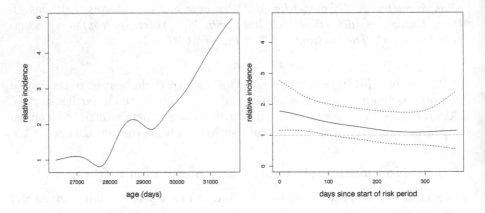

FIGURE 6.13
Nonparametric SCCS model for initiation of antidepressants and hip fractures. Left: age effect. Right: exposure effect (full line) with 95% pointwise confidence bands (dashed lines). The horizontal dotted line is at $RI = 1$.

smooth exposure effect suggests that the effect is highest immediately after the initiation of treatment with antidepressants, then declines to a roughly constant value close to 1 over the remainder of the 12-month period of exposure. The pointwise 95% confidence bands lie above 1 up to about 100 days after the initiation of treatment.

These results broadly match those obtained with the standard SCCS model and the spline SCCS model for age. Arguably, however, the parametric representations of the exposure effect used in those models provide a sharper description of the risk profile in the period of primary interest, which immediately follows the initiation of treatment.

6.3.6 Further material on spline-based models*

In many respects, the SCCS models with spline-based exposure effect are similar to the SCCS model with spline-based age effect. Thus the material in Section 6.2.5 will be referred to in the present section. We focus here on some key differences, notably likelihood contributions, choice of smoothing parameter or parameters, and calculation of approximate pointwise confidence bands for the exposure-related relative incidence function.

Likelihood contributions

We consider first the model with piecewise constant age effect. Suppose that case i experiences n_i events at ages t_{ij}, $j = 1, \ldots, n_i$, and has exposure period $(d_{i1}, d_{i2}]$. Let $D_i(t)$ denote the indicator function for $(d_{i1}, d_{i2}]$, equal to 1 if $d_{i1} < t \leq d_{i2}$ and equal to 0 otherwise, for t in $(a_i, b_i]$, the observation period for case i. The likelihood contribution for case i is:

$$L_i = \prod_{j=1}^{n_i} \frac{\psi(t_{ij}) \left(\sum_{s=1}^{S} \beta_s^2 M_s(t_{ij} - d_{i1}) \right)^{D_i(t_{ij})}}{\int_{a_i}^{b_i} \psi(t) \left(\sum_{s=1}^{S} \beta_s^2 M_s(t - d_{i1}) \right)^{D_i(t)} dt}.$$

Suppose now that $\psi(t)$ is piecewise constant. Then there are cutpoints c_{ir}, $r = 1, \ldots, R_i$ including $\{d_{i1}, d_{i2}\}$ and with $c_{i0} = a_i$ and $c_{iR_i} = b_i$ such that $\psi(t)$ is constant with value $\exp(\alpha_{h(i,r)})$ on $(c_{ir-1}, c_{ir}]$. Also, suppose that event time t_{ij} lies in $(c_{ir_j-1}, c_{ir_j}]$ so that $\psi(t_{ij}) = \exp(\alpha_{h(i,r_j)})$. The likelihood contribution L_i of case i may then be written:

$$\prod_{j=1}^{n_i} \frac{\exp(\alpha_{h(i,r_j)}) \left(\sum_{s=1}^{S} \beta_s^2 M_s(t_{ij} - d_{i1}) \right)^{D_i(t_{ij})}}{\sum_{r=1}^{R_i} \exp(\alpha_{h(i,r)}) e_{ir}^{1-D_{ir}} \left(\sum_{s=1}^{S} \beta_s^2 [I_s(c_{ir} - d_{i1}) - I_s(c_{ir-1} - d_{i1})] \right)^{D_{ir}}},$$

where $e_{ir} = c_{ir} - c_{ir-1}$ and $D_{ir} = D_i(c_{ir})$, which is equal to 1 if $(c_{ir-1}, c_{ir}]$ is contained within $(d_{i1}, d_{i2}]$ and 0 otherwise. The functions $I_s(t)$ in the denominator are the cubic I-spline basis functions, described in Section 6.2.5.

When $\psi(t)$ is itself a spline, with $\psi(t) = \sum_{s=1}^{S_1} \alpha_s^2 M_{1s}(t)$, the exposure-related relative incidence function being $\rho(u) = \sum_{s=1}^{S_2} \beta_s^2 M_{2s}(u)$, the likelihood contribution is:

$$L_i = \prod_{j=1}^{n_i} \frac{\sum_{s=1}^{S_1} \alpha_s^2 M_{1s}(t_{ij}) \left(\sum_{s=1}^{S_2} \beta_s^2 M_{2s}(t_{ij} - d_{i1}) \right)^{D_i(t_{ij})}}{\int_{a_i}^{b_i} \sum_{s=1}^{S_1} \alpha_s^2 M_{1s}(t) \left(\sum_{s=1}^{S_2} \beta_s^2 M_{2s}(t - d_{i1}) \right)^{D_i(t)} dt}.$$

The denominator involves integrals of products of cubic M-spline basis functions. These may be obtained explicitly using integration by parts. The denominator turns out to involve I-splines and their first, second and third integrals.

---

* This section may be skipped.

The calculations, though not difficult, are unenlightening and are not included. Full details may be found in Ghebremichael-Weldeselassie et al. (2017b).

Choice of smoothing parameter(s)
For the SCCS model with spline-based exposure effect and piecewise constant age effect, the selection of the smoothing parameter closely follows the procedure described in Section 6.2.5, with the roles of parameter vectors α and β switched. Thus, the cross-validation score is now defined as

$$V(\lambda) = \sum_{i=1}^{N} \log L_i(\hat{\boldsymbol{\beta}}_{-i}),$$

where $L_i(\boldsymbol{\beta})$ is the contribution of case i to the SCCS likelihood and $\hat{\boldsymbol{\beta}}_{-i}$ is the maximum penalised likelihood estimate obtained when case i is removed, both with $\boldsymbol{\alpha} = \mathbf{0}$.

The only difference is that there is no constraint on the parameters β_s. Thus, in the last step of the calculation in which the matrix $\mathbf{P}$ is obtained, we set $\mathbf{P} = \mathbf{P}^+$, where $\mathbf{P}^+$ is defined in Section 6.2.5.

For the nonparametric SCCS model, both procedures are used: the method described in Section 6.2.5 is used to obtain λ_1, the smoothing parameter associated with the age effect, and the procedure just described is used to obtain λ_2, the smoothing parameter associated with the exposure effect.

Calculation of confidence bands
Approximate pointwise 95% confidence bands for the exposure-related relative incidence function $\rho(u)$ may be obtained as follows. Let $\hat{\mathbf{V}}$ denote the approximate covariance of $\hat{\boldsymbol{\beta}}$, obtained from the negative of the inverted Hessian of the penalised likelihood $PL(\hat{\boldsymbol{\alpha}}, \hat{\boldsymbol{\beta}})$ evaluated at the penalised maximum log likelihood estimates. Then

$$\hat{\mathbf{W}} = 4 \operatorname{diag}(\hat{\boldsymbol{\beta}}) \hat{\mathbf{V}} (\operatorname{diag}(\hat{\boldsymbol{\beta}}))^T$$

is the approximate covariance matrix of $\hat{\boldsymbol{\beta}}^2$. Let

$$\mathbf{M}_2(u)^T = (M_{21}(u), \ldots, M_{2S_2}(u)).$$

The approximate confidence bands on $\rho(u) = \sum_{s=1}^{S_2} \beta_s^2 M_{2s}(u)$, for u in $(0, d]$, are

$$\hat{\rho}(u) \pm 1.96 \sqrt{\mathbf{M}_2(u)^T \hat{\mathbf{W}} \mathbf{M}_2(u)}.$$

Alternatively, to ensure the confidence bands lie above zero, they can be calculated on the log scale as

$$\hat{\rho}(u) \exp\left(\pm 1.96 \hat{\rho}(u)^{-1} \sqrt{\mathbf{M}_2(u)^T \hat{\mathbf{W}} \mathbf{M}_2(u)} \right).$$

6.4 SCCS model for multi-type events

All SCCS models described so far have been for events of a single type. In this section, we consider models for events that may be classified as belonging to one of several exclusive types: we refer to these as multi-type events. Multi-type events may arise, for example, when events occur with distinct clinical presentations. The analysis of non-recurrent multi-type events is usually referred to as competing risks (Aalen et al., 2008, pages 114–117). Most commonly, competing risks analysis is used to analyse deaths, the different types corresponding to mutually exclusive causes of death. With greater relevance to the SCCS method, one can also envisage non-terminal competing risks, such as the first occurrence of a potentially recurrent multi-type event.

In Section 6.4.1 we discuss standard SCCS models for multi-type events. Examples of these models are described in Sections 6.4.2 and 6.4.3. Starred Section 6.4.4 contains some more technical material on these models, including competing risks, and may be skipped.

6.4.1 Modelling multi-type events

Suppose that the event of interest can take one of several, mutually exclusive types labelled $r = 1, \ldots, R$. We assume to begin with that, for each individual i, the R event types are potentially recurrent, and arise independently within the individual's observation period $(a_i, b_i]$ according to Poisson processes. (This assumption will subsequently be relaxed.) Thus, an individual i may experience more than one event type over the observation period.

Suppose that an individual i experiences n_{ir} events of type r in $(a_i, b_i]$. The total number of events experienced by individual i is $n_i = \sum_{r=1}^{R} n_{ir}$. A case is now defined as an individual with $n_i \geq 1$. This means that for some, but not necessarily all, $r = 1, \ldots, R$, $n_{ir} \geq 1$. Suppose that there are N cases, and define

$$E_r = \{i : n_{ir} > 0, i = 1, \ldots, N\}.$$

Thus, E_r is the subset of cases who have experienced one or more events of type r. The sets E_r may overlap, since a case may experience more than one event type, but the union of the E_r is just the set of cases: $\bigcup_{r=1}^{R} E_r = \{1, \ldots, N\}$.

The derivation of the SCCS likelihood for multi-type events closely follows that for events of a single type, described in Chapter 3, Section 3.8. The main difference is that, rather than conditioning on the overall number of events n_i for individual i, we condition on the numbers of events of each type for that individual, contained in the vector $(n_{i1}, \ldots, n_{iR})$. The multi-type SCCS likelihood then turns out to be the product of the SCCS likelihoods for each event type taken separately. Thus, if L_{ir} is the SCCS likelihood contribution of an individual i in E_r, that is, of a type r case, then the overall multi-type

SCCS likelihood is

$$L = \text{constant} \times \prod_{r=1}^{R} \prod_{i \in E_r} L_{ir}.$$

The multi-type SCCS likelihood is derived in Section 6.4.4. The practical consequence of the fact that the multi-type SCCS likelihood is just the product of the SCCS likelihoods for the individual event types is that the multi-type model may be fitted in much the same way as a single type SCCS model.

To keep matters simple, we shall assume that the standard SCCS model applies to each event type – and thus, that the incidence rate is piecewise constant on pre-determined age and exposure intervals. In a simple model with no fixed covariates, the incidence rate kernel of event type r for an individual i at age level j and exposure level k is:

$$\nu_{ijkr} = \exp(\alpha_{jr} + \beta_{kr}). \tag{6.4}$$

The age and exposure intervals can differ for different event types, though this is not usually needed: it is much simpler to use the same intervals for all event types, if necessary by subdividing them. The age and exposure parameters, however, will typically differ between event types, and investigating such differences constitutes the main focus of the multi-type analysis.

The standard multi-type SCCS model is fitted in a similar way to the single type model, with a new R-level factor for event type, which may be treated as a time-invariant covariate. A sequence of models may then be fitted, to include interactions with event type if required.

The baseline model is $\nu_{ijkr} = \exp\{\alpha_j + \beta_k\}$, represented by the model formula

Age + Exposure

which implies $\alpha_{jr} = \alpha_j$ and $\beta_{kr} = \beta_k$ for all j, k, r – that is, no effect of type on the age or exposure effects. Variation of the age effect according to event type may be investigated by fitting the model $\nu_{ijkr} = \exp\{\alpha_{jr} + \beta_k\}$ with model formula

Age + Exposure + Age.Type

where Age.Type represents the interaction between Age and Type. The main effect of Type is not included as it is time-invariant and so cannot be estimated in the SCCS model. Similarly, variation of the exposure effect according to event type corresponds to the model $\nu_{ijkr} = \exp\{\alpha_j + \beta_{kr}\}$ with model formula

Age + Exposure + Exposure.Type.

The full model in Equation 6.4 allows variation in both age and exposure effect by event type, with model formula

Age + Exposure + Age.Type + Exposure.Type.

This model is equivalent to fitting separate models for each of the R different event types. The main advantage of the multi-type formulation is that it enables formal significance tests to be undertaken, using the likelihood ratio test, to compare the different models.

This framework for the multi-type SCCS model applies to recurrent events of different types that are independent within individuals. It encompasses situations in which there is clustering of events within individuals, and hence marginal dependence in the event-type counts n_{ir}. This framework may also be used for competing risks analyses when all event types are rare. More contrived circumstances, in which the event types of interest are rare, but competing events not of primary interest are not rare, may also be treated in this framework, provided that such incidental events are unrelated to the exposure of interest. Further details of all these scenarios are provided in starred Section 6.4.4.

Summary

- The multi-type SCCS model provides a framework for analysing events that arise in several, mutually exclusive types.

- The multi-type SCCS likelihood is the product of the SCCS likelihoods for the individual event types.

- Multi-type analyses using the standard SCCS model involve interactions between a factor representing the different event types and the age and exposure effects.

- The model may be used when recurrences of the various event types are independent within individuals, or for competing events when the event types potentially associated with the exposure of interest are rare.

6.4.2 Febrile and non-febrile convulsions

This example uses new data on convulsions and MMR vaccine in the second year of life (366 to 730 days of age). The risk period of interest spans the first two weeks after vaccination: $[0, 7]$ and $[8, 14]$ days. The jittered data, in data frame febdat, comprise 988 convulsions, including 894 first events and 94 recurrences. The convulsions are classified in one of two exclusive types, in variable type: non-febrile convulsions (type $= 1$) and febrile convulsions (type $= 2$).

There are 119 non-febrile convulsions and 869 febrile convulsions. Figure 6.14 shows the age distribution of the two event types. There are no striking differences in the age distribution of febrile and non-febrile convulsions: a more detailed, model-based analysis is required. Figure 6.15 shows the centred event and observation plots. The bin size for the centred event plot

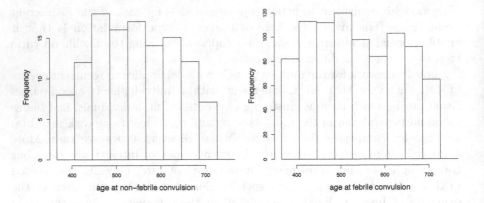

FIGURE 6.14
Age at convulsion (days). Left: non-febrile convulsions. Right: febrile convulsions.

is 20 days. There is a clear trough in the period immediately prior to MMR vaccination, so we shall use a pre-exposure risk period of 21 days.

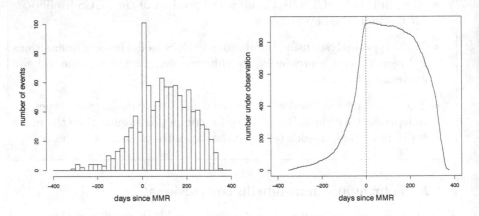

FIGURE 6.15
Centred plots for convulsions. Left: event plot. Right: observation plot.

Figure 6.15 was obtained with the following code:

```
par(mfrow=c(1,2), mar=c(4.1,4.1,1,1), cex.lab=1.4)
mmrx <- ifelse(febdat$mmr<366-15|febdat$mmr>730, NA, febdat$mmr)
timint <- febdat$conv - mmrx
timhis <- hist(timint, breaks=seq(-400,400,20), xlab=
          "days since MMR", ylab="number of events",
          main=NULL)
```

```
xtime <- seq(min(febdat$sta-mmrx,na.rm=T), max(febdat$end-mmrx,
        na.rm=T), 1)
ytime <- NULL
for (i in 1:length(xtime)){
ytime[i] <- sum((febdat$sta-mmrx<=xtime[i])*
        (xtime[i]<=febdat$end-mmrx), na.rm=T)
}
plot(xtime, ytime,type="s", xlim=c(-400,400),
    xlab="days since MMR", ylab="number under observation")
abline(v=0, lty=2)
```

The baseline model, with a common exposure and age effect for the two event types, is specified as follows with six age groups of approximately two month durations.

```
ageg <- c(426,486,546,606,666)
feb.mod1 <- standardsccs(event~mmr+age, indiv=case, astart=sta,
            aend=end, aevent=conv, adrug=mmr, aedrug=mmr+14,
            expogrp=c(-21,0,8), agegrp=ageg, data=febdat)
```

This produces the following exposure effect estimates.

```
> feb.mod1
.....
      exp(coef) exp(-coef) lower .95 upper .95
mmr1    0.5997    1.6676    0.4144    0.8678
mmr2    1.0341    0.9670    0.6720    1.5913
mmr3    3.0686    0.3259    2.3273    4.0460
```

The pre-exposure risk period effect is statistically significant. There is no marked effect in the $[0, 7]$ day risk period (relative incidence 1.03, 95% CI $(0.67, 1.59)$, but a clearly elevated relative incidence in the $[8, 14]$-day period: $RI = 3.07$, 95% $(2.33, 4.05)$. This is apparent in the centred event plot of Figure 6.15.

To investigate the multi-type SCCS model proper, we now fit a sequence of models with interactions with the variable type. Model feb.mod2 allows for separate exposure effects for the two event types, model feb.mod3 for separate age effects, and model feb.mod4 for separate exposure and age effects.

```
feb.mod2 <- standardsccs(event~factor(type)/mmr+age, indiv=case,
            astart=sta, aend=end, aevent=conv, adrug=mmr,
            aedrug=mmr+14, expogrp=c(-21,0,8), agegrp=ageg,
            data=febdat)
feb.mod3 <- standardsccs(event~mmr+factor(type)/age, indiv=case,
            astart=sta, aend=end, aevent=conv, adrug=mmr,
            aedrug=mmr+14, expogrp=c(-21,0,8), agegrp=ageg,
            data=febdat)
```

```
feb.mod4 <- standardsccs(event~factor(type)/(mmr+age),
           indiv=case, astart=sta, aend=end, aevent=conv,
           adrug=mmr, aedrug=mmr+14, expogrp=c(-21,0,8),
           agegrp=ageg, data=febdat)
```

In the full model, feb.mod4, the exposure effects are as follows.

```
> feb.mod4
.....
                      exp(coef) exp(-coef) lower .95 upper .95
factor(type)2              NA         NA         NA         NA
factor(type)1:mmr1    0.3298     3.0321    0.08024     1.3557
factor(type)2:mmr1    0.6329     1.5800    0.43109     0.9292
factor(type)1:mmr2    1.2190     0.8204    0.38119     3.8980
factor(type)2:mmr2    1.0072     0.9928    0.63330     1.6019
factor(type)1:mmr3    2.7366     0.3654    1.18176     6.3371
factor(type)2:mmr3    3.1071     0.3218    2.31760     4.1655
```

The relative incidences associated with the $[0, 7]$-day risk period are, respectively, 1.22 and 1.01 for non-febrile and febrile convulsions, both statistically non-significant. The relative incidences for the $[8, 14]$-day risk period are 2.74, 95% CI $(1.18, 6.34)$ for non-febrile convulsions, and 3.11, 95% CI $(2.32, 4.17)$ for febrile convulsions.

The estimates obtained using the full model feb.mod4 are the same as would have been obtained if separate analyses had been undertaken of febrile and non-febrile convulsions. The advantage of the multi-type analysis, however, is that it provides a framework in which to test whether any differences in exposure effects between event types are statistically significant. This may be done using likelihood ratio tests.

```
> lrtsccs(feb.mod1,feb.mod2)
   test df pvalue
  1.347  3  0.718
> lrtsccs(feb.mod1,feb.mod3)
   test df pvalue
  4.839  5 0.4358
> lrtsccs(feb.mod1,feb.mod4)
   test df pvalue
  5.917  8 0.6565
```

These three likelihood ratio tests yield p-values well above 0.05, and so there is little evidence to reject the null hypothesis that age and exposure effects are identical for febrile and non-febrile convulsions. Thus, the estimates obtained from the baseline model feb.mod1 may validly be used to summarise the results.

6.4.3 Antidiabetic drugs and fracture site

In Chapter 4, Section 4.8.1, we discussed a SCCS analysis of the association between antidiabetics and fracture. In the present example, we revisit this application, focusing on fracture site.

Fracture sites are in variable type, and are coded type = 1 for foot, ankle, wrist or hand fractures, type = 2 for hip fractures, and type = 3 for spine fractures. The data, which are simulated based on Douglas et al. (2009), include 2000 cases. Only first fractures are included, so the event types compete.

Note that, in principle (though not in our data), fracture sites need not be exclusive: for example, a double fracture might occur in two different sites. There are several ways to handle such multiple type events. One is to define a hierarchy of types and always allocate multiple types to the highest in the hierarchy. Another is to create a new category for multiple types. Finally, in some circumstances it may be appropriate to count a multiple type event as several distinct events, one for each type.

In the present data, in data frame adidat, the type frequencies are as follows:

```
> table(adidat$type)

   1    2    3
1596  262  142
```

Thus, fractures of the limb extremities (type = 1) are much more frequent than hip or spine fractures.

In the previous analysis in Chapter 4, Section 4.8.1, we used 40 age groups defined by the quantiles of frac, the age at fracture. In the present analysis, using such a large number of age groups would produce large numbers of empty multinomial categories for the less frequent event types (notably those for spine fracture, of which there are only 142). In consequence, many type-specific age parameters would lie on the boundary of the parameter space. This in turn may affect the validity of the asymptotic p-values from likelihood ratio tests. To mitigate this problem, we shall reduce the number of age groups to 20.

The baseline model, with common exposure and age effects for the three event types, but now with only 20 age groups, is specified as follows.

```
ageq2 <- quantile(adidat$frac,seq(0.05,0.95,0.05), names=F)
adi.mod5 <- standardsccs(event~adi+age, indiv=case,
            astart=sta, aend=end, aevent=frac, adrug=
            adi, aedrug=end, expogrp=0, agegrp=ageq2,
            data=adidat)
```

The effect estimate from this model is common to the three types of fractures, and is as follows.

```
> adi.mod5
.....
        exp(coef)  exp(-coef)  lower .95  upper .95
adi1     1.5608      0.6407     1.3581      1.794
```

The relative incidence is 1.56, 95% CI $(1.36, 1.79)$, which differs little from that obtained in Chapter 4, Section 4.8.1, namely $RI = 1.56$, with 95% CI $(1.35, 1.80)$. Thus reducing the number of age groups does not introduce any appreciable bias.

We now fit a sequence of multi-type SCCS models to investigate any differences in the age and exposure effects according to event type.

```
adi.mod6 <- standardsccs(event~factor(type)/adi+age,
            indiv=case, astart=sta, aend=end, aevent=frac,
            adrug=adi, aedrug=end, expogrp=0, agegrp=ageq2,
            data=adidat)
adi.mod7 <- standardsccs(event~adi+factor(type)/age,
            indiv=case, astart=sta, aend=end, aevent=frac,
            adrug=adi, aedrug=end, expogrp=0, agegrp=ageq2,
            data=adidat)
adi.mod8 <- standardsccs(event~factor(type)/(adi+age),
            indiv=case, astart=sta, aend=end, aevent=frac,
            adrug=adi, aedrug=end, expogrp=0, agegrp=ageq2,
            data=adidat)
```

Model `adi.mod6` allows the exposure effect to vary with event type. Model `adi.mod7` allows the age effect to vary between types. And model `adi.mod8` allows both exposure and age effects to vary. These elaborations of the baseline model may then be investigated by likelihood ratio tests (models `adi.mod7` and `adi.mod8` each have a single empty age group, but this will not unduly influence the tests).

```
> lrtsccs(adi.mod5,adi.mod6)
   test df    pvalue
  13.62  2 0.001103
> lrtsccs(adi.mod5,adi.mod7)
  test df pvalue
  46.4 38 0.1646
> lrtsccs(adi.mod5,adi.mod8)
   test df pvalue
  48.06 40 0.1787
```

The *p*-value of 0.0011 for the comparison between `adi.mod5` and `adi.mod6` is highly statistically significant, suggesting that the exposure effects differ according to event type. The other comparisons yield *p*-values in excess of 0.15. Thus, it would appear reasonable to summarise the data with model `adi.mod6`.

```
> adi.mod6
. . . . .
                  exp(coef) exp(-coef) lower .95 upper .95
. . . . .
factor(type)1:adi1    1.4016     0.7134    1.2055    1.630
factor(type)2:adi1    2.3777     0.4206    1.7519    3.227
factor(type)3:adi1    2.2253     0.4494    1.4908    3.322
```

According to this model, the antidiabetic drugs studied are positively associated with fractures at all three sites, though the association is strongest with hip and spine fractures. For foot, ankle, wrist or hand fractures, the relative incidence is 1.40, with 95% CI $(1.21, 1.63)$. For hip fractures, $RI = 2.38$, 95% CI $(1.75, 3.23)$. And for spine fractures, $RI = 2.23$, 95% CI $(1.49, 3.32)$.

As found in Chapter 4, Section 4.8.1, the relative incidence varies by time since the beginning of treatment. It is of interest to describe the trajectories for the different event types. This may be done as follows, using the same variable exint as used in Chapter 4, Section 4.8.1.

```
exint <- c(0,366,731,1096,1461,1826,2191)
adi.mod9 <- standardsccs(event~factor(type)/adi+age,
            indiv=case, astart=sta, aend=end, aevent=frac,
            adrug=adi, aedrug=end, expogrp=exint, agegrp=ageq2,
            data=adidat)
```

The parameters from this model may be used to obtain Figure 6.16, which shows the relative incidence by time since start of treatment for the three event types (R code not shown). There is a similar pattern for the three event types: a rise, followed by a drop. All three trajectories begin at a similar level, but the subsequent rise appears steeper for spine and (especially) hip fractures.

6.4.4   SCCS likelihoods for multi-type events*

We provide details of the derivation of the multi-type SCCS likelihood, under the assumptions described in Section 6.4.1.

Marginally independent recurrent event types
In this setting the type-specific event processes are independent non-homogeneous Poisson processes. Let $\lambda_{ir}(t|x_i, y_i)$ denote the incidence of events of type r for an individual i over the observation period $(a_i, b_i]$. As usual, x_i is the exposure and observation history over $(a_i, b_i]$ and y_i is a set of time-invariant covariates; we assume without loss of generality that these covariates are the same for all event types. The incidence of events, irrespective of type, is

$$\lambda_{i+}(t|x_i, y_i) = \sum_{r=1}^{R} \lambda_{ir}(t|x_i, y_i).$$

---

* This section may be skipped.

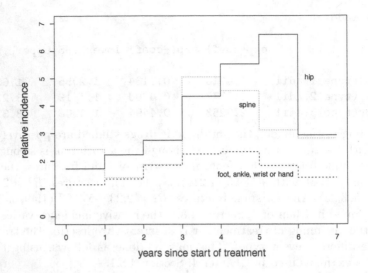

FIGURE 6.16
Relative incidence of fracture by time since start of treatment, by fracture type.

If individual i experiences $n_{ir} > 0$ events of type r in $(a_i, b_i]$, let t_{irs}, $s = 1, \ldots, n_{ir}$ denote the event times. The cohort likelihood contribution for individual i is then

$$L_{ci} = \prod_{r=1}^{R} \prod_{s=1}^{n_{ir}} \lambda_{ir}(t_{irs}|x_i, \boldsymbol{y}_i) \exp\left(-\int_{a_i}^{b_i} \lambda_{i+}(t|x_i, \boldsymbol{y}_i) dt \right),$$

with the convention that if $n_{ir} = 0$ then the corresponding term in the product is replaced by 1. Conditioning on the total number of events of each type experienced by individual i, that is, on the vector $(n_{i1}, \ldots, n_{iR})$, yields the following conditional likelihood contribution:

$$L_i = \text{constant} \times \prod_{r=1}^{R} \frac{\prod_{s=1}^{n_{ir}} \lambda_{ir}(t_{irs}|x_i, \boldsymbol{y}_i)}{\left(\int_{a_i}^{b_i} \lambda_{ir}(t|x_i, \boldsymbol{y}_i) dt \right)^{n_{ir}}}.$$

The overall multi-type SCCS likelihood is the product of these contributions for the N cases:

$$
\begin{aligned}
L &= \text{constant} \times \prod_{i=1}^{N} \prod_{r=1}^{R} \frac{\prod_{s=1}^{n_{ir}} \lambda_{ir}(t_{irs}|x_i, \boldsymbol{y}_i)}{\left(\int_{a_i}^{b_i} \lambda_{ir}(t|x_i, \boldsymbol{y}_i) dt \right)^{n_{ir}}} \\
&= \text{constant} \times \prod_{r=1}^{R} \prod_{i \in E_r} \frac{\prod_{s=1}^{n_{ir}} \lambda_{ir}(t_{irs}|x_i, \boldsymbol{y}_i)}{\left(\int_{a_i}^{b_i} \lambda_{ir}(t|x_i, \boldsymbol{y}_i) dt \right)^{n_{ir}}}, \quad (6.5)
\end{aligned}
$$

where E_r is the set of individuals experiencing one or more events of type r, defined in Section 6.4.1. This last expression is the product, over the different types, of the type-specific SCCS likelihoods. Note that if the overall number of events n_i were conditioned upon for each individual, an extra term would appear in the conditional likelihood, corresponding to the relative marginal abundances of the different types.

Marginally dependent recurrent event types
In this setting, the marginal counts n_{ir} of the different event types are dependent, but the type-specific event times remain independent within individuals. In such a scenario it is commonly assumed that, for individual i, events of type r arise according to a non-homogeneous Poisson process with rate

$$\mu_{ir}(t|x_i, y_i, U_{ir}) = U_{ir}\lambda_{ir}(t|x_i, y_i),$$

where U_{ir} is a positive random variable, $r = 1, \ldots, R$, and $U_i = (U_{i1}, \ldots, U_{iR})$ is sampled from some R-variate density. Conditioning on U_i as well as $(n_{i1}, \ldots, n_{iR})$, the frailty terms U_{ir} factor out and we retrieve Expression 6.5.

Competing risks: all event types are rare
We now suppose that the event of interest is non-recurrent. Thus, the event types compete, in the sense that occurrence of one event types precludes any other from occurring. Let t_i denote the unique event time for individual i. The cohort likelihood contribution of individual i is then

$$L_{ci} = \prod_{r=1}^{R} \lambda_{ir}(t_i|x_i, y_i)^{n_{ir}} \exp\left(-\int_{a_i}^{t_i} \lambda_{i+}(t|x_i, y_i)dt\right).$$

Conditioning on $(n_{i1}, \ldots, n_{iR})$ yields the conditional likelihood contribution

$$L_i = \frac{\prod_{r=1}^{R} \lambda_{ir}(t_i|x_i, y_i)^{n_{ir}} \exp\left(-\int_{a_i}^{t_i} \lambda_{i+}(t|x_i, y_i)dt\right)}{\int_{a_i}^{b_i} \prod_{r=1}^{R} \lambda_{ir}(s|x_i, y_i)^{n_{ir}} \exp\left(-\int_{a_i}^{s} \lambda_{i+}(t|x_i, y_i)dt\right)ds}. \tag{6.6}$$

If all event types are rare, we apply a similar argument as in Chapter 3, Section 3.8. We write the overall hazard as

$$\lambda_{i+}(t|x_i, y_i) = \phi\nu_{i+}(t|x_i, y_i),$$

where the functions ν_{i+} are bounded, and consider the limit of the conditional likelihood as $\phi \to 0$. The exponentiated terms in Equation 6.6 tend to 1, and so the multi-type SCCS likelihood contribution is retrieved. Thus, in this limit, the overall multi-type SCCS likelihood is

$$L = \prod_{r=1}^{R} \prod_{i \in E_r} \frac{\lambda_{ir}(t_i|x_i, y_i)}{\int_{a_i}^{b_i} \lambda_{ir}(t|x_i, y_i)dt},$$

which is of the same form as Expression 6.5.

Competing risks: only event types of interest are rare
In this final scenario, we distinguish between event types of interest, which are those potentially associated with the exposure, and event types that are not of primary interest, which can safely be assumed not to be associated with the exposure. Only the events of interest are sampled. Events not of primary interest are referred to as incidental events.

We assume that only the events of interest are rare: the incidental event types may not be rare. This setting might apply, for example, in elderly populations with the incidental competing events representing deaths unrelated to the exposure. We assume that the event types of interest are labelled $r = 1, \ldots, R_0$, where $R_0 < R$; event types $R_0 + 1, \ldots, R$ are the incidental events, which are not sampled and may not be rare. Define

$$\lambda_{i++}(t|\boldsymbol{y}_i) = \sum_{r=R_0+1}^{R} \lambda_{ir}(t|\boldsymbol{y}_i)$$

to be the total hazard for the incidental event types. Note that, by assumption, this does not involve the exposure history in x_i. For the rare event types $r = 1, \ldots, R_0$, for which $\sum_{r=1}^{R_0} n_{ir} = 1$, we write

$$\lambda_{ir}(t|x_i, \boldsymbol{y}_i) = \phi\nu_{ir}(t|x_i, \boldsymbol{y}_i).$$

Now let ϕ tend to zero. Then $\lambda_{i+}(t|x_i, \boldsymbol{y}_i) \to \lambda_{i++}(t|\boldsymbol{y}_i)$. Thus, in this limit, the SCCS likelihood contribution of case i becomes

$$L_i = \frac{\prod_{r=1}^{R_0} \lambda_{ir}(t_i|x_i, \boldsymbol{y}_i)^{n_{ir}} \exp\left(-\int_{a_i}^{t_i} \lambda_{i++}(t|\boldsymbol{y}_i)dt\right)}{\int_{a_i}^{b_i} \prod_{r=1}^{R_0} \lambda_{ir}(s|x_i, \boldsymbol{y}_i)^{n_{ir}} \exp\left(-\int_{a_i}^{s} \lambda_{i++}(t|\boldsymbol{y}_i)dt\right)ds}. \tag{6.7}$$

The exponentiated terms do not disappear in the rare events limit because the incidental event types are not rare. Suppose now that, for the event types $r = 1, \ldots, R_0$ of interest,

$$\lambda_{ir}(t|x_i, \boldsymbol{y}_i) = \mu_{ir}(t|\boldsymbol{y}_i)\rho(t|x_i, \boldsymbol{y}_i).$$

Define

$$\lambda_{ir}^*(t|x_i, \boldsymbol{y}_i) = \mu_{ir}^*(t|\boldsymbol{y}_i)\rho(t|x_i, \boldsymbol{y}_i),$$

with

$$\mu_{ir}^*(t|\boldsymbol{y}_i) = \mu_{ir}(t|\boldsymbol{y}_i)\exp\left(-\int_0^t \lambda_{i++}(s|\boldsymbol{y}_i)ds\right).$$

With this substitution, the SCCS likelihood contribution of case i from Equation 6.7 may be written

$$L_i = \frac{\prod_{r=1}^{R_0} \lambda_{ir}^*(t_i|x_i, \boldsymbol{y}_i)^{n_{ir}}}{\int_{a_i}^{b_i} \prod_{r=1}^{R_0} \lambda_{ir}^*(s|x_i, \boldsymbol{y}_i)^{n_{ir}}ds}.$$

The overall SCCS likelihood is

$$
\begin{aligned}
L &= \prod_{i=1}^{N} \frac{\prod_{r=1}^{R_0} \lambda_{ir}^*(t_i|x_i, \boldsymbol{y}_i)^{n_{ir}}}{\int_{a_i}^{b_i} \prod_{r=1}^{R_0} \lambda_{ir}^*(s|x_i, \boldsymbol{y}_i)^{n_{ir}} ds} \\
&= \prod_{r=1}^{R_0} \prod_{i \in E_r} \frac{\lambda_{ir}^*(t_i|x_i, \boldsymbol{y}_i)}{\int_{a_i}^{b_i} \lambda_{ir}^*(s|x_i, \boldsymbol{y}_i) ds}.
\end{aligned}
$$

This takes the multi-type SCCS likelihood form of Equation 6.5. The exposure effects are unaffected: the estimates therefore retain their original interpretation. The age effects, however, have a different interpretation: they describe the baseline hazards of the events of interest, conditional on no incidental events occurring.

6.5 SCCS models for quantitative individual exposures

All the SCCS models so far described have involved a binary exposure, that is, an exposure that at any one time is either present or absent. This reflects the fact that most applications of the SCCS method, notably in pharmacoepidemiology, involve binary exposures.

However, there is nothing about the SCCS method that intrinsically requires exposures to be binary. In this section, we consider quantitative exposures, that is, exposures that are measured on a continuous scale. In Section 6.5.1 the SCCS model for individual quantitative exposures is discussed. This model requires a different data format from those used previously, but in all other respects it is very similar to the SCCS models described so far. Section 6.5.2 describes an application with individual quantitative exposures.

6.5.1 Modelling quantitative exposures

Suppose that individual i experiences a quantitative exposure $x_i(t)$ at age (or time) t, and is observed over the observation period $(a_i, b_i]$. In practice, $x_i(t)$ is not measured continuously. We assume throughout this section that $x_i(t)$ is measured at successive time points, expressed in days, hours, or some other appropriate time unit. In this section, all times, including the observation period endpoints a_i and b_i, are assumed to be expressed as integer values in these units. For consistency with other sections of the book, we refer to these time units as days.

Let $d_i = b_i - a_i$ denote the number of days of observation for individual i. The exposure variable $x_i(t)$ is assumed to be roughly constant on each day, taking the value x_{ij} on the jth day of observation for individual i, that is, over the time interval $(a_i + j - 1, a_i + j]$, for $j = 1, \ldots, d_i$. The temporal effect can be age, calendar time, day of the week, day of observation, or some other relevant time variable. The incidence rate kernel ν_{ij} for a simple model with temporal effect parameterised by α and exposure effect parameterised by β is

$$\nu_{ij} = \exp(\alpha_{h(i,j)} + \beta x_{ij}),$$

where $h(i,j)$ is the level of the temporal effect for case i on day j of observation. This may be compared to the standard SCCS model described in Chapter 4, Section 4.1. The main difference is that β is the coefficient of a quantitative exposure, rather than a factor level. It represents the log of the relative incidence associated with a 1 unit increase in exposure.

Let n_i denote the total number of events experienced by individual i over the observation period $(a_i, b_i]$, and let n_{ij} denote the number of events on day j of observation. The SCCS likelihood contribution of a case i with $n_i > 0$ is then

$$L_i = \text{constant} \times \prod_{j=1}^{d_i} \left(\frac{\nu_{ij}}{\sum_{j=1}^{d_i} \nu_{ij}} \right)^{n_{ij}}.$$

This is similar to a likelihood contribution for the standard SCCS model obtained in Chapter 3, Equation 3.1. There are two main differences. First, the risk periods, previously indexed by k, no longer feature; second, the time period durations (previously e_{ijk}) no longer feature explicitly, because each exposure level x_{ij} now lasts for 1 day.

Owing to these similarities with the standard SCCS model, the SCCS model for quantitative exposures may be fitted using similar methods. However, the data format is different to accommodate the exposure variable, which must now be specified on each day of observation for each case. Accordingly, the observation periods for all cases are concatenated into a single column.

Thus, for SCCS analyses with quantitative exposures, the data are arranged with a column `indiv` for individual case identifiers $i = 1, \ldots, N$, replicated d_i times; a column `day` for day of observation $j = 1, \ldots, d_i$ for individual i; a column for event counts n_{ij}; and further columns for exposures x_{ij} and temporal variables. Each row represents a different day of observation; there are $D = \sum_{i=1}^{N} d_i$ rows. Here is an example with $d_1 = 4$, $d_2 = 3$ and $d_3 \geq 2$, a single quantitative exposure variable `expo`, and a day-of-week variable `dow` (1 for Monday, 2 for Tuesday, etc):

indiv	day	event	expo	dow
1	1	0	1.276	5
1	2	1	2.417	6
1	3	0	1.863	7
1	4	1	1.980	1
2	1	0	0.428	3
2	2	1	0.329	4
2	3	0	0.875	5

```
3       1     1      0.979    2
3       2     0      1.032    3
.....
```

The SCCS model for quantitative exposures is fitted using function `quantsccs` within the R package SCCS.

Summary

- The SCCS method may be used to study quantitative exposures – that is, exposures expressed on a continuous scale – measured at successive time points within the observation period of each case.

- Accommodating quantitative exposures requires a different data format, in which exposures are concatenated into a single column.

6.5.2 Headaches and blood pressure

A cohort study has suggested that high systolic blood pressure may be negatively associated with headaches, in the sense that individuals with high blood pressure are less likely to experience headaches than individuals with normal blood pressure (Hagen et al., 2002). A rather different question is whether transient high (or low) blood pressure is a trigger for headaches. In the present example, we illustrate how a SCCS analysis with quantitative blood pressure data could help, in principle, throw light on this question.

The design involves individuals taking twice daily (early morning and late afternoon) systolic and diastolic blood pressure readings for 7 successive days, and recording any headaches arising between these readings. The data include 71 headaches (the occurrences of which were simulated at random) in 64 individuals. The data are in data frame `bpdat` and include the variables `case`, numbered 1 to 64, `time` for time of day (1: am, 2: pm), `dow` for day of the week (1: Monday, 2: Tuesday, ..., 7: Sunday), `sys` for systolic blood pressure, `dia` for diastolic blood pressure, and `head` taking the value 1 if the individual experienced a headache starting between this blood pressure reading and the next (or during the 12 hours following the final reading). The time unit in this analysis is a half day.

The data comprise $64 \times 7 \times 2 = 896$ rows, with one column per variable. Figure 6.17 shows the distribution of diastolic and systolic blood pressures, together with those values for which a headache was recorded. This figure was obtained using the following code:

```
par(mfrow=c(1,2), mar=c(4.1,4.1,1,1), cex.lab=1.4)
hist(bpdat$dia, xlab="diastolic pressure", main=NULL)
rug(bpdat$dia[bpdat$head==1])
hist(bpdat$sys, xlab="systolic pressure", main=NULL)
rug(bpdat$sys[bpdat$head==1])
```

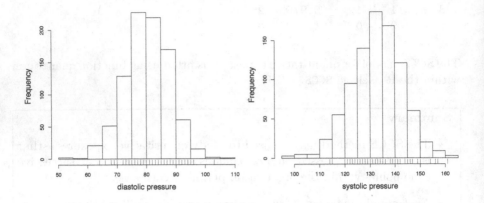

FIGURE 6.17
Distribution of blood pressure (mmHg). The rugs below each histogram indicate at what pressures a headache was recorded.

The rugs below the histograms in Figure 6.17 do not suggest that headaches cluster within the tails of the distributions. A SCCS model for these data with just the two blood pressure variables is as follows:

```
bp.mod1 <- quantsccs(event~sys+dia, indiv=case, event=head,
          data=bpdat)
```

This yields:

```
> bp.mod1
.....
    exp(coef) exp(-coef) lower .95 upper .95
sys    1.024     0.9761     0.9894     1.061
dia    1.008     0.9920     0.9637     1.054
```

The relative incidence is 1.02 for systolic blood pressure, 95% CI $(0.99, 1.06)$, and 1.01 for diastolic blood pressure, 95% CI $(0.96, 1.05)$. Thus, an increase of 1 unit in systolic (respectively, diastolic) blood pressure is associated with an increase in the incidence of headache in the following period of 2% (respectively, 1%). However, these increases are not statistically significant, as the 95% confidence intervals for the relative incidences include 1.

Model `bp.mod1` does not adjust for time-of-day or day-of-week variation, which may be associated with headache and thus may be a confounder. Adjustment of the variation in headache incidence owing to time of day and day of week may be achieved by including the `time` by `dow` interaction in the model, with both variables entered as factors:

```
bp.mod2 <- quantsccs(event~sys+dia+factor(time)*factor(dow),
          indiv=case, event=head, data=bpdat)
```

This yields:

```
> bp.mod2
.....
      exp(coef) exp(-coef) lower .95 upper .95
sys      1.0258    0.97485   0.99040      1.062
dia      1.0114    0.98875   0.96664      1.058
```

There is little change from model bp.mod1. Other variables of interest may be created by grouping values of dow. For example, to contrast working week and weekend effects, a new factor wend may be created and fitted as follows:

```
wend <- cut(bpdat$dow, breaks=c(0,5,7))
bp.mod3 <- quantsccs(event~sys+dia+wend, indiv=case,
           event=head, data=bpdat)
```

The new variable wend is a factor taking level 1 on Monday to Friday (corresponding to values of dow in $(0,5]$), and level 2 on Saturday and Sunday (values of dow in $(5,7]$). This yields:

```
> bp.mod3
.....
           exp(coef) exp(-coef) lower .95 upper .95
sys           1.025     0.9756    0.9899      1.061
dia           1.006     0.9942    0.9613      1.052
wend(5,7]     0.745     1.3422    0.4253      1.305
```

Thus, headaches are less frequent at weekends (relative incidence $RI = 0.75$), but this effect is not statistically significant as the 95% confidence interval $(0.43, 1.31)$ includes 1.

When reporting relative incidences associated with quantitative exposures, it is sometimes convenient to use unit multiples. For example, in the models described here, the relative incidences of headaches are calculated for an increase of 1 unit in blood pressure. If the relative incidences relating to an increase in 10 units were required, the blood pressure data should be scaled (divided by 10) prior to fitting the model, or the RI estimates relating to an increase in 1 unit should be raised to the power 10. The relative incidence of headaches associated with a rise of 10 units in systolic blood pressure, estimated from model bp.mod3, is $RI = 1.28$, 95% $(0.90, 1.81)$. Whether or not multiple units are used, it is essential to specify explicitly what units the relative incidences relate to.

6.6   SCCS models for environmental exposures

The timings and levels of all exposures so far considered have been specific to each individual, and thus typically vary between individuals. In some applications, however, the exposure is population-wide and exogenous. Such population exposures arise notably in environmental epidemiology: for example, an entire population may experience the same air quality, the same weather extremes, or the same pollution levels.

Several methods of analysis of such data have been suggested which, owing to the conditioning involved, are instances of the SCCS method. These include the full-stratum bidirectional case-crossover method (Navidi, 1998), the time-stratified case-crossover method (Lumley and Levy, 2000), and the conditional Poisson method (Armstrong et al., 2014). The terminology commonly used in this area is a little confusing, since case-crossover studies relate to a different study design. Some further discussion is provided in Section 6.7.

In Section 6.6.1 we describe the SCCS model for environmental exposures, and illustrate its application in Sections 6.6.2 and 6.6.3. The model is formulated within the context of Poisson generalised linear models, which provide a general and flexible modelling environment in this setting.

6.6.1 SCCS likelihood for environmental exposure data

Suppose that all individuals are observed over the same time period $(a, b]$ and experience the same population exposures. In line with many environmental epidemiology applications, we shall assume that these exposures are quantitative, though the model also applies to binary exposures. As in Section 6.5.1, we assume that exposures are measured at d successive intervals of one time unit, which we shall refer to as days. All individuals are observed from days 1 to $d = b - a$.

In such a setting, the exposure effect is completely confounded with the age or time effect, because there is no between-individual variation in exposure. In order to control for temporal variation in the incidence of the events of interest, we subdivide the overall observation period into short time windows, over which it is reasonable to assume that there is little temporal variation. The SCCS analysis is then undertaken within these short time windows, conditionally on the total numbers of events observed within each window.

For notational convenience, we shall assume that there are K such time windows of equal duration J, so that $d = J \times K$ (in practice the windows need not be of equal length). Let x_{jk} denote the exposure on day j of time window k, and let n_{ijk} denote the number of events experienced by individual i on day j of time window k.

The incidence rate kernel for an individual i on day j in time window k is

$$\nu_{ijk} = \exp(\alpha_k + \beta x_{jk}),$$

where α_k is the time (or age) effect, which we have assumed to be constant on window k. This model can easily be extended to include additional time-varying covariates measured at the same time points. Let n_{ik} denote the number of events experienced by case i within time window k. Thus,

$$n_{ik} = \sum_{j=1}^{J} n_{ijk},$$

for $k = 1, \ldots, K$. The SCCS likelihood contribution L_i for case i is obtained as described in Chapter 3, by conditioning on the subtotals n_{ik} for case i, rather than on the overall total n_i. The benefit of this is that the age effects $\exp(\alpha_k)$ are time-invariant within each segment, and therefore cancel out of the likelihood. Thus, the likelihood contribution for case i is:

$$L_i = \text{constant} \times \prod_{k=1}^{K} \prod_{j=1}^{J} \left\{ \frac{\exp(\beta x_{jk})}{\sum_r \exp(\beta x_{rk})} \right\}^{n_{ijk}}.$$

The overall SCCS likelihood $L = L_1 \times L_2 \times \cdots \times L_N$ is thus

$$L = \text{constant} \times \prod_{k=1}^{K} \prod_{j=1}^{J} \left\{ \frac{\exp(\beta x_{jk})}{\sum_r \exp(\beta x_{rk})} \right\}^{n_{jk}}, \tag{6.8}$$

where

$$n_{jk} = \sum_{i=1}^{N} n_{ijk}$$

is the total number of events observed on day j of time window k. Note that all reference to the individual cases indexed by i has disappeared in Equation 6.8. Thus, the data required for a SCCS analysis in this setting is just the time series of event counts aggregated over all cases, cross-classified by time windows k, $k = 1, \ldots, K$, together with the exposures. This SCCS model is identical to the time-stratified case-crossover model.

Since the data now comprise event counts, rather than the timings of individual events within cases, the R functions used up till now no longer apply. However, it turns out in any case to be more fruitful to exploit the equivalence between SCCS models, which are product multinomial, and Poisson models via the so-called Poisson trick, described in Chapter 4, Section 4.2. The SCCS model is fitted using a Poisson generalised linear model with the daily event count as response, log link, and a factor for the K time windows:

$$n_{jk} \sim \text{P}(\nu_{jk}),$$
$$\log(\nu_{jk}) = \beta x_{jk} + \gamma_k.$$

The γ_k are incidental parameters that ensure that the Poisson and SCCS likelihoods coincide. (Specifically, the incidental parameters constrain the fitted total number of events in each time window to match the observed total.) Only the parameter β is of interest, though it is essential to include the time window indicators as a factor.

Fitting the SCCS model via the associated Poisson model suffers the disadvantage of having to estimate large numbers of incidental parameters, though in some software implementations it is possible to eliminate these parameters. However, in the present setting, using the associated Poisson model does also have certain advantages.

One advantage is that the Poisson model lies within the much richer class of time series models. Should the SCCS model prove to be inappropriate (for example, owing to the presence of overdispersion or autocorrelation), time series models may provide a more suitable modelling environment. Unlike data on individual cases with individual exposures, data on shared population exposures are often not sparse – that is, the event variable does not consist primarily of 0's and 1's. This makes it possible to use standard tools for checking assumptions in generalised linear models, notably plots of residuals and asymptotic goodness of fit methods. These may be of benefit to assess the presence of overdispersion and autocorrelation and the validity of the Poisson and other assumptions, along with the potential impact of any failure of assumptions.

Given that the data are presented as a time series, one might ask why bother at all with the SCCS model? One advantage of using the SCCS framework is that it requires the investigator to focus on which time windows to use so as to minimise confounding by temporal effects. This may be of benefit when the effects of interest are small compared to those associated with temporal variation, as is often the case in studies of air pollution. Keeping within the SCCS modelling framework also has the advantage that time-invariant multiplicative confounders are automatically controlled. But if the Poisson assumption does not hold, for example if there is non-ignorable overdispersion, it cannot be assumed that such confounding is eliminated in this way; see Chapter 3, Section 3.7.2 for a counter-example.

Checking goodness of fit may be done by computing the Pearson residuals

$$r_{jk} = \frac{(n_{jk} - \hat{\nu}_{jk})}{\sqrt{\hat{\nu}_{jk}}},$$

where the $\hat{\nu}_{jk}$ are the fitted values of the ν_{jk}. The Pearson chi-square statistic χ^2 and associated dispersion parameter ϕ may also be obtained:

$$\chi^2 = \sum_{j,k} r_{jk}^2,$$

$$\hat{\phi} = \chi^2/\mathrm{df},$$

where df is the residual degrees of freedom of the model; in the setup presented in this section (K windows of equal duration J, and just one covariate), df $=$ $KJ - K - 1$. Under the null hypothesis that the correct model has been fitted (and hence that the data conform to the Poisson distribution), χ^2 is asymptotically distributed according to the chi-squared distribution with df degrees of freedom, and $\phi = 1$. In R, these analyses may be undertaken using the function `glm`. Alternatively, the R package `gnm` may be used (Turner and Firth, 2015); this has an absorption facility with the advantage that incidental parameters may be eliminated, and is therefore considerably more efficient. For more details on Poisson generalised linear models, see McCullagh and Nelder (1989).

Should the SCCS method fail, owing to the fact that no time windows can be found in which the underlying incidence can be assumed to be constant, the investigator can consider time series models for count data that generalise the Poisson model but which lie beyond the SCCS modelling framework.

Summary

- In applications involving population exposures, all cases are observed over the same period and experience the same exposures. Time and exposure effects are then confounded.

- A SCCS analysis may be undertaken provided that the exposure period can be subdivided into short time windows over which temporal variation may be ignored. The analysis proceeds conditionally within these time windows.

- The SCCS model may be implemented by fitting a Poisson generalised linear model to the time series data, with incidental parameters for the time windows. This model can be used to check the Poisson assumption directly.

6.6.2 Air pollution and asthma

Hospital admissions for asthma in Nottingham were recorded on successive days over 8 years, starting in September 1996. Daily air pollution levels in Nottingham over the same period were also recorded. In this example, we focus on PM_{10} levels, which are the concentrations in $\mu g/m^3$ of particulate matter less than $10\mu m$ in diameter. These data are also described in Farrington and Whitaker (2006). The question of interest is whether PM_{10} levels are associated with asthma admissions.

The data frame `pmdat` contains three variables: `day`, taking values 1 to 2922; `asma`, containing the count of hospital admissions for asthma during the course of that day (ranging from 0 to 14); and `pm10`, the PM_{10} concentration for that day.

The data are all from the same location, so there is no between-individual variation in exposures. Thus, the temporal effect is confounded with the exposure. However, provided that the temporal effect may be regarded as constant on short time intervals, a SCCS analysis may be undertaken.

The total number of admissions for asthma is 3264. The cumulative number of asthma cases from day 1 may be plotted as follows:

```
par(mar=c(4.1,4.1,1,1), cex.lab=1.4)
plot(pmdat$day, cumsum(pmdat$asma), type="l",
     xlab="time (days)", ylab="cumulative asthma admissions")
```

The plot, shown in Figure 6.18, is roughly linear. This suggests a broadly constant rate of accrual: there is no substantial systematic variation in the daily incidence of asthma. This in turn suggests that it is reasonable to ignore temporal effects on short time scales. We shall use time windows of 7 days.

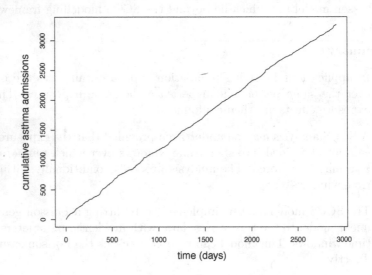

FIGURE 6.18
Cumulative number of hospital admissions for asthma over time.

There are 418 successive time windows: 417 7-day windows, and one final 3-day window. These windows are in variable **week** defined as follows:

```
week <- ceiling(pmdat$day/7)
```

We shall also control for day of week, to allow for any day-of-week variation in admission patterns for asthma. To this end, we shall create a new variable **dow** with the labels 1: Monday, ..., 7: Sunday. The first day of the series is a Wednesday, so the variable is obtained with the following code:

```
dow <- rep(c(3,4,5,6,7,1,2), length.out=length(pmdat$day))
```

As outlined in Section 6.6.1, the SCCS model is fitted via an associated Poisson generalised linear model with incidental parameters for the time windows:

```
pm.mod1 <- glm(asma~pm10+factor(dow)+factor(week),
           family=poisson, data=pmdat)
```

This model has 425 parameters: the intercept, the PM_{10} coefficient β, the 6 day-of-week contrasts, and the 417 window contrasts. Only the parameter corresponding to pm10 and the 6 parameters for dow are of interest; the rest are incidental parameters and (with the exception of the intercept) are not reproduced here:

```
> summary(pm.mod1)
.....
                  Estimate Std. Error z value Pr(>|z|)
(Intercept)       1.327164   0.232793   5.701 1.19e-08 ***
pm10             -0.002346   0.002601  -0.902 0.367170
factor(dow)2     -0.015603   0.062446  -0.250 0.802695
factor(dow)3     -0.080737   0.063566  -1.270 0.204043
factor(dow)4     -0.250825   0.066459  -3.774 0.000161 ***
factor(dow)5     -0.192846   0.065407  -2.948 0.003194 **
factor(dow)6     -0.207213   0.065623  -3.158 0.001591 **
factor(dow)7     -0.027328   0.063043  -0.433 0.664670
```

The rightmost column contains approximate p-values. The effect of PM_{10} is not statistically significant ($p = 0.37$). Asthma admissions are statistically significantly less frequent on Thursdays, Fridays and Saturdays (dow = 4, 5 or 6) than on Mondays (the reference category).

The parameter estimates (listed in the first column) and their standard errors (second column) are on the log scale, and need to be transformed to obtain relative incidences and confidence intervals. The relative incidence in asthma admissions associated with an increase in PM_{10} levels of 10 $\mu g/m^3$ (note the unit multiplier 10 here) is

$$RI = \exp(10 \times -0.002346) \simeq 0.98$$

and the 95% confidence limits are

$$RI^- = \exp(10 \times -0.002346 - 1.96 \times 10 \times 0.002601) \simeq 0.93$$
$$RI^+ = \exp(10 \times -0.002346 + 1.96 \times 10 \times 0.002601) \simeq 1.03$$

As noted in Section 6.6.1, the associated Poisson model in this setting makes it possible to check for overdispersion. The Pearson chi-square statistic and degrees of freedom are obtained as follows:

```
pearson <- sum((pmdat$asma-pm.mod1$fitted.values)^2/
              pm.mod1$fitted.values)
df <- pm.mod1$df.residual
```

These may be used to test the null hypothesis that the model provides an adequate fit to the data:

```
> pchisq(pearson, df, lower.tail=F)
[1] 0.01649165
```

The *p*-value is 0.016. Thus there is evidence that the Poisson model does not provide an adequate fit. However, the degrees of freedom are large (df = 2497), so the test is likely to pick up even a small departure from the Poisson assumption. The key question is whether this departure from the Poisson assumption is of practical importance. We obtain the estimated dispersion parameter:

```
> pearson/df
[1] 1.06129
```

The dispersion parameter is 1.06, which is very close to 1, the value expected under the Poisson assumption. Such a small departure from assumptions is unlikely to be of material importance. We conclude that inferences from the SCCS model are reliable for these data.

The R function `glm` provides no facility for eliminating the incidental parameters, and so is relatively inefficient (and produces reams of redundant output). The model may be fitted much more efficiently using R package `gnm` for generalised nonlinear models, which has an **eliminate** option. After loading the package, the model is fitted as follows:

```
library(gnm)
pm.mod2 <- gnm(asma~pm10+factor(dow), eliminate=factor(week),
          family=poisson, data=pmdat)
```

The incidental parameters are not estimated explicitly. Only the parameters of interest are displayed in the summary output:

```
> summary(pm.mod2)
.....
               Estimate Std. Error z value Pr(>|z|)
pm10          -0.002346   0.002601  -0.902 0.367170
factor(dow)2  -0.015603   0.062446  -0.250 0.802695
factor(dow)3  -0.080737   0.063566  -1.270 0.204043
factor(dow)4  -0.250825   0.066459  -3.774 0.000161 ***
factor(dow)5  -0.192846   0.065407  -2.948 0.003194 **
factor(dow)6  -0.207213   0.065623  -3.158 0.001591 **
factor(dow)7  -0.027328   0.063043  -0.433 0.664670
```

These parameters are the same as those from model `pm.mod1`.

6.6.3   Ambient temperature and RSV

In this section we present an example which is more challenging, owing to severe confounding between seasonal and exposure effects. The data relate to respiratory syncytial virus (RSV), a common respiratory infection, in England and Wales. RSV displays regular seasonal variation of great regularity and amplitude, the cause of which is poorly understood. One question of interest is whether ambient temperature plays any role in such fluctuations, independently of any seasonal effect. An intrinsic difficulty in such an analysis is that temperature and seasonality are strongly correlated.

The data comprise weekly laboratory reports of RSV isolates obtained over 7 years, 1996 to 2003. The data were described in Whitaker et al. (2007). The data frame `rsvdat` comprises the variables `year`, the year of report; `win`, a vector of indicators for 91 successive 4-week windows; `week`, denoting week of the year, numbered 1 to 52; `rsv`, the count of RSV isolates in that week; and `temp`, the average temperature over the previous week in Central England. The previous week's temperature is used (rather than the current week's) to allow for the incubation period of RSV.

Figure 6.19 shows the time series of RSV counts. The time series displays

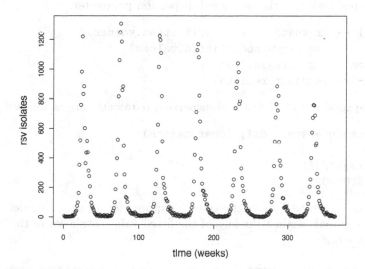

FIGURE 6.19
Number of RSV isolates over time.

very marked seasonality, peaking in the winter weeks, and dropping close to zero in summer. The minimum weekly count over the period is 1; the maximum is 1306. The amplitude of the seasonal fluctuations varies from year to year.

It is apparent from Figure 6.19 that no choice of time window based on successive weeks is likely to be appropriate for a SCCS model in this application. This is because the seasonality is so pronounced that the baseline incidence cannot be regarded as constant within such a window. For example, suppose we fit a SCCS model with 4-week windows:

```
rsv.mod1 <- glm(rsv~temp+factor(win),
          family=poisson, data=rsvdat)
```

Alternatively, function `gnm` may be used, as described in Section 6.6.2. This yields the following output (ignoring the intercept and the incidental parameters corresponding to factor win):

```
> summary(rsv.mod1)
.....
             Estimate Std. Error z value Pr(>|z|)
temp        -0.030737   0.002211 -13.901  < 2e-16 ***
```

According to this model, there is a statistically highly significant negative association between temperature and RSV: the relative incidence associated with a 10^oC increase in average ambient temperature is $RI = 0.74$, 95% CI $(0.70, 0.77)$. However, the model is inadequate in several respects, as revealed by the residuals and the estimated dispersion parameter.

```
resid1 <- (rsvdat$rsv-rsv.mod1$fitted.values)/
          sqrt(rsv.mod1$fitted.values)
pearson1 <- sum(resid1^2)
df1 <- rsv.mod1$df.residual
```

The goodness of fit test and dispersion parameter are as follows:

```
> pchisq(pearson1, df1, lower.tail=F)
[1] 0
> pearson1/df1
[1] 18.09202
```

Thus, $\hat{\phi} = 18.1$, well above the value 1 required for a Poisson model. The plot of the residuals against the logs of the fitted values is shown in the left panel of Figure 6.20.

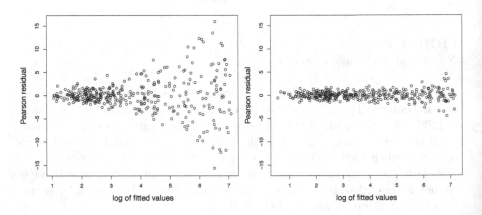

FIGURE 6.20
Residual plots for RSV models. Left: with windows comprising 4 adjacent weeks. Right: with week-of-year windows and year adjustment.

The plot's funnel shape provides clear evidence that the residual variance is not constant. Thus, a different approach is required.

There is nothing in SCCS theory described in Section 6.6.1 that requires the time windows within which the analysis is conditioned to comprise adjacent weeks. The only requirement is that the windows should be non-overlapping and not determined by events. An alternative strategy, which may provide better control of seasonality, is to use week of year to define the windows. For example, the first window comprises week 27 in the seven years 1996 to 2002; the next window comprises week 28 in these years, and so on. Thus, there are 52 7-week windows. As evident from Figure 6.19, there is clear year-to-year variation in RSV counts, and this needs to be taken into account. In the present SCCS context, with week-of-year windows, year becomes a time-varying covariate, which can be controlled in the SCCS model. Ideally, the year effect would be allowed to differ for each week-of-year: however, owing to the lack of replication (we have only the one time series), this would leave no information to estimate the temperature effect, which is completely confounded with the temporal effect. Instead, we use the next best thing, which is to group week-of-year into pairs, and fit the interaction between year and this grouped variable. This pairing is defined as follows:

```
gwk <- cut(rsvdat$week, seq(0,52,2))
```

Variable gwk is a factor with 26 levels: level 1 for weeks 1 and 2, level 2 for weeks 3 and 4, and so on. We now fit the SCCS model with time windows defined by week. The time-varying covariates are temperature, and the year by grouped week interaction:

```
rsv.mod2 <- glm(rsv~temp+factor(year)*gwk+factor(week),
                family=poisson, data=rsvdat)
```

This yields the following estimate for the temperature effect:

```
> summary(rsv.mod2)
.....
         Estimate Std. Error z value Pr(>|z|)
temp     -0.006065   0.003501  -1.732 0.083202 .
```

The association with temperature is no longer statistically significant, the relative incidence associated with a 10°C increase in temperature being $RI = 0.94$, 95% CI $(0.88, 1.01)$. The residuals and dispersion parameter are obtained as follows.

```
resid2 <- (rsvdat$rsv-rsv.mod2$fitted.values)/
          sqrt(rsv.mod2$fitted.values)
pearson2 <- sum(resid2^2)
df2 <- rsv.mod2$df.residual
```

This yields:

```
> pearson2/df2
[1] 2.229287
```

The estimated dispersion parameter is thus $\hat{\phi} = 2.23$. This is much closer to 1, though still indicative of overdispersion. The residual plot is shown in the right panel of Figure 6.20. The funnel shape has largely disappeared, and the residual variance is plausibly constant, aside from a few outliers for some weeks with large fitted values. Figure 6.20 was obtained using the following code:

```
par(mfrow=c(1,2), mar=c(4.1,4.1,1,1), cex.lab=1.4)
plot(log(rsv.mod1$fitted.values), resid1, ylim=c(-16,16),
     xlab="log of fitted values", ylab="Pearson residual")
plot(log(rsv.mod2$fitted.values), resid2, ylim=c(-16,16),
     xlab="log of fitted values", ylab="Pearson residual")
```

In fact, all but 11 residuals have absolute values less than 2. Our final model excludes these 11 outliers in case they should unduly influence the results:

```
wt <- as.numeric(resid2^2<4)
rsv.mod3 <- glm(rsv~temp+factor(year)*gwk+factor(week),
            family=poisson, weights=wt, data=rsvdat)
```

The estimate of the temperature effect is now as follows:

```
> summary(rsv.mod3)
.....
            Estimate Std. Error z value Pr(>|z|)
temp        -0.000556   0.003667  -0.152 0.879490
```

The corresponding relative incidence for an increase in $10^\circ C$ is $RI = 0.99$, 95% CI $(0.93, 1.07)$. The overdispersion is still statistically significant (the Pearson chi-square test gives $p = 0.0006$). However, the estimated dispersion parameter for this final model is $\hat{\phi} = 1.42$, which is indicative of rather mild overdispersion. This is unlikely to invalidate inferences from this model.

We therefore conclude that there is little evidence to support an association between temperature and RSV, independently of the seasonal effect. However, the SCCS model cannot resolve entirely the confounding of temperature and temporal effects, which could in principle be achieved by using disaggregated data from distinct geographical areas.

6.7   Bibliographical notes and further material

The semiparametric SCCS model was proposed in Farrington and Whitaker (2006). The SCCS model with spline-based age effect was described in

Ghebremichael-Weldeselassie et al. (2014), and the model with spline-based exposure effect in Ghebremichael-Weldeselassie et al. (2016). The nonparametric SCCS model, in which both age and exposure effects are spline-based, was published in Ghebremichael-Weldeselassie et al. (2017b).

The SCCS model with spline-based age effect overcomes some of the limitations of the semiparametric model – namely, its potential lack of efficiency and its high computational cost, both of which are due to the possibly large number of age-related parameters to be estimated. Lee and Carlin (2014) proposed a different strategy to tackle the same issues, based on fractional polynomials rather than splines. In their model, the relative age effect is piecewise constant as in the standard SCCS model, but the step heights at the age group midpoints are represented by a fractional polynomial of low dimension.

The multi-type SCCS model for recurrent events and competing risks was described in Ghebremichael-Weldeselassie et al. (2017a). The applicability of the SCCS model to competing risks was originally raised by Andersen (2006). A bivariate copula-based SCCS model for studying the dependence between two distinct events or event types has been developed by Hocine et al. (2005), and applied to an investigation of antibiotic resistance.

The time-stratified case-crossover method was developed by Lumley and Levy (2000), in order to correct biases that had become apparent in applications of case-crossover methodology to environmental time series data. The full-stratum bidirectional case-crossover method proposed by Navidi (1998) is a special case of the time-stratified case-crossover method, with a single stratum. Note that other, more standard, case-crossover designs used for environmental time series data are not equivalent to the SCCS method owing to differences in the sampling scheme. These differences were alluded to in Chapter 3, Section 3.9. The relationship between case-crossover methods and the SCCS method is discussed more fully in Vines and Farrington (2001) and Whitaker et al. (2007).

Several other SCCS models have been proposed, relating to adverse event surveillance or signal detection in pharmacoepidemiology. These include sequential versions of the SCCS model, applied using the sequential probability ratio test (Hocine et al., 2009) or cumulative sum charts (Musonda et al., 2008a). Another is the Multiple SCCS (or MSCCS) model described by Simpson et al. (2013). This was developed to analyse data on a given event in longitudinal observational databases, so as to account simultaneously for the potential effect of large numbers of different drugs. In this model, the SCCS log likelihood is supplemented by a shrinkage penalty on the drug-related parameters. A further development is the Factorised SCCS (or FSCCS) model, in which a hierarchical SCCS model is used to study large numbers of event types as well as large numbers of drugs, using latent variables to link related drugs or outcomes (Moghaddass et al., 2016). Both the MSCCS and FSCCS models may be formulated in a Bayesian framework; see also Shaddox et al. (2016). A SCCS model incorporating the effect of cumulative exposures and other features relevant to long-term use of pharmaceutical drugs has been

developed by Schuemie et al. (2016). A further special SCCS model is that
applied by Escolano et al. (2011) to intussusception and rotavirus vaccine,
and described in greater detail by Escolano et al. (2013). This model may be
used in some circumstances to investigate spontaneous reports of potentially
vaccine-associated adverse events, with the aim of enhancing the investigation
of vaccine safety signals.

7

Extensions of the SCCS model

In earlier chapters we described several versions of the SCCS model, all of which were based on the SCCS likelihood derived in Chapter 3. In the present chapter we move outside this framework, with the aim of weakening some of the assumptions of the SCCS method.

In Section 7.1 we develop a SCCS model to handle event-dependent exposures. These are exposures that may be influenced by prior events, thus violating a key assumption. This takes us away from likelihood-based methods altogether, and into the realm of estimating equations.

In Section 7.2 we describe a SCCS model to handle event-dependent observation periods, specifically in the situation where occurrence of an event may precipitate the end of observation, thus violating another key assumption. The approach we propose requires an additional modelling step to obtain weights with which the SCCS likelihood is then adjusted.

Finally, in Section 7.3 we discuss more specifically the application of the SCCS method when the event of interest is death. In this situation both the observation period and the exposure are event-dependent in an extreme sense.

The models described in Sections 7.1 and 7.2 require some sustained mathematical arguments. For both models, we have sought to provide heuristic accounts of the key ideas that underpin the mathematics which, as elsewhere in the book, are developed in starred sections which may be skipped.

7.1 SCCS for event-dependent exposures

In this section we describe a SCCS model which, under some assumptions, is appropriate even when the exposure of interest may depend on prior events. The assumptions are that the event is non-recurrent and rare, that the observation period for each case is not influenced by the event, that the exposure periods are not indefinite, and that the intended duration of each exposure period is known from the outset once it begins. The latter assumption applies, for example, to risk periods following a point exposure such as a vaccination, and to drug treatment periods determined by prescription. When the event is rare but potentially recurrent, the method may be applied to first events.

Event-dependent exposures may arise in different ways. For example, occurrence of an event may preclude any subsequent exposure. This occurs in pharmacoepidemiology when the event of interest is a contra-indication to treatment. An example is rotavirus vaccination and intussusception: rotavirus vaccine is unlikely to be administered to a child who has experienced an intussusception. Thus, rotavirus vaccination is an event-dependent exposure when intussusception is the event. Conversely, events may precipitate exposures that would not otherwise have occurred. For example, sustaining an injury in a car accident may result in being prescribed opioid analgesics. Thus, treatment with opioid analgesics is an event-dependent exposure when car accident injuries are the events of interest. Event-dependence of exposures may also arise owing to idiosyncracies in the ascertainment of exposures: for example, if exposure histories are collected at the time of event, then post-event exposures will be undocumented. Finally, occurrence of an event may affect the timing of subsequent exposures. For example, occurrence of an adverse health event may delay a routine vaccination.

Whatever its manifestation, event-dependence of exposures means that post-event exposure data cannot validly be conditioned upon to obtain the SCCS likelihood, as outlined in Chapter 3, Section 3.7. A SCCS analysis that ignores the issue may yield biased estimates. The direction of bias is predictable: if the event precludes (or reduces the frequency of) subsequent exposures, the relative incidence will be biased upwards. On the other hand, if the event precipitates (or increases the frequency of) subsequent exposures, the relative incidence will be biased downwards towards zero.

As seen in Chapter 5, Section 5.4, including a pre-exposure risk period can sometimes reduce the bias resulting from a short-term reduction in exposure frequency following an event. However, other methods are required to handle more prolonged event-dependence.

Our approach in the rest of this section is to set aside any exposures arising after the occurrence of an event, as they may be affected by the event. Thus, without loss of generality, we focus on the situation in which post-event exposures are suppressed, for whatever reason, and adjust the analysis in an appropriate way. In Section 7.1.1 we seek to convey in non-technical terms the ideas behind this extension of the SCCS model, in particular the notion of a counterfactual. Four applications are provided in Sections 7.1.2 to 7.1.5. Results obtained with the modified and the standard SCCS models are contrasted in Section 7.1.4. The technical machinery used, which involves estimating equations, is developed in a special case in Section 7.1.6; the general method is described in Section 7.1.7. Both these sections are starred, and may be skipped.

7.1.1 Estimating equations and counterfactual exposures

The SCCS likelihood framework described in Chapter 3 cannot be used when the information on exposures is event-dependent. Instead of maximum likelihood estimation, we use the more general framework provided by the theory of estimating equations.

Suppose that α and β are the parameters for age and exposure effects. Throughout, we take the primary time line to be age, but it could be calendar time. An elementary unbiased estimating function for case i is a function $M_{ir}(t_i; \alpha, \beta)$ of the age at event t_i for case i, with zero mean under the correct model. Suppose that there are J free age parameters and K free exposure parameters. We need as many distinct estimating functions as there are free parameters, so $r = 1, 2, \ldots, J + K$. The parameter estimates are obtained by solving the system

$$\sum_{i-1}^{N} M_{ir}(t_i; \alpha, \beta) = 0, \quad r = 1, 2, \ldots, J + K$$

for α and β. The method of estimating equations generalises maximum likelihood estimation: in maximum likelihood, the elementary unbiased estimating functions are the likelihood scores (the derivatives of the log likelihood contribution for each case with respect to the parameters). The advantage is that estimating equations may be used even when the likelihood is unavailable. Further details on the theory of estimating equations may be obtained from Jesus and Chandler (2011).

In the present section, we shall describe very informally the ideas behind the construction of suitable unbiased estimating functions in a special case. The estimating equations for this special case are derived in Section 7.1.6.

Suppose, for the time being, that the exposure of interest occurs at most twice, and that no exposures can occur (or be observed) after an event. We consider a case with observation period $(a, b]$. Note that, whatever the event age t, the observation period remains $(a, b]$: this is because we have assumed that the observation period is not influenced by the event. (This and other assumptions were set out at the start of Section 7.1.) This two-exposure scenario applies, for example, to two-dose vaccines, with events whose occurrence constitutes a contra-indication to vaccination.

To begin with, consider only cases for which the age at event occurs after the start of a second exposure at age c_2, the first exposure having occurred at age $c_1 < c_2$. There are two possible scenarios, according to the age at occurrence of the event, represented in Figure 7.1.

In scenario 1 of Figure 7.1, the event occurs at age t in the age interval $(d_2, b]$, after the end of the second risk period $(c_2, d_2]$. Because no individual can experience more than two exposures, we know that no further exposures could occur after d_2, whatever the value of t. Similarly, in scenario 2 of Figure 7.1, if the event occurs at an age t during the second risk period $(c_2, d_2]$, the exposure history is also known after t, since by assumption the end of exposure d_2 is determined by c_2, and the duration of the risk period is known a priori.

Thus, provided the event occurs after a second exposure, the exposure

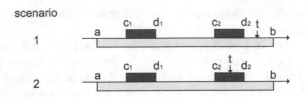

FIGURE 7.1
Scenarios for a case with event after the start of the second exposure. Age t is the age at event, $(c_1, d_1]$ is the first risk period and $(c_2, d_2]$ is the second risk period.

history up to b is known, and is unaffected by the age at event t. In other words, for this subset of cases, exposures are not event-dependent. Hence we can use the estimating equation derived from the SCCS likelihood for cases with observation periods $(c_2, b]$ to estimate the parameter β_2 associated with second exposures. This argument has made use of the assumption that exposures can occur at most twice. In fact, it turns out (as will be explained in Section 7.1.6) that this assumption can be weakened: it's enough to assume that, in our dataset, the exposure occurs at most twice for any case.

Suppose now that we try to apply a similar argument to cases for which the event occurs after the start of the first exposure at age c_1. There are now four possible scenarios, represented in Figure 7.2.

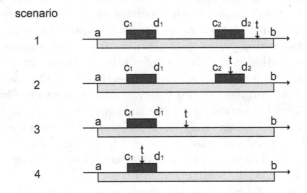

FIGURE 7.2
Scenarios for a case with event after the start of the first exposure. Age t is the age at event, $(c_1, d_1]$ is the first risk period and $(c_2, d_2]$ is the second risk period.

In each of the four scenarios in Figure 7.2, we know that the case experiences a first exposure, with risk period ending at age d_1. Thereafter, the observed exposure history depends on the event age t: in scenarios 1 and 2 a second exposure is observed, while in scenarios 3 and 4, no further exposure is observed. In these last two scenarios, had the event not occurred, the case might have experienced no further exposure, or might have experienced a second exposure. We call the exposure history that would have arisen, had the event not occurred, the counterfactual exposure history.

To estimate the parameter β_1 associated with the first exposure, we cannot apply the SCCS likelihood directly, even with the observation period $(c_1, b]$, because the observed exposure history between d_1 and b depends on when the event arises. Thus, the conditioning argument upon which the SCCS likelihood depends can no longer be used.

In order to get round this difficulty, we shall derive an estimating equation based on a counterfactual exposure history in which no second exposure ever occurs. This counterfactual exposure history is, by definition, unaffected by the event age t after c_1 since, whatever t, there is no second exposure. Thus, for cases arising after a first exposure, that is, for which the event occurs at an age t in $(c_1, b]$, we use an estimating procedure derived from the SCCS likelihood with observation period $(c_1, b]$, based on there being no further exposures after c_1. The obvious difficulty with this approach is that we might observe second exposures for some cases, as in scenarios 1 and 2 in Figure 7.2. In order to conform to our counterfactual, we reduce the expected number of events by the factor $\exp(\beta_2)$ in second risk periods when a second exposure happens to be observed. This correction factor is illustrated in Figure 7.3. This approach, once formalised appropriately, as will be described in Section 7.1.6, offers a

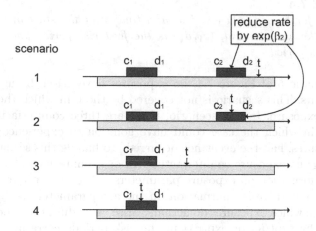

FIGURE 7.3
Adjustment to the second risk period when a second exposure is observed. Age t is the age at event, $(c_1, d_1]$ is the first risk period and $(c_2, d_2]$ is the second risk period.

way of estimating β_2 based on cases with events occurring after c_2, and β_1 using cases with events occurring after c_1. Information on the age parameters α may also be derived from these cases in a similar manner.

We have so far considered cases for which the event arises after one or two exposures. What about cases for which the event age t does not necessarily arise after any exposure? These comprise all cases arising in $(a, b]$. There are now five scenarios, shown in Figure 7.4.

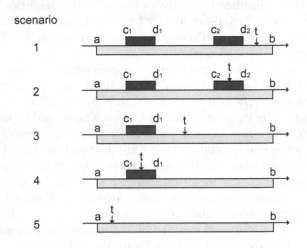

FIGURE 7.4

Scenarios for a case with event at any time after the start of observation a. Age t is the age at event, $(c_1, d_1]$ is the first risk period and $(c_2, d_2]$ is the second risk period.

In scenario 5 of Figure 7.4, no exposures have arisen by age t when the event occurs. This scenario is not covered by those in which the event arises after an exposure. In this scenario, there are three counterfactual exposure histories, in which the case could have gone on to experience zero, one or two exposures, had the event not occurred. To handle this scenario, we again impose our no exposure counterfactual. In our counterfactual world, there is now no information on exposure parameters (since no exposures are deemed to occur), but there is information on the age parameters α. To handle the scenarios in which exposures do actually arise, we reduce the expected number of events by $\exp(\beta_1)$ or $\exp(\beta_2)$ in the risk periods corresponding to those exposures that happen to be observed. These correction factors are illustrated in Figure 7.5.

This discussion of counterfactuals has purposefully avoided any technicalities, aiming only to provide a flavour of the method, which is distinctly non-standard. The estimating equations for the special case of up to two exposures and two age groups are derived in Section 7.1.6. The estimating equations for

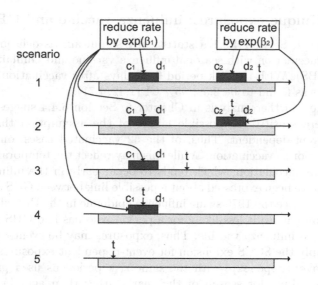

FIGURE 7.5
Adjustment to the first and second risk periods when observed. Age t is the age at event, $(c_1, d_1]$ is the first risk period and $(c_2, d_2]$ is the second risk period.

the general method, with an arbitrary number of exposures and age groups, are given in Section 7.1.7. In this section we also describe how to obtain confidence intervals for the parameters, and we outline how to fit the model. Both these sections involve substantial technicalities; accordingly, they are starred and may be skipped.

The method is implemented in the R package SCCS by the function eventdepenexp. In the next four sections we describe some examples of its application.

Summary

- An extension of the SCCS model is available for rare non-recurrent events when exposures are event-dependent.

- Observation periods are assumed not to be event-dependent. The risk periods must be of finite duration. The duration of each risk period is assumed to be known once it begins.

- The model parameters are obtained by solving a system of estimating equations. The corresponding estimating functions are obtained using counterfactual exposure histories.

7.1.2 Unique exposures: influenza vaccine and GBS

In Chapter 4, Section 4.9.1 a statistically significant association was found between vaccination with seasonal influenza vaccine and Guillain–Barré syndrome (GBS). With the risk period 0–42 days after vaccination, the relative incidence was found to be 2.58, 95% CI $(1.42, 4.71)$.

However, further analysis in Chapter 5, Section 5.4.4 suggested that the results were sensitive to possible failure of the assumption that exposures are not event-dependent. Thus, of the 52 vaccinated cases, only one event occurred prior to vaccination. While this may reflect the temporal distribution of influenza vaccination, which tends to occur early in the influenza season, concerns have been expressed about a possible link between GBS and influenza vaccination since the 1976 swine influenza epidemic in the United States. Such concerns may make it less likely for a person who has had GBS subsequently to receive an influenza vaccine. Thus, exposures may be event-dependent.

We apply the SCCS extension for event-dependent exposures using the R function `eventdepenexp`, with the same risk period as used previously. As before, we adjust for season of the year (rather than age) in six monthly categories:

```
seas  <- cumsum(c(31,30,31,31,28,31))
gbs.mod5 <- eventdepenexp(indiv=case, astart=sta, aend=end,
           aevent=gbs, adrug=flu, aedrug=flu+42, agegrp=seas,
           data=gbsdat)
```

This yields:

```
> gbs.mod5
......
       exp(coef) exp(-coef) lower .95 upper .95
flu1     1.8573    0.5384     0.9965    3.4619
age2     1.4179    0.7053     0.8190    2.4549
age3     1.2864    0.7774     0.7081    2.3370
age4     1.9158    0.5220     1.1022    3.3298
age5     1.8529    0.5397     1.0411    3.2980
age6     0.6757    1.4799     0.3370    1.3547
age7     0.4286    2.3332     0.2029    0.9053
```

Thus, the relative incidence is 1.86 with 95% confidence interval $(1.00, 3.46)$. The relative incidence is lower than when the standard SCCS model is used, and is now only borderline statistically significant. Owing to the lack of robustness of the standard model, these results are to be preferred to those from Chapter 4, Section 4.9.1.

Note that the syntax of function `eventdepenexp` is similar to that of function `standardsccs`, except that the model formula is not specified explicitly. This model formula is always of the form

```
Exposure + Age
```

where age is specified by `agegrp`. Age could be replaced by calendar time, but the model can only handle a single time-varying exposure. For the GBS data, the age variable is replaced by time of year, in variables `seas`. In order to fit a model with just the exposure, then use `agegrp=NULL` as follows:

```
gbs.mod6 <- eventdepenexp(indiv=case, astart=sta, aend=end,
             aevent=gbs, adrug=flu, aedrug=flu+42, agegrp=NULL,
             data=gbsdat)
```

This yields:

```
> gbs.mod6
......
     exp(coef) exp(-coef) lower .95 upper .95
flu1    2.332     0.4289     1.337     4.068
```

The *RI* without adjustment for time of year is markedly higher: time of the year is a time-varying confounder and should be included in the model. Note, however, that unlike models obtained with `standardsccs`, nested models obtained using `eventdepenexp` cannot be compared formally using a likelihood ratio test. This is because this SCCS extension does not use a likelihood.

7.1.3   Multiple doses: rotavirus vaccine and intussusception

The first vaccine against rotavirus infection was withdrawn after case-control and SCCS studies showed it to be associated with a substantial increase in the risk of intussusception in infants (Murphy et al., 2001). Subsequently, other rotavirus vaccines were developed with an improved safety profile, and routine vaccination against rotavirus was introduced in the United Kingdom in 2013. The vaccine is given to infants under six months of age in a 2-dose schedule. Rotavirus vaccination is contra-indicated for children who have had an intussusception. A SCCS study was undertaken in the United Kingdom to assess the safety of the vaccine (Stowe et al., 2016). This example includes the data from this study, with ages jittered to preserve confidentiality.

The data are in format `multi` in data frame `rotdat`. There are 566 cases. Of these, 79 occurred after the first dose and 49 occurred after the second dose of rotavirus vaccine. The age at intussusception is in variable `intus`. The ages at first and second doses of vaccine are in `rv` and `rvd2`, respectively. Cases were ascertained between the ages of 42 and 183 days. The distributions of age at vaccination (both doses combined) and intussusception in these cases is shown in Figure 7.6. The bimodal distribution of age at vaccination reflects the recommended age at vaccination: 2 months for dose 1, 3 months for dose 2. Most observation periods stretch from 42 to 183 days; Figure 7.6 suggests that the risk of intussusception increases with age over the first six months of life.

Since intussusception is a contra-indication for rotavirus vaccination, the standard SCCS model cannot be applied as exposures are event-dependent.

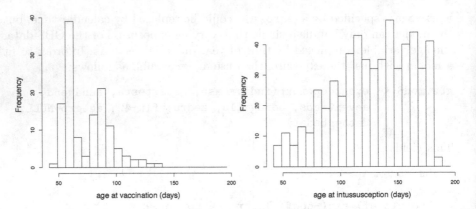

FIGURE 7.6
Left: age at rotavirus vaccination (both doses combined). Right: age at intussusception.

Thus, we use the SCCS extension for event-dependent exposures. The risk period of interest is [1, 21] days post-vaccination. The day of vaccination (day 0) is excluded: this was to compare with results from other studies. In the first model, we assume that the vaccine effect is the same at both vaccine doses. We use 14-day age groups.

```
age <- seq(56,168,14)
rot.mod1 <- eventdepenexp(indiv=case, astart=sta, aend=end,
            aevent=intus, adrug=cbind(rv,rvd2), expogrp=1,
            aedrug=cbind(rv+21,rvd2+21), agegrp=age,
            dataformat="multi", data=rotdat)
```

The estimated vaccine-related relative incidence from this model is as follows.

```
> rot.mod1
......
      exp(coef) exp(-coef) lower .95 upper .95
rv1       3.601     0.2777    2.1897     5.923
```

Thus, $RI = 3.60$, 95% CI $(2.19, 5.92)$, both doses combined, indicating a statistically significant association. To investigate this association in more detail, we fit a second model in which the risk period is partitioned into two intervals, [1, 7] days and [8, 21] days:

```
rot.mod2 <- eventdepenexp(indiv=case, astart=sta, aend=end,
            aevent=intus, adrug=cbind(rv,rvd2),
            aedrug=cbind(rv+21,rvd2+21), expogrp=c(1,8),
            agegrp=age, dataformat="multi", data=rotdat)
```

The results from this model are as follows.

```
> rot.mod2
......
      exp(coef) exp(-coef) lower .95 upper .95
rv1       6.318    0.1583    3.4855    11.453
rv2       2.505    0.3993    1.3921     4.506
```

Thus, $RI = 6.32$ in the 1–7 day risk period and $RI = 2.51$ in the 8–21 day risk period, both being statistically significantly greater than 1. We now obtain separate estimates for each of the two vaccine doses, by specifying sameexpopar=F as follows.

```
rot.mod3 <- eventdepenexp(indiv=case, astart=sta, aend=end,
              aevent=intus, adrug=cbind(rv,rvd2),
              aedrug=cbind(rv+21,rvd2+21), expogrp=c(1,8),
              sameexpopar=F, agegrp=age, dataformat="multi",
              data=rotdat)
```

This yields the following parameter estimates (including the age-related relative incidences):

```
> rot.mod3
......
       exp(coef) exp(-coef) lower .95 upper .95
rv1     14.2298    0.07027    7.2815    27.809
rv2      1.6014    0.62447    0.5966     4.299
rv3      2.2446    0.44551    0.8604     5.856
rv4      2.8918    0.34580    1.5016     5.569
age2     0.9137    1.09445    0.4610     1.811
age3     1.8442    0.54224    0.9851     3.452
age4     3.2021    0.31230    1.7880     5.734
age5     3.2830    0.30459    1.8329     5.881
age6     5.3504    0.18690    3.0360     9.429
age7     4.5672    0.21895    2.5891     8.057
age8     5.1603    0.19379    2.9271     9.097
age9     5.9376    0.16842    3.3913    10.396
age10    4.5282    0.22084    2.5879     7.923
```

These results indicate that the association relates primarily to the first week after the first dose: $RI = 14.2$, 95% CI $(7.28, 27.8)$. In contrast, the relative incidence for the 8–21 day risk period after the first dose is 1.60, 95% CI $(0.60, 4.30)$ and thus not statistically significantly raised. After the second dose, the relative incidences are 2.24 for the 1–7 day risk period and 2.89 for the 8–21 day risk period, only the second of these being statistically significant, 95% CI $(1.50, 5.57)$. The age-related relative incidences indicate a sharp rise in incidence with age over the first six months of life. The estimated age profile is displayed in Figure 7.7, which was obtained as follows.

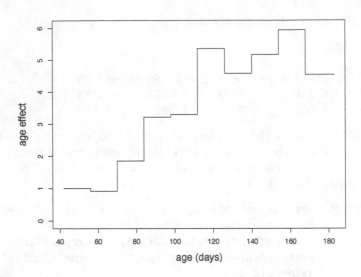

FIGURE 7.7
Intussusception: estimated relative age profile.

```
par(mar=c(4.1,4.1,1,1), cex.lab=1.4)
ari <- c(1, rot.mod3$coef[5:13,2], rot.mod3$coef[13,2])
ageg <- c(42,age,183)
plot(ageg, ari, type="s", ylim=c(0,6), xlab="age (days)",
    ylab="age effect")
```

In conclusion, administration of this rotavirus vaccine is associated with an increased risk of intussusception, primarily in the first week after the first dose. The first dose is administered at an early age (2 months), at which the incidence of intussusception is low.

7.1.4   Model comparisons: OPV and intussusception

In this example we use data on oral polio vaccine (OPV) and intussusception in the United Kingdom (Andrews et al., 2001) to compare models, in two different ways. Intussusception is not a contra-indication to OPV vaccination, so the standard SCCS model can be used. Our first model comparison is to analyse these data with both the standard SCCS model, and the extension of the SCCS model for event-dependent exposures. This type of comparison can be used informally when it is unclear whether results may be sensitive to the assumption that exposures are not event-dependent.

The second comparison involves comparing subgroups of cases. In the standard SCCS model, this is most easily achieved using a likelihood ratio test, as described in Chapter 4, Section 4.6. However, the SCCS extension for event-dependent exposures does not involve a likelihood (the method is based on estimating equations). Nevertheless, results obtained in non-overlapping subgroups of cases can be compared using a chi-squared test.

The data, in data format `multi`, are in data frame `opvdat`. The observation period for this study was 27 to 365 days of age. There are 207 cases, each with one intussusception. The age at intussusception is in variable `intus`. Each case received up to 3 doses of OPV vaccine; the ages at vaccination are in `opv`, `opvd2` and `opvd3`. 614 doses were administered before age 365 days. The distribution of age at vaccination (all doses combined) up to 365 days of age, and of age at intussusception, are in Figure 7.8. The distribution of ages

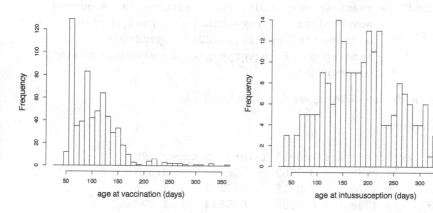

FIGURE 7.8
Left: age at OPV (all doses combined). Right: age at intussusception.

at vaccination reflects the recommended 2-, 3-, 4-month vaccination schedule for oral polio vaccine. The incidence of intussusception peaks at 5 to 7 months of age.

Comparing SCCS methods
Since intussusception is not a contra-indication for OPV, there is no reason a priori not to use the standard SCCS method. We use the risk period 0–20 days after each dose, and 30-day age groups. Allowing a different parameter at each dose, the model is specified as follows:

```
ageg <- seq(60,330,30)
opv.mod1 <- standardsccs(event~opv+age, indiv=case,
            astart=sta, aend=end, aevent=intus,
            adrug=cbind(opv,opvd2,opvd3),
            aedrug=cbind(opv+20,opvd2+20,opvd3+20),
            sameexpopar=F, agegr=ageg, dataformat="multi",
            data=opvdat)
```

The vaccine-associated relative incidences are as follows:

```
> opv.mod1
......
        exp(coef)  exp(-coef)  lower .95  upper .95
opv1    1.3008      0.7688      0.5694      2.971
opv2    0.5454      1.8334      0.2671      1.114
opv3    1.2238      0.8171      0.7400      2.024
```

We now apply the SCCS extension for event-dependent exposures. In this model, the 98 post-event exposures are set aside (they are recoded as missing). The model is as follows:

```
opv.mod2 <- eventdepenexp(indiv=case, astart=sta, aend=end,
            aevent=intus, adrug=cbind(opv,opvd2,opvd3),
            aedrug=cbind(opv+20,opvd2+20,opvd3+20),
            sameexpopar=F, agegrp=ageg, dataformat="multi",
            data=opvdat)
```

This yields the following vaccine-associated RIs:

```
> opv.mod2
......
        exp(coef)  exp(-coef)  lower .95  upper .95
opv1    1.3068      0.7652      0.5933      2.878
opv2    0.4825      2.0725      0.2272      1.025
opv3    1.1368      0.8796      0.6814      1.897
```

The estimates from models `opv.mod1` and `opv.mod2`, and their confidence intervals, are very similar. This kind of informal comparison is useful when there is some doubt about whether the assumption that exposures are not event-dependent is satisfied. For these data, neither model suggests there is evidence of an association between OPV and intussusception, for any vaccine dose.

Finally, it is instructive to apply the standard SCCS model to the data with post-event exposures removed, in order to display the bias resulting from event-dependent exposures. First, we obtain the censored exposures:

```
copv <- ifelse(opvdat$opv>opvdat$intus, NA, opvdat$opv)
copvd2 <- ifelse(opvdat$opvd2>opvdat$intus, NA, opvdat$opvd2)
copvd3 <- ifelse(opvdat$opvd3>opvdat$intus, NA, opvdat$opvd3)
```

The standard SCCS model applied to these censored exposures is:

```
opv.mod3 <- standardsccs(event~copv+age, indiv=case,
            astart=sta, aend=end, aevent=intus,
            adrug=cbind(copv,copvd2,copvd3),
            aedrug=cbind(copv+20,copvd2+20,copvd3+20),
            sameexpopar=F, agegr=ageg, dataformat="multi",
            data=opvdat)
```

which yields:

```
> opv.mod3
......
         exp(coef)  exp(-coef)  lower .95  upper .95
copv1      1.595      0.6269      0.6744      3.773
copv2      0.781      1.2804      0.3719      1.640
copv3      1.939      0.5157      1.1463      3.280
```

The estimates are higher than those from opv.mod1 and opv.mod2. In particular, the relative incidence after the third dose is 1.94, 95% CI (1.15, 3.28) and therefore appears statistically significant. These results are biased owing to failure of the assumption that exposures are not event-dependent. Model opv.mod2, which is obtained using the same censored exposures, successfully corrects this bias.

Comparing subgroups
Does gender modify the relative incidence associated with OPV? In the standard SCCS model, this may be investigated by fitting the interaction between gender and exposure, and using a likelihood ratio test. With the SCCS extension for event-dependent exposures, this is not possible as no likelihood has been defined. However, a chi-squared test is possible, based on the parameter estimates and standard errors obtained from males and females separately. Suppose that the estimated parameter is $\hat{\beta}_m$ for males and $\hat{\beta}_f$ for females, with standard errors s_m and s_f respectively. The test statistic is

$$U = \frac{(\hat{\beta}_m - \hat{\beta}_f)^2}{s_m^2 + s_f^2}.$$

Under the null hypothesis that $\beta_m = \beta_f$, U is approximately distributed as chi-squared on 1 degree of freedom in large samples.

To apply this to the OPV and intussusception data, we first fit the SCCS extension to males and females separately, with doses combined using sameexpopar=T (this is the default, and is only included for emphasis). Gender is in variable sex, coded 1 for males and 2 for females.

```
opv.mod4 <- eventdepenexp(indiv=case, astart=sta, aend=end,
              aevent=intus, adrug=cbind(opv,opvd2,opvd3),
              aedrug=cbind(opv+20,opvd2+20,opvd3+20),
              sameexpopar=T, agegrp=ageg, dataformat="multi",
              data=subset(opvdat,sex==1))

opv.mod5 <- eventdepenexp(indiv=case, astart=sta, aend=end,
              aevent=intus, adrug=cbind(opv,opvd2,opvd3),
              aedrug=cbind(opv+20,opvd2+20,opvd3+20),
              sameexpopar=T, agegrp=ageg, dataformat="multi",
              data=subset(opvdat,sex==2))
```

The estimates for males and females, respectively, are as follows:

```
> opv.mod4
......
        exp(coef) exp(-coef) lower .95 upper .95
opv1       1.089      0.9181    0.6342      1.870
```

```
> opv.mod5
......
        exp(coef) exp(-coef) lower .95 upper .95
opv1      0.6602     1.51477   0.32636     1.335
```

Thus, the *RIs* are 1.09 for males and 0.66 for females. The test statistic and *p*-value are obtained as follows:

```
num <- coef(opv.mod4)[1,1]-coef(opv.mod5)[1,1]
var <- coef(opv.mod4)[1,3]^2+coef(opv.mod5)[1,3]^2
test <- num^2/var
pval <- pchisq(test, df=1, lower.tail=F)
```

The test statistic is in `test` and its *p*-value is in `pval`:

```
> c(test, pval)
[1] 1.2208747 0.2691891
```

Thus, the test statistic is 1.22, and the *p*-value is 0.27: there is very little evidence of a statistically significant difference between the relative incidences for males and females.

7.1.5   Multiple exposures: respiratory infections and MI

All three examples presented so far in this section have involved one or more doses of vaccine. The present application involves multiple exposures of the same type. The exposures of interest are respiratory tract infections, and the event is myocardial infarction (MI). The data are simulated, based on data from the Clinical Practice Research Datalink published in Smeeth et al. (2004b).

The data comprise 940 first myocardial infarctions in patients aged 65 to 80 years of age with at least one recorded respiratory tract infection in that time. The data are in data frame `midat` and are organised in format `stack`, with one line per exposure. Age at myocardial infarction is in variable `mi`, age at infection is in `rti`. The variable `cen` indicates whether or not the observation period was terminated early, taking the value 1 if it was and 0 if not.

To avoid any issues relating to event-dependent observation periods (which will be addressed in Section 7.2), we restrict attention to the 454 cases whose observation period was not curtailed. Experiencing a myocardial infarction may alter the subsequent risk of infection: it may increase it, if the MI or treatment for it impairs the patient's immune system; or it may reduce it, if precautionary measures to avoid infections are taken. Our interest is in assessing whether such an effect, if present, affects the association between respiratory tract infection and MI.

Figure 7.9 shows the observation periods for these 454 cases. The appear-

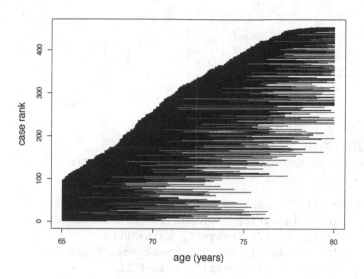

FIGURE 7.9
Observation periods for 454 cases of myocardial infarction.

ance of the plot at the edges results from the fact that the data were abstracted from a larger dataset. This figure was obtained as follows.

```
unin <- (1-duplicated(midat$case))*(midat$cen==0)
par(mar=c(4.1,4.1,1,1), cex.lab=1.4)
usta <- midat$sta[unin==1]
uend <- midat$end[unin==1]
os <- order(usta)
plot(c(min(usta)/365.25,max(uend)/365.25), c(1,length(os)),
    type="n", xlab="age (years)", ylab="case rank")
segments(usta[os]/365.25, 1:length(os), uend[os]/365.25,
    1:length(os))
```

These 454 cases experienced 1077 respiratory tract infections; 233 had 1, 106 had 2. One had 29.

Figure 7.10 shows the age distributions for respiratory tract infections and MIs. Interpretation of the graphs is complicated by the variation in observation periods. One noteworthy feature is that, above 75 years of age, the frequency of respiratory infections drops but that of MIs remains high. Figure 7.10 was obtained using the following code.

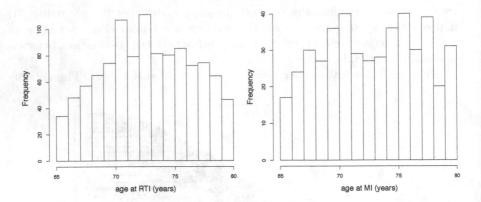

FIGURE 7.10
Left: age at respiratory tract infection. Right: age at MI.

```
par(mfrow=c(1,2), mar=c(4.1,4.1,1,1), cex.lab=1.4)
hist(midat$rti[midat$cen==0]/365.25, breaks=seq(65,80,1),
    xlab="age at RTI (years)", main=NULL)
hist(midat$mi[unin==1]/365.25, breaks=seq(65,80,1),
    xlab="age at MI (years)", main=NULL)
```

To evaluate the association between respiratory tract infections and MI, we first fit a standard SCCS model with risk periods 0–7 and 8–14 days post-infection. We use age groups defined by the 0.1-quantiles of age at MI.

```
ageq <- floor(quantile(midat$mi[unin==1], seq(0.1,0.9,0.1),
    names=F))
mi.mod1 <- standardsccs(event~rti+age, indiv=case, astart=sta,
    aend=end, aevent=mi, adrug=rti, aedrug=rti+14,
    expogrp=c(0,8), agegr=ageq, dataformat="stack",
    data=subset(midat,cen==0))
```

This produces the following estimates for the exposure effect.

```
> mi.mod1
......
      exp(coef) exp(-coef) lower .95 upper .95
rti1    4.958     0.2017    3.1347     7.843
rti2    1.415     0.7065    0.5831     3.436
```

Thus the relative incidence for the [0, 7] day risk period is 4.96, with 95% CI (3.13, 7.84): there is a strong association between infection and MI. There is no statistically significant association in the risk period [8, 14] days. But might the 0–7 day risk period estimate be biased owing to event-dependent exposures? For example, if infections tended to occur less frequently after an MI, perhaps owing to precautionary measures, the RI would be biased upwards.

To investigate this we can use the SCCS extension for event-dependent exposures. This ignores the post-event exposure history of each case, which therefore cannot affect the results. The model is applied as follows.

```
mi.mod2 <- eventdepenexp(indiv=case, astart=sta, aend=end,
             aevent=mi, adrug=rti, aedrug=rti+14, expogrp=c(0,8),
             agegrp=ageq, dataformat="stack",
             data=subset(midat,cen==0))
```

As in the specification of `mi.mod1`, we include `dataformat="stack"` just for emphasis: as for function `standardsccs`, this is the default so is not strictly required.

This model yields

```
> mi.mod2
......
      exp(coef) exp(-coef) lower .95 upper .95
rti1     4.073    0.2455    2.4575     6.750
rti2     1.219    0.8205    0.4790     3.101
```

The estimates are lower than those for `mi.mod1`. However the differences are not important in practicat terms: in the $[0, 7]$-day risk period, $RI = 4.07$ with 95% CI $(2.46, 6.75)$. The substantive conclusions from this analysis are that there is indeed a genuine association between respiratory tract infections and MI in the week after an infection, and that this is not a spurious effect resulting from event-dependent exposures.

7.1.6 SCCS for event-dependent exposures: a special case*

In this section we derive the estimating equations for the parameters α and β in a special case, in which at most two exposures can arise, each corresponding to a single risk period, and in which there are just two age groups. Thus there are three parameters to estimate: one age-related parameter α, and the two exposure-related parameters β_1 and β_2, corresponding to the first and second exposures, respectively. The ages at first and second exposure for case i are denoted c_{i1} and c_{i2}, respectively; the corresponding risk periods (expressed in mathematical notation) are $(c_{i1}, d_{i1}]$ and $(c_{i2}, d_{i2}]$. We define elementary estimating functions M_{i1}, M_{i2} and M_{i3} for α, β_1 and β_2, respectively.

The observation period $(a_i, b_i]$ of a case i is partitioned by the exposures into five successive exposure intervals, indexed by $k = 1, 2, \ldots, 5$. The two age groups are indexed by $j = 0, 1$. One such configuration is shown in Figure 7.11. Note that the indices k code the exposure history, and do not uniquely correspond to exposure levels. Thus in Figure 7.11, $k = 1, 3, 5$ all correspond to the

---

* This section may be skipped.

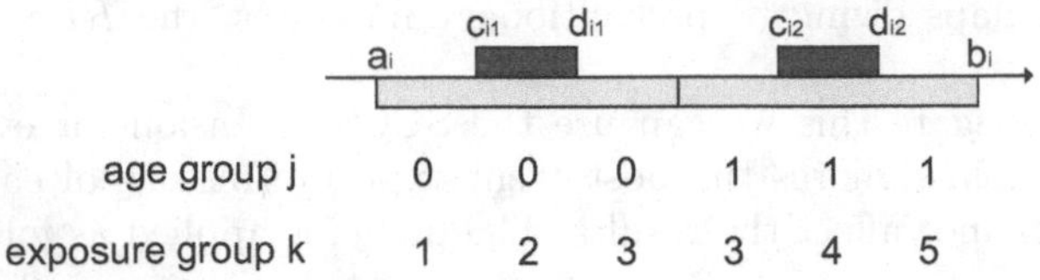

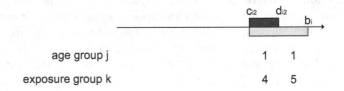

| age group j | 0 | 0 | 0 | 1 | 1 | 1 |
| exposure group k | 1 | 2 | 3 | 3 | 4 | 5 |

FIGURE 7.11

Illustration: one configuration for two exposures and two age groups. The intervals $(c_{i1}, d_{i1}]$ and $(c_{i2}, d_{i2}]$ are the first and second risk periods, respectively.

unexposed level. In this particular configuration, the cutpoint separating the two age groups occurs between the two exposure periods, but it could occur at any time in relation to either exposure, or not at all. For simplicity, we shall assume that, for all i, $a_i < c_{i1}$, $d_{i1} < c_{i2}$ and $d_{i2} \leq b_i$. In the general case described in Section 7.1.7 these restrictions are not necessary, and arbitrary numbers of risk periods may be used after each exposure.

When individual i is a case, some or all of these exposures may not be observed: they are then counterfactual, that is, they are the exposures that would have been observed, had that individual not been a case.

Let $e_{ijk} \geq 0$ denote the duration of the time spent by case i, really or counterfactually, in age group j and in exposure interval k, and n_{ijk} the number of events (0 or 1, by assumption) experienced by case i in this interval. The total number of events experienced by case i is $n_i = 1$.

Suppose now that the event for case i occurs after the second exposure. In this scenario, both exposures are observed. We proceed using the standard SCCS method, using the observation period $(c_{i2}, b_i]$. This is illustrated in Figure 7.12 for the configuration described in Figure 7.11. The standard SCCS

| age group j | 1 | 1 |
| exposure group k | 4 | 5 |

FIGURE 7.12

Illustration: standard SCCS method applied to the observation period $(c_{i2}, b_i]$.

likelihood contribution for case i, using the observation period $(c_{i2}, b_i]$ is:

$$L_i(\alpha, \beta_2) = \text{constant} \times$$
$$\frac{(e^{\beta_2} e_{i04})^{n_{i04}} \times (e^{\alpha+\beta_2} e_{i14})^{n_{i14}} \times (e_{i05})^{n_{i05}} \times (e^{\alpha} e_{i15})^{n_{i15}}}{\{e^{\beta_2}(e_{i04} + e^{\alpha} e_{i14}) + (e_{i05} + e^{\alpha} e_{i15})\}^{(n_{i04}+n_{i14}+n_{i05}+n_{i15})}}.$$
$$(7.1)$$

The first derivative of $\log(L_i)$ with respect to β_2 gives the elementary likelihood score function for β_2:

$$M_{i3}(\alpha, \beta_2) = n_{i.4} - (n_{i.4} + n_{i.5}) \frac{e^{\beta_2}(e_{i04} + e^{\alpha} e_{i14})}{e^{\beta_2}(e_{i04} + e^{\alpha} e_{i14}) + (e_{i05} + e^{\alpha} e_{i15})}.$$

In this expression, the dots represent sums over $j = 0, 1$, so for example $n_{i.4} = n_{i04} + n_{i14}$. The estimating equation for β_2 is then

$$\sum_{i=1}^{N} M_{i3}(\alpha, \beta_2) = 0.$$

To obtain an unbiased estimating function for β_1, we consider a case i with event arising after the first exposure. The exposure history after the event represented by the partitioning illustrated in Figure 7.11 is now counterfactual: it is the exposure history which would have been observed had the event not occurred; alternatively, it is the exposure history that would have been observed, had the event not affected subsequent exposures. Based on this partly counterfactual exposure history, the elementary likelihood score function for β_1, obtained by differentiating the standard SCCS likelihood contribution for that case with the observation period $(c_{i1}, b_i]$, would be

$$n_{i.2} - (n_{i.2} + n_{i.3} + n_{i.4} + n_{i.5}) \times$$
$$\frac{e^{\beta_1}(e_{i02} + e^{\alpha} e_{i12})}{e^{\beta_1}(e_{i02} + e^{\alpha} e_{i12}) + (e_{i03} + e^{\alpha} e_{i13}) + e^{\beta_2}(e_{i04} + e^{\alpha} e_{i14}) + (e_{i05} + e^{\alpha} e_{i15})}.$$
$$(7.2)$$

However, this likelihood score function cannot usually be evaluated, since the intervals e_{ij3}, e_{ij4} and e_{ij5}, for $j = 0, 1$, may not be observed. To get round this difficulty, we modify this score function to conform with a counterfactual in which no exposures occur after the first. This involves removing the term e^{β_2} in Expression 7.2. Also, the count $n_{i.4}$ must be divided by e^{β_2} to ensure that the expected value conforms with our imposed counterfactual. This adjustment is illustrated in Figure 7.13 for the configuration described in Figure 7.11.

These modifications result in the following elementary estimating function for β_1:

$$M_{i2}(\alpha, \beta_1, \beta_2) = n_{i.2} - (n_{i.2} + n_{i.3} + n_{i.4}e^{-\beta_2} + n_{i.5}) \times$$
$$\frac{e^{\beta_1}(e_{i02} + e^{\alpha} e_{i12})}{e^{\beta_1}(e_{i02} + e^{\alpha} e_{i12}) + (e_{i03} + e^{\alpha} e_{i13}) + (e_{i04} + e^{\alpha} e_{i14}) + (e_{i05} + e^{\alpha} e_{i15})}.$$
$$(7.3)$$

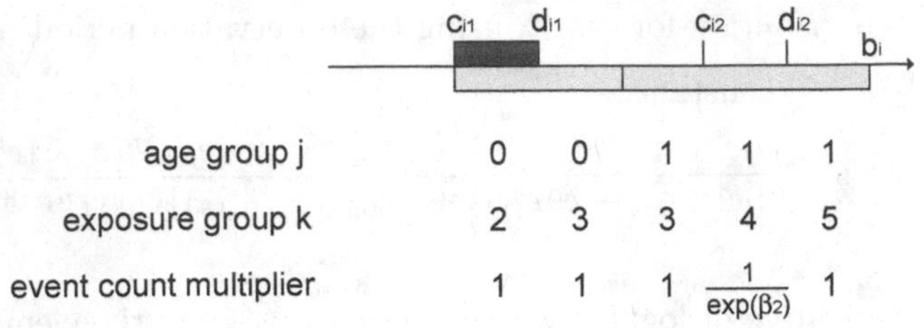

age group j	0	0	1	1	1
exposure group k	2	3	3	4	5
event count multiplier	1	1	1	$\dfrac{1}{\exp(\beta_2)}$	1

FIGURE 7.13
Illustration: adjustment to event count in second risk period.

This elementary estimating function can always be evaluated, even if the event occurs before a second exposure has arisen, since in this case $n_{i.4} = n_{i.5} = 0$ and $e_{i.3} + e_{i.4} + e_{i.5} = b_i - d_{i1}$, and the subdivision of this interval by age is known. Thus, $e_{i03} + e_{i04} + e_{i05}$ and $e_{i13} + e_{i14} + e_{i15}$ are known. Our estimating equation for β_1 is then

$$\sum_{i=1}^{N} M_{i2}(\alpha, \beta_1, \beta_2) = 0.$$

It remains to construct an unbiased estimating function for α. This comprises three components, which are added together. The first component comes from the SCCS likelihood contribution in Equation 7.1. The first derivative of the log likelihood contribution with respect to α yields the following elementary likelihood score function for α:

$$(n_{i14} + n_{i15}) - (n_{i.4} + n_{i.5}) \times \frac{e^{\alpha}(e^{\beta_2} e_{i14} + e_{i15})}{(e^{\beta_2} e_{i04} + e_{i05}) + e^{\alpha}(e^{\beta_2} e_{i14} + e_{i15})}. \quad (7.4)$$

This is the first component.

The second component is derived in a similar way to M_{i2} in Equation 7.3. We start with the elementary likelihood score function for α, derived from the standard SCCS likelihood contribution for that case with the observation period $(c_{i1}, b_i]$. This is

$$(n_{i12} + n_{i13} + n_{i14} + n_{i15}) - (n_{i.2} + n_{i.3} + n_{i.4} + n_{i.5}) \times$$
$$\frac{e^{\alpha}(e^{\beta_1} e_{i12} + e_{i13} + e^{\beta_2} e_{i14} + e_{i15})}{(e^{\beta_1} e_{i02} + e_{i03} + e^{\beta_2} e_{i04} + e_{i05}) + e^{\alpha}(e^{\beta_1} e_{i12} + e_{i13} + e^{\beta_2} e_{i14} + e_{i15})}.$$

We then modify this score function in line with our imposed counterfactual. Thus, as before, we remove the e^{β_2} and adjust n_{i14} and $n_{i.4}$. This yields the second component:

$$(n_{i12} + n_{i13} + n_{i14}e^{-\beta_2} + n_{i15}) - (n_{i.2} + n_{i.3} + n_{i.4}e^{-\beta_2} + n_{i.5}) \times$$
$$\frac{e^{\alpha}(e^{\beta_1} e_{i12} + e_{i13} + e_{i14} + e_{i15})}{(e^{\beta_1} e_{i02} + e_{i03} + e_{i04} + e_{i05}) + e^{\alpha}(e^{\beta_1} e_{i12} + e_{i13} + e_{i14} + e_{i15})}. \quad (7.5)$$

The third component is derived from the elementary likelihood score function for α obtained from the standard SCCS likelihood with observation period $(a_i, b_i]$. This score function is

$$\frac{(n_{i11} + n_{i12} + n_{i13} + n_{i14} + n_{i15}) - (n_{i.1} + n_{i.2} + n_{i.3} + n_{i.4} + n_{i.5}) \times}{E_0(\beta_1, \beta_2) + e^\alpha E_1(\beta_1, \beta_2)} \frac{e^\alpha(e_{i11} + e^{\beta_1} e_{i12} + e_{i13} + e^{\beta_2} e_{i14} + e_{i15})}{}, \tag{7.6}$$

where

$$E_j(\beta_1, \beta_2) = e_{ij1} + e^{\beta_1} e_{ij2} + e_{ij3} + e^{\beta_2} e_{ij4} + e_{ij5}, \quad j = 0, 1.$$

As before, we modify this score function to accord with our no exposures counterfactual. Thus, we remove the terms e^{β_1} and e^{β_2} in Expression 7.6, multiply n_{i02} and n_{i12} by $e^{-\beta_1}$, and multiply n_{i04} and n_{i14} by $e^{-\beta_2}$. This is illustrated in Figure 7.14 for the configuration described in Figure 7.11.

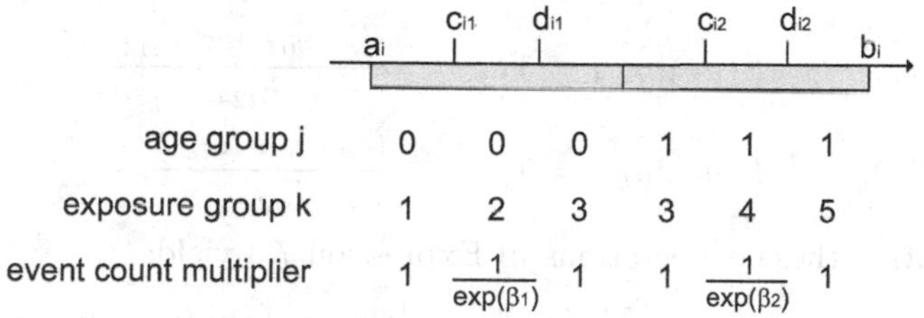

	c_{i1}	d_{i1}		c_{i2}	d_{i2}	
age group j	0	0	0	1	1	1
exposure group k	1	2	3	3	4	5
event count multiplier	1	$\frac{1}{\exp(\beta_1)}$	1	1	$\frac{1}{\exp(\beta_2)}$	1

FIGURE 7.14
Illustration: adjustments to event counts in first and second risk periods.

These adjustments yield

$$(n_{i11} + n_{i12}e^{-\beta_1} + n_{i13} + n_{i14}e^{-\beta_2} + n_{i15}) -$$
$$(n_{i.1} + n_{i.2}e^{-\beta_1} + n_{i.3} + n_{i.4}e^{-\beta_2} + n_{i.5}) \times \frac{e^\alpha e_{i1.}}{e_{i0.} + e^\alpha e_{i1.}}, \tag{7.7}$$

where $e_{ij.} = e_{ij1} + e_{ij2} + e_{ij3} + e_{ij4} + e_{ij5}$ for $j = 0, 1$. This is our third component. The elementary estimating function $M_{i1}(\alpha, \beta_1, \beta_2)$ for α is the sum of the three components in Expressions 7.4, 7.5 and 7.7. The estimating equation for α is

$$\sum_{i=1}^{N} M_{i1}(\alpha, \beta_1, \beta_2) = 0.$$

The elementary estimating functions $M_{ir} \equiv M_{ir}(\alpha, \beta_1, \beta_2)$ are unbiased, that is, have zero expectation under the correct model. This is immediate for $r = 3$ since M_{i3} is an elementary likelihood score function. We show unbiasedness for $r = 2$; the case $r = 1$ proceeds component-wise under similar lines.

Since individual i is a case, and events are non-recurrent, then $n_i = 1$. It follows that either $n_{i.1} = 0$ or $n_{i.1} = 1$. Now, we have

$$E(M_{i2}) = E(M_{i2}|n_{i.1} = 1)P(n_{i.1} = 1) + E(M_{i2}|n_{i.1} = 0)P(n_{i.1} = 0).$$

But $M_{i2} = 0$ when $n_{i.1} = 1$, since then $n_{i.2} = \cdots = n_{i.5} = 0$. And if $n_{i.1} = 0$, then $n_{i2+} = n_{i.2} + n_{i.3} + n_{i.4} + n_{i.5} = 1$. So it suffices to show that M_{i2} has zero expectation when $n_{i2+} = 1$. Let

$$E_{i2+} = e^{\beta_1}(e_{i02} + e^\alpha e_{i12}) + (e_{i03} + e^\alpha e_{i13}) + e^{\beta_2}(e_{i04} + e^\alpha e_{i14}) + (e_{i05} + e^\alpha e_{i15}).$$

The conditional expectations of the n_{ijk}, for $k \geq 2$, are

$$E(n_{i.2}|n_{i2+} = 1) = \frac{e^{\beta_1}(e_{i02} + e^\alpha e_{i12})}{E_{i2+}},$$

$$E(n_{i.3}|n_{i2+} = 1) = \frac{(e_{i03} + e^\alpha e_{i13})}{E_{i2+}},$$

$$E(n_{i.4}|n_{i2+} = 1) = \frac{e^{\beta_2}(e_{i04} + e^\alpha e_{i14})}{E_{i2+}},$$

$$E(n_{i.5}|n_{i2+} = 1) = \frac{(e_{i05} + e^\alpha e_{i15})}{E_{i2+}}.$$

Substituting these expectations in Expression 7.3 yields

$$E[M_{i2}(\alpha, \beta_1, \beta_2)|n_{i2+} = 1] = 0,$$

as required.

The restriction that a case can experience at most two exposures can be relaxed: it is only necessary that no case in the data set at hand experiences more than two exposures. To see this, suppose that, in principle, a case could experience three exposures, but that no case actually does. The third exposure, which in these data is always counterfactual and is never actually observed, could be represented by a further risk period $(c_{i3}, d_{i3}]$. The likelihood score equation is then altered as before in line with our no further exposure counterfactual. But since no event occurs after c_{i3} for any i, the inclusion of this additional counterfactual risk period does not affect the evaluation of any of the equations. Unsurprisingly, since third exposures are not observed, the corresponding parameter β_3 does not appear in the estimating functions, and is not estimable from these data. Thus, such hypothetical additional exposure intervals can simply be ignored.

7.1.7 General method for event-dependent exposures*

In this section we consider the general case when there are an arbitrary number of age groups, exposures, and risk periods. We also give some further

---

* This section may be skipped.

details about the calculation of standard errors and confidence limits, and outline a model fitting strategy.

Estimating equations in the general case
In this section, we state the unbiased estimating functions for α and β when there is an arbitrary number J of age-related parameters (and so $J+1$ age groups) and an arbitrary number of exposures, each contributing one or several contiguous risk periods, for example corresponding to distinct vaccine doses, or repeated treatment with the same drug. The derivation of these functions is similar to that presented in Section 7.1.6.

We suppose to start with that a case i experiences up to R distinct exposure episodes of the same exposure (for example the same drug) at ages c_{ir}, $r = 1, \ldots, R$. We assume that each exposure gives rise to S contiguous risk periods $(d_{ir}^{s-1}, d_{ir}^{s}]$, $s = 1, \ldots, S$, with $d_{ir}^{0} = c_{ir}$. The log relative incidence associated with risk period s after exposure r is β_{rs}; there are in all $R \times S$ risk periods. We assume for the time being that the corresponding $R \times S$ relative incidences may be distinct. It will be explained later how to obtain a common estimate when $\beta_{rs} = \beta_{s}$ for all r. Let α_j denote the log relative incidence associated with age group j relative to age group 0, for $j = 1, \ldots, J$.

For each case i, with observation period $(a_i, b_i]$, the indices $k = 1, \ldots K$ for $K = R \times (S+1) + 1$ count the successive exposure intervals from a_i to b_i. The first $(k = 1)$ is $(a_i, c_{i1}]$; the second is $(c_{i1}, d_{i1}^{1}]$; and so on. These intervals are further subdivided by age. The interval for case i corresponding to age group j and exposure interval k has length $e_{ijk} \geq 0$. If an interval does not arise then its length is set to zero; k represents the same position relative to successive exposures for all cases. The number of events (zero or one) arising in interval ijk is n_{ijk}.

To move between the interval counter k and the risk periods defined by the indices r and s we shall use the following three functions, defined for $r = 1, \ldots, R$, $s = 1, \ldots, S$ and $k = 1, \ldots, K$:

$$r(k) = \begin{cases} r, & \text{if } (r-1)(S+1) + 2 \leq k \leq r(S+1), \\ 0, & \text{otherwise}; \end{cases}$$

$$s(k) = \begin{cases} s, & \text{if } r(k) \geq 1 \text{ and } \{r(k) - 1\}(S+1) + 1 + s = k, \\ 0, & \text{otherwise}; \end{cases}$$

$$k(r, s) = (r-1)(S+1) + 1 + s.$$

In some applications, for example those involving vaccines, it is important to distinguish between doses. The notation introduced above allows for observation periods starting after the first dose: in this case e_{ijk} is set to zero for the missing intervals. The key point is that k represents the same position relative to successive doses for all cases.

Now define, for $r = 0, 1, \ldots, R$ (note the inclusion of $r = 0$ here),

$$
w_{ijk}^{(r)} = \begin{cases} 0, & \text{if } k \le (r-1)(S+1)+1, \\ 1, & \text{if } r = r(k) \text{ or } k = r'(S+1)+1 \text{ for some } r' \ge r, \\ \exp(-\beta_{r's}), & \text{if } k = k(r',s) \text{ for some } r' > r \text{ and some } s. \end{cases}
$$

In this definition, the subscripts i and j are redundant but are retained for consistency in what follows. Set $\beta_{0s} = 0$ for all $s = 0, 1, \ldots, S$. Now define the following subsets of cases:

$$
\mathfrak{S}_0 = \{i : a_i \notin \cup_{r=1}^{R} (c_{ir}, d_{ir}^S]\},
$$

and, for $r = 1, \ldots, R$,

$$
\mathfrak{S}_r = \{i : (c_{ir}, d_{ir}^S] \cap (a_i, b_i] \ne \emptyset\}.
$$

Note that unexposed cases, if present, are included in $\mathfrak{S}_0$. With this notation, the elementary estimating function for α_j, $j = 1, \ldots, J$ is

$$
M_{i,j}(\boldsymbol{\alpha}, \boldsymbol{\beta}) = \sum_{r=0}^{R} M_{ij}^r(\boldsymbol{\alpha}, \boldsymbol{\beta}),
$$

where, if $i \in \mathfrak{S}_r$,

$$
M_{i,j}^r(\boldsymbol{\alpha}, \boldsymbol{\beta}) = \sum_{k=1}^{K} w_{ijk}^{(r)} n_{ijk} - \left(\sum_{j=0}^{J} \sum_{k=1}^{K} w_{ijk}^{(r)} n_{ijk} \right) \times
$$
$$
\frac{\sum_{k=1}^{K} w_{ijk}^{(r)} e^{\alpha_j + \beta_{r(k)s(k)}} e_{ijk}}{\sum_{j=0}^{J} \sum_{k=1}^{K} w_{ijk}^{(r)} e^{\alpha_j + \beta_{r(k)s(k)}} e_{ijk}}, \tag{7.8}
$$

and $M_{i,j}^r(\boldsymbol{\alpha}, \boldsymbol{\beta}) = 0$ if $i \notin \mathfrak{S}_r$. Note that $\beta_{00} = 0$. The notations $M_{i,j}$ and M_{ij} are equivalent – the comma separating the indices here is used for greater clarity.

The elementary estimating function for β_{rs}, $r = 1, \ldots, R$, for $i \in \mathfrak{S}_r$, is

$$
M_{i,(r-1)S+s}(\boldsymbol{\alpha}, \boldsymbol{\beta}) = \sum_{j=0}^{J} n_{ijk(r,s)} - \left(\sum_{j=0}^{J} \sum_{k=1}^{K} w_{ijk}^{(r)} n_{ijk} \right) \times
$$
$$
\frac{\sum_{j=0}^{J} w_{ijk(r,s)}^{(r)} e^{\alpha_j + \beta_{rs}} e_{ijk(r,s)}}{\sum_{j=0}^{J} \sum_{k=1}^{K} w_{ijk}^{(r)} e^{\alpha_j + \beta_{r(k)s(k)}} e_{ijk}}. \tag{7.9}
$$

If $i \notin \mathfrak{S}_r$ then $M_{i,(r-1)S+s}^r(\boldsymbol{\alpha}, \boldsymbol{\beta}) = 0$.

Note that the terms $w_{ijk}^{(r)} e^{\beta_{r(k)s(k)}}$ in the expressions on the right-hand side of Equations 7.8 and 7.9 are

$$
w_{ijk}^{(r)} e^{\beta_{r(k)s(k)}} = \begin{cases} 0, & \text{if } k \le (r-1)(S+1)+1, \\ \exp(\beta_{rs}), & \text{if } r = r(k) \text{ and } s = s(k), \\ 1, & \text{if } k = r'(S+1)+1 \text{ for some } r' \ge r, \\ 1, & \text{if } k = k(r',s) \text{ for some } r' > r \text{ and some } s. \end{cases}
$$

The system of $J + RS$ estimating equations for $(\boldsymbol{\alpha}, \boldsymbol{\beta})$ is

$$\sum_{i=1}^{N} M_{i,m}(\boldsymbol{\alpha}, \boldsymbol{\beta}) = 0, \quad m = 1, \ldots, J + RS.$$

The estimators $\hat{\boldsymbol{\alpha}}$, $\hat{\boldsymbol{\beta}}$ are the solutions of this system of equations.

If the parameters β_{rs} are equal at different doses, so that $\beta_{rs} = \beta_s$ for $r = 1, \ldots, R$, there are only S exposure parameters to be estimated. The elementary estimating functions for β_{rs} are added over $r = 1, \ldots, R$. The elementary estimating function for β_s is then

$$M_{i,J+s}(\boldsymbol{\alpha}, \boldsymbol{\beta}) = \sum_{r=1}^{R} M_{i,(r-1)S+s}(\boldsymbol{\alpha}, \beta, \ldots, \beta)$$

where $\boldsymbol{\beta} = (\beta_1, \ldots, \beta_S)$ and the dots on the right of the equation represent R repeats.

Approximate confidence intervals

Confidence intervals for the parameters may be obtained using standard results from the theory of estimating equations (Jesus and Chandler, 2011). Let $\mathbf{V}(\boldsymbol{\theta})$ denote the observed covariance matrix of the vector of unbiased estimating functions, with components $\sum_{i=1}^{N} M_{im}(\boldsymbol{\theta})$, where $\boldsymbol{\theta}$ is the parameter vector $(\boldsymbol{\alpha}, \boldsymbol{\beta})^T$. Let $\mathbf{H}(\boldsymbol{\theta})$ denote the Jacobian of the vector of estimating functions. Thus, $\mathbf{V}(\boldsymbol{\theta})$ and $\mathbf{H}(\boldsymbol{\theta})$ are $(J + RS) \times (J + RS)$ matrices with (u, v) elements

$$V_{uv}(\boldsymbol{\theta}) = \sum_{i=1}^{N} M_{iu}(\boldsymbol{\theta}) M_{iv}(\boldsymbol{\theta}),$$

$$H_{uv}(\boldsymbol{\theta}) = \sum_{i=1}^{N} \frac{\partial M_{iu}(\boldsymbol{\theta})}{\partial \theta_v}.$$

The covariance matrix $\text{cov}(\hat{\boldsymbol{\theta}})$ may be estimated using the sandwich estimator $\mathbf{H}(\hat{\boldsymbol{\theta}})^{-1} \mathbf{V}(\hat{\boldsymbol{\theta}}) \mathbf{H}(\hat{\boldsymbol{\theta}})^{-1T}$. This may then be used to obtain confidence intervals for $\boldsymbol{\theta}$.

Fitting the model

In the final part of this section we give some brief indications about how to fit the model. The key is to note that the elementary estimating equations for $i \in \mathfrak{S}_r$, $r = 0, 1, \ldots, R$, may be interpreted as score equations from a pseudo-Poisson model. For a count n and a weight w with $0 \leq w \leq 1$, let the expression $wn \sim P(\mu)$ denote a likelihood contribution proportional to $e^{-\mu} \mu^{wn}$ when $w \neq 0$ and equal to 1 when $w = 0$. This model is called pseudo-Poisson because the response variable wn need not be an integer.

The elementary estimating equations derived for $i \in \mathfrak{S}_0$ may equivalently be obtained as elementary score equations from the pseudo-Poisson model

$$w_{ijk}^{(0)} n_{ijk} \sim P(\lambda_{ijk}^{(0)} e_{ijk})$$
$$\log(\lambda_{ijk}^{(0)}) = \phi_i^{(0)} + \alpha_j.$$

Similarly, the elementary estimating equations for $i \in \mathfrak{S}_r$ correspond to elementary score equations from the pseudo-Poisson model

$$w_{ijk}^{(r)} n_{ijk} \sim P(\lambda_{ijk}^{(r)} e_{ijk})$$
$$\log(\lambda_{ijk}^{(r)}) = \phi_i^{(r)} + \alpha_j + \beta_{rs} I(k(r,s) = k),$$

with $I(.)$ the indicator function.

To fit the model, we first stack the $R + 1$ data subsets $\mathfrak{S}_0, \mathfrak{S}_1, \ldots, \mathfrak{S}_R$, with distinct individual identifiers for each stack level $r = 0, 1, \ldots, R$, and with covariate vectors to match the submodels described above. For an initial choice of parameters β_{rs}, the $w_{ijk}^{(r)} n_{ijk}$ are defined as response variables. The model is fitted iteratively, alternatively maximising the pseudo-Poisson likelihood for given weights $w_{ijk}^{(r)}$ and then updating the weights $w_{ijk}^{(r)}$ using the latest parameter estimates of the β_{rs}, until a convergence criterion is met.

Note that the elementary estimating functions in Expressions 7.8 and 7.9, when evaluated at the observed values n_{ijk} for $i \in \mathfrak{S}_r$, take the form of the residual $y - \nu\pi$. Thus, y is $0, 1$ or $\exp(-\beta_{r's})$ for some $r' > r$ and some s (since $n_i = 1$); ν similarly involves $\exp(-\beta_{r's})$; and π may involve the age parameters α_j and the parameters relating to exposure r, $\beta_{r1}, \ldots, \beta_{rS}$.

The elementary estimating functions for each parameter may be obtained from the converged pseudo-Poisson model by summing the residuals corresponding to the cells indexed by that parameter. The matrix $\mathbf{V}$ is then calculated directly from these elementary estimating functions.

To obtain the matrix of derivatives $\mathbf{H}$, note that the partial derivatives are of the form

$$\frac{\partial}{\partial \theta}(y - \nu\pi) = \left(\frac{\partial y}{\partial \theta} - \frac{\partial \nu}{\partial \theta}\pi\right) - \nu\frac{\partial \pi}{\partial \theta}. \tag{7.10}$$

The first bracket on the right-hand side of Equation 7.10 is either of the form $-(y - \nu\pi)$, if $\theta = \beta_{r's}$, or 0 otherwise. The last term on the right-hand side of Equation 7.10 is a contribution to the Hessian of the pseudo-Poisson model.

Thus, the matrix $\mathbf{H}$ may be obtained from the Hessian of the converged pseudo-Poisson model and its residuals. The sandwich variance estimator may then be obtained from $\mathbf{V}$ and $\mathbf{H}$ as described above.

Some details about the about the model fitting procedure may be obtained by specifying `verbose=T` in function `eventdepenexp`. For example, with the rotavirus and intussusception data of Section 7.1.3,

```
rot.mod2 <- eventdepenexp(indiv=case, astart=sta, aend=end,
```

```
                    aevent=intus, adrug=cbind(rv,rvd2),
                    aedrug=cbind(rv+21,rvd2+21), expogrp=c(1,8),
                    sameexpopar=T, agegrp=age, dataformat="multi",
                    data=rotdat, verbose=T)
```

produces the following output:

```
No. exposures after first event (treated as missing): 0
No. events included at stack level 0: 566
No. events included at stack level 1: 79
No. events included at stack level 2: 49
iteration: 1
beta: 1 1.57803590021434 beta: 2 0.699352762537988
iteration: 2
beta: 1 1.81714591093924 beta: 2 0.892285864427605
......
iteration: 10
beta: 1 1.84341970787888 beta: 2 0.918140503166051
```

The first line indicates that 0 cases received rotavirus vaccination after intussusception; if some cases had, these post-event exposures would have been
recoded as missing. The next three lines describe the construction of the data
stack: at stack level 0, all 566 events are included. At stack level 1, the 79
events after the first dose of vaccine are included. At stack level 2 the 49 post
second dose events are included. Finally, some details of the iterative fit are
provided: in this case, the fitting process was deemed to have converged at
the 10th iteration.

7.2 SCCS for event-dependent observation periods

We now turn to an extension of the SCCS model that applies when observation
periods are influenced by events. We consider one specific context, in which
events may bring forward the end of observation. This arises, for example,
when the event of interest is associated with high mortality. The extension
is required when the methods described in Chapter 5, Section 5.3, suggest
that this type of event-dependence could bias the estimated associations of
interest in a standard SCCS model. This bias may be in either direction; and
it is possible that violation of the assumption produces no bias, as shown in
Chapter 5, Section 5.3.4.

The standard SCCS model applies when the observation periods extend
to the planned end of the study. It also applies if the observation periods are
censored at random (Kalbfleisch and Prentice, 2002, page 53), as may occur if
observation is curtailed owing to circumstances unconnected with the event.

The extension to the standard SCCS model requires information on whether the observation period for each case has been censored. It applies to rare non-recurrent events (if the event is recurrent, the method should be applied to first occurrences). Exposures within the observation period are assumed not to be event-dependent. The method requires two additional assumptions. First, censoring may be influenced by, but should not necessarily coincide with, the event of interest. Second, given the event history, the censoring process should not depend on the exposure history.

The practical implications of these assumptions merit some further consideration. Regarding the first assumption, note that the event of interest must not itself censor observation, as is the case with death. (The use of SCCS methods when death is the event of interest is discussed in Section 7.3.) For example, suppose that censoring occurs owing to death caused by stroke, the event of interest. Stroke increases the risk of death, so censoring through death is event-dependent, but stroke does not always result in death.

The second assumption holds provided the exposure is not an independent risk factor for censoring. In the stroke example, the assumption means that any death caused by the exposure must be due to a stroke caused by the exposure, and not some other exposure-induced pathology. In other words, stroke must lie on any causal pathway that may exist between exposure and death. For most applications in pharmacoepidemiology, this assumption is unlikely to be unduly restrictive. However, if deaths directly induced by a drug are of concern, then death would most likely be the event of interest in the analysis. In this case, the methods described in Section 7.3 should be used.

The extension of the standard SCCS model involves a two-stage modelling approach, described in Section 7.2.1. Three applications are described, in Sections 7.2.2 to 7.2.4. Fitting the model can require some experimentation with initial parameter values, aspects of which are considered in Section 7.2.5. Further details of the model are provided in Sections 7.2.6 and 7.2.7. These sections are starred and may be skipped.

7.2.1 A two-stage modelling approach

In this section we describe informally how the SCCS likelihood described in Chapter 3, Section 3.5, must be modified to take account of event-dependent observation periods. Technical details of the derivation are in starred Section 7.2.6.

We suppose that each case i experiences a single event at age t_i. Let a_i denote the start of observation for individual i, and b_i^* the *planned* end of observation. In practice, the observation period might end earlier than planned, at some age $c_i < b_i^*$. If this occurs, then we say that the observation period is censored. If the observation period is not censored, we write $c_i \geq b_i^*$. The actual observation period is $(a_i, b_i]$, where

$$b_i = \min\{c_i, b_i^*\}.$$

This notation was introduced in Chapter 5, Section 5.3. We shall also use the censoring indicator previously defined in that section:

$$I_i = 1 \text{ if } b_i < b_i^*, 0 \text{ if } b_i = b_i^*. \tag{7.11}$$

We assume that the value of I_i is available for each case.

Two key changes to the standard SCCS likelihood are required; both of these involve the censoring process – that is, the process that may lead to early termination of the observation period. The exposure history is x_i, and is unaffected by prior events; the observation history is now modelled explicitly.

First, let $S_i(t)$ denote the probability that censoring has not occurred by age t for case i, in the absence of an event. To derive the SCCS likelihood, we condition on the number of events (0 or 1, in our case) that have occurred for individual i during their observation period. Suppose that one event occurs, at age t_i. It then follows that individual i was not censored before age t_i, which occurs with probability $S_i(t_i)$. The event intensity function $\lambda_i(t|x_i)$ must be adjusted to take account of the thinning effect of censoring. To this end, we replace $\lambda_i(t|x_i)$ in the SCCS likelihood by

$$\lambda_i^*(t|x_i) = \lambda_i(t|x_i) \times S_i(t).$$

Since, by assumption, $S_i(t)$ does not involve the exposure history x_i, inclusion of this term will only alter the relative age effect, and not the exposure effect which is generally of primary interest. The relative age effect estimated from the extended SCCS model will thus incorporate the thinning effect of censoring. This modification only really involves a change in interpretation of the age effects, and does not require any alteration to the model.

The second change to the SCCS likelihood that is required to accommodate the effect of event-dependent observation periods is more fundamental. It turns out that event times must be weighted in a particular manner. The weight for a case i turns out to be, essentially, the probability that the observation period ended at b_i, given t_i and the indicator I_i.

The reason why such weights must be introduced may be explained informally as follows. If occurrence of an event precipitates the end of observation, then conditioning on – informally, fixing – the end of observation affects the distribution of the event time. To illustrate this, suppose that the event of interest is stroke, which carries relatively high short-term mortality. Suppose that case i suffered a stroke in the age interval $(a_i, b_i]$. Without further information, age is the only factor available to us which influences the timing of the stroke within this interval. However, if it is also known that case i *died of stroke* at age b_i (so that $I_i = 1$), then it becomes much more likely that the stroke occurred shortly before b_i, since many deaths from stroke occur shortly after the stroke. Thus, this extra information affects the distribution of age at stroke for this case: the distribution must be weighted towards b_i. The amount of weighting depends on the distribution of the interval between stroke and death. If such a weighting is not introduced, the clustering of events shortly before b_i, if it occurs, may incorrectly be ascribed to age or exposure effects. This may produce biased estimates of these effects.

Let $w_i(b_i|t, I_i)$ denote the weight function for case i, where I_i is the censoring indicator. The modified SCCS likelihood contribution for a case i with a single event at t_i turns out to be

$$L_i = \frac{\lambda_i^*(t_i|x_i) \times w_i(b_i|t_i, I_i)}{\int_{a_i}^{b_i} \lambda_i^*(t|x_i) \times w_i(b_i|t, I_i)dt}. \tag{7.12}$$

The derivation is provided in Section 7.2.6. Expression 7.12 may be contrasted with the corresponding likelihood contribution for the standard SCCS model:

$$L_i = \frac{\lambda_i(t_i|x_i)}{\int_{a_i}^{b_i} \lambda_i(t|x_i)dt},$$

where all event times have the same weight of 1.

As with the standard SCCS model, time-invariant covariates acting multiplicatively on the incidence rate drop out of the likelihood, though interactions with exposure or age effects may be estimated. In addition, and unlike the standard SCCS model, time-invariant covariates y_i may also influence the weight functions which are then written $w_i(t|b_i, I_i, y_i)$.

Fitting the model is done in two stages. In the first stage, the weight functions $w_i(t|b_i, I_i)$ are estimated by modelling the distributions of the intervals from the event times t_i to the end of observation b_i, given I_i. In the second stage, the standard SCCS model is used to obtain the parameters for the age effect (which adjust for the impact of censoring) and the exposure effects, using the weights estimated in the first stage. This is the approach used with the function **eventdepenobs** in R package SCCS: four different weight models are fitted automatically, and the best-fitting is used to calculate the weights.

These weight models are mixture models. Fitting them is not straightforward, and may require some experimentation with initial parameter values. However, the results obtained from the SCCS model at the second stage are not unduly sensitive to the values of the weights. Further details of the weight models, the fitting procedure, and the convergence problems that may be encountered are discussed in starred Section 7.2.7.

Summary

- An extension of the SCCS model is available for rare non-recurrent events when observation periods are censored after the event by a process that depends on the event, but not on the exposure.

- In this extended SCCS model, event times are weighted by a function that depends on the time interval from event to end of observation.

- The model is fitted in two stages. In stage one, the weights are estimated. In stage two, a standard SCCS model is fitted using these weights.

7.2.2 Nicotine replacement therapy and MI

We return to the application on nicotine replacement therapy (NRT) and first myocardial infarction (MI), first discussed in Chapter 4, Section 4.8.3. There we fitted a standard SCCS model, with a planned (or nominal) observation period ending 365 days after NRT initiation. Then in Chapter 5, Section 5.3.2 we discussed using the actual observation period rather than the planned period. Some of the actual observation periods end early, possibly owing to death of the patient resulting from their MI: an instance of event-dependent observation periods.

The results obtained from the two analyses are summarised in Table 7.1. The relative incidences obtained with actual observation periods are much

TABLE 7.1

Results from two SCCS analyses of the NRT and MI data.

Risk period	Planned obs period		Actual obs period	
	RI	95% CI	RI	95% CI
0–7 days	1.69	0.69 – 4.12	0.89	0.34 – 2.31
8–14 days	1.93	0.79 – 4.71	1.01	0.39 – 2.63
15–21 days	1.16	0.37 – 3.63	0.68	0.21 – 2.19
22–28 days	1.16	0.37 – 3.63	0.74	0.23 – 2.36

lower than those obtained with planned observation periods. That these differences may be due to event-dependent observation periods is suggested by Figure 7.15, in which the distributions of the intervals from MI to actual end of observation are plotted separately for censored and uncensored intervals. The mode close to zero in censored individuals suggests that some of these individuals may have died from their MI.

To explore this further we use the SCCS extension for event-dependent observation periods, implemented in R function eventdepenobs. The model requires the censoring indicator, which is in variable cen. This takes the value 1 if the observation period was censored (so the actual end of observation is earlier than planned) and 0 otherwise.

The model is specified as follows:

```
nrt.mod6 <- eventdepenobs(event~nrt, indiv=case, astart=nrt,
          aend=act, aevent=mi, adrug=nrt, aedrug=nrt+28,
          censor=cen, expogrp=c(0,8,15,22), agegrp=NULL,
          data=nrtdat)
```

Most of the arguments of function eventdepenobs are the same as for standardsccs. The only new argument used here is censor=cen to specify the censoring variable.

The resulting (edited) output is as follows.

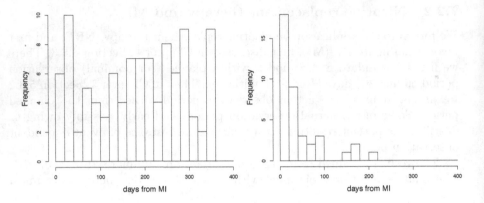

FIGURE 7.15
Distribution of interval from MI to actual end of observation for NRT data.
Left: uncensored values. Right: censored values.

```
> nrt.mod6
......
              EWA        EWI        EGA        EGI
Loglik  -28.57869  -25.40956  -28.59141  -25.64863
AIC      65.15738   58.81912   65.18282   59.29725
......
        exp(coef)  exp(-coef)  lower .95  upper .95
nrt1       1.928      0.5188     0.7666      4.847
nrt2       2.007      0.4984     0.7729      5.209
nrt3       1.244      0.8039     0.3795      4.077
nrt4       1.343      0.7446     0.4193      4.302
```

The first part of the output provides details of the four inbuilt parametric models used to obtain the weights. These are exponential–Weibull (EWA and EWI) and exponential–gamma (EGA and EGI) mixture models, to be described in Section 7.2.7. The model with the best fit, that is the lowest value of the Akaike Information Criterion (AIC), is selected: in this case it is model EWI, with $AIC = 58.82$.

The last part of the output gives the SCCS model parameters obtained using these weights. For example, for the risk period 0–7 days after NRT, $RI = 1.93$ with 95% CI $(0.77, 4.85)$. These estimates are corrected for the effect of event-dependence of observation periods. These corrected estimates may be compared to those in Table 7.1. They are quite close to those obtained using the planned observation periods.

These results were obtained using default initial values for the parameters of the weight models. The choice of initial values is important for these models, and is discussed further in Section 7.2.5.

7.2.3 Respiratory tract infections and MI

We return to the data on respiratory tract infections (RTI) and myocardial infarction (MI) discussed in Section 7.1.5. The data comprise 940 cases of first MI. Of these, 486 were censored: the observation period ended before the planned end of the study. Some of the censoring may be unrelated to the MI; but it is likely that in some cases occurrence of an MI resulted in death.

Figure 7.16 shows the distribution of intervals from MI to end of observation in censored and uncensored cases. Both distributions display a mode

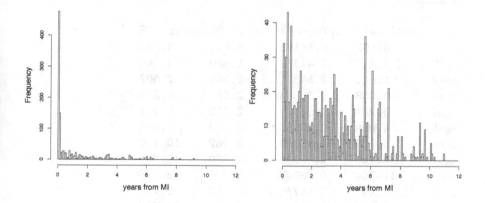

FIGURE 7.16
Distribution of interval from MI to end of observation for RTI data. Left: censored values. Right: uncensored values.

close to zero, but it is very much more pronounced in the censored cases, as would be expected if censoring was event-dependent.

To investigate the potential impact of event-dependent observation periods, we test the interaction between the exposure effect and the censoring indicator, as described in Chapter 5, Section 5.3.1. First, we obtain the standard SCCS models without and with interaction, as follows.

```
uni <- (1-duplicated(midat$case))
ageq <- floor(quantile(midat$mi[uni==1], seq(0.1,0.9,0.1),
        names=F))
mi.mod3 <- standardsccs(event~rti+age, indiv=case, astart=sta,
            aend=end, aevent=mi, adrug=rti, aedrug=rti+14,
            expogrp=c(0,8), agegr=ageq, data=midat)
mi.mod4 <- standardsccs(event~factor(cen)/rti+age, indiv=case,
            astart=sta, aend=end, aevent=mi, adrug=rti,
            aedrug=rti+14, expogrp=c(0,8), agegr=ageq,
            data=midat)
```

These models have two risk periods, as in Section 7.1.5: 0–7 days and 8–14 days after each infection. We now compare these models using the likelihood ratio test:

```
> lrtsccs(mi.mod3,mi.mod4)
   test df  pvalue
  5.233   2 0.07306
```

The interaction is marginally statistically non-significant. Ignoring any impact of event-dependent observation periods, the estimated parameters are:

```
> mi.mod3
......
```

	exp(coef)	exp(-coef)	lower .95	upper .95
rti1	6.195	0.16143	4.748	8.082
rti2	2.417	0.41374	1.560	3.745
age2	1.841	0.54321	1.300	2.607
age3	3.088	0.32384	2.095	4.551
age4	3.231	0.30951	2.112	4.943
age5	4.859	0.20580	3.109	7.594
age6	6.344	0.15764	3.962	10.156
age7	9.766	0.10240	5.980	15.949
age8	11.304	0.08847	6.790	18.818
age9	17.421	0.05740	10.209	29.727
age10	39.885	0.02507	22.861	69.587

Parameters `rti1` and `rti2` relate to the exposure effect. They suggest there is a large effect, $RI = 6.20$ with 95% CI $(4.75, 8.08)$ in the 0–7 day risk period after each respiratory tract, reducing to $RI = 2.42$, 95% CI $(1.56, 3.75)$ in the period 8–14 days after infection. The age effect is markedly increasing.

To investigate whether these estimates are subject to bias resulting from event-dependent observation periods, we now fit the SCCS extension.

```
mi.mod5 <- eventdepenobs(event~rti+age, indiv=case, astart=sta,
           aend=end, aevent=mi, adrug=rti, aedrug=rti+14,
           expogrp=c(0,8), agegrp=ageq, censor=cen, data=midat,
           initval=rep(1.1,4))
```

Each of the weight models has four parameters. Here, we have specified initial values for these parameters with `initval=rep(1.1,4)`. The choice of initial values, and their impact on results, is discussed further in Section 7.2.5.

This model yields the following output.

```
> mi.mod5
......
```

	EWA	EWI	EGA	EGI
Loglik	−640.6667	−648.9525	−700.9147	−648.9943
AIC	1289.3335	1305.9049	1409.8294	1305.9887

```
......
```

	exp(coef)	exp(-coef)	lower .95	upper .95
rti1	6.4503	0.1550	4.8688	8.546
rti2	2.4445	0.4091	1.5595	3.832
age2	1.0358	0.9654	0.7334	1.463
age3	1.1243	0.8894	0.7743	1.632
age4	0.9643	1.0370	0.6491	1.433
age5	0.9564	1.0456	0.6288	1.455
age6	0.9340	1.0707	0.6033	1.446
age7	1.0680	0.9364	0.6770	1.685
age8	0.9283	1.0772	0.5791	1.488
age9	0.8724	1.1462	0.5315	1.432
age10	1.1123	0.8990	0.6623	1.868

Weight model EWA, with $AIC - 1289.33$, provides the best fit, so the weights obtained with this model are used. The estimated relative incidences corrected for event-dependence of observation periods are $RI = 6.45$ with 95% CI $(4.87, 8.55)$ for the 0–7 day risk period, and $RI = 2.44$, 95% CI $(1.56, 3.83)$ for the 8 14 day risk period. These estimates are not very different from those from model mi.mod3 obtained with the standard SCCS method.

The estimated age effects, however, have changed considerably. The age-related relative incidences obtained for models mi.mod5 and mi.mod3 are shown (on the log scale) in Figure 7.17. The age-related trends are clearly very different for the two models.

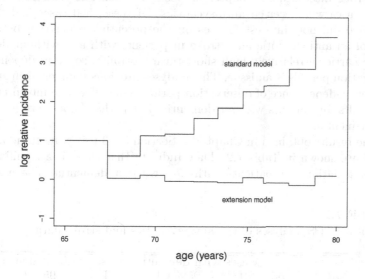

FIGURE 7.17
Estimated age-related log relative incidences. Top graph: model mi.mod3. Bottom graph: model mi.mod5.

This graph was obtained using the following code.

```
ari.mod3 <- c(1, mi.mod3$coef[3:11,1], mi.mod3$coef[11,1])
ari.mod5 <- c(1, mi.mod5$summary$coef[3:11,1],
              mi.mod5$summary$coef[11,1])
age.x <- c(65, ageq/365.25, 80)
par(mar=c(4.1,4.1,1,1), cex.lab=1.4)
plot(c(65,80), c(-1,4), type="n", xlab="age (years)",
     ylab="log relative incidence")
lines(age.x, ari.mod3, type="s")
lines(age.x, ari.mod5, type="s")
text(75, 3, "standard model")
text(75, -0.5, "extension model")
```

There are two reasons for the difference between the two estimated age effects. First, they represent different quantities: that for model `mi.mod5` incorporates the thinning effect of censoring. Second, the age effect estimated in model `mi.mod3` is likely to be biased at older ages, owing to the curtailment of observation periods due to event-dependent censoring.

7.2.4 Antipsychotics and stroke

In this application, we continue the investigation of the data on antipsychotics and stroke discussed in Chapter 5, Section 5.3.3. The data comprise 2000 stroke cases who received antipsychotics. Of these, 500 cases had dementia and 1500 did not. Interest focuses on the potential association between receipt of an antipsychotic and stroke in patients with and without dementia. Stroke carries a relatively high short-term mortality, so event-dependence of observation periods is an issue. The analyses previously undertaken suggested that event-dependence of observation periods may affect the interpretation of the results for patients without dementia, but perhaps not those for patients with dementia.

The results obtained in Chapter 5, Section 5.3.3 using the standard SCCS model are shown in Table 7.2. They indicate that there is a significant positive association, for patients with and without dementia. The association

TABLE 7.2
Standard SCCS analyses of the antipsychotics and stroke data.

	Cases with dementia		Cases without dementia	
Risk period	RI	95% CI	RI	95% CI
On drug	2.96	2.25 − 3.90	1.43	1.21 − 1.71
Washout 1	2.91	2.17 − 3.89	1.45	1.20 − 1.76
Washout 2	1.98	1.28 − 3.06	1.14	0.85 − 1.52

is stronger for patients with dementia, with $RI = 2.96$, 95% CI $(2.25, 3.90)$ while on drug for patients with dementia compared to $RI = 1.43$, 95% CI $(1.21, 1.71)$ for patients without dementia. But are these estimates reliable?

To obtain corrected estimates we use the SCCS extension for event-dependent observation periods, with the same age and exposure groups as in previous analyses. We begin by analysing cases with and without dementia separately. After a little experimentation with the initial values specified in initval, the model for cases with dementia is as follows.

```
agedem <- floor(seq(70,95,5)*365.25)
ap.mod7 <- eventdepenobs(event~ap+age, indiv=case, astart=sta,
          aend=end, aevent=stro, adrug=ap, aedrug=endap,
          washout=c(1,92,182), agegrp=agedem, censor=cen,
          data=subset(apdat,dem==1), initval=rep(0.9,4))
```

This yields:

```
> ap.mod7
......
          EWA       EWI       EGA       EGI
Loglik -385.108 -387.2556 -392.9409 -387.3082
AIC     778.216  782.5112  793.8818  782.6163
......
     exp(coef) exp(-coef) lower .95 upper .95
ap1   2.49383    0.4010   1.889246    3.2919
ap2   1.78342    0.5607   1.318000    2.4132
ap3   1.19219    0.8388   0.758056    1.8749
```

Weight model EWA is selected as the best-fitting, with $AIC = 778.22$. The estimated relative incidences are a little lower than those in Table 7.2: while on drug, $RI = 2.49$ with 95% CI $(1.89, 3.29)$, and is thus statistically significantly elevated. The relative incidence subsequently declines to a non-significant value in the second washout period.

For cases without dementia, the model is:

```
agenod <- floor(seq(45,95,5)*365.25)
ap.mod8 <- eventdepenobs(event~ap+age, indiv=case, astart=sta,
          aend=end, aevent=stro, adrug=ap, aedrug=endap,
          washout=c(1,92,182), agegrp=agenod, censor=cen,
          data=subset(apdat,dem==0), initval=rep(0.9,4))
```

This model gives the following results.

```
> ap.mod8
......
           EWA        EWI        EGA        EGI
Loglik -2022.713 -2115.370 -2122.568 -2115.369
AIC     4053.426  4238.739  4253.135  4238.738
```

```
......
      exp(coef) exp(-coef) lower .95 upper .95
ap1      1.0602     0.9433    0.89396     1.2573
ap2      0.8560     1.1683    0.70619     1.0375
ap3      0.7808     1.2807    0.57768     1.0554
```

Weight model EWA again gives the best fit, with $AIC = 4053.43$. The relative incidences are lower than those reported for non-dementia cases in Table 7.2, and are now close to or less than 1 and not statistically significant, providing little evidence of an association between antipsychotics and stroke. Thus, event-dependence of observation periods does materially affect the conclusions to be drawn for patients without dementia.

So far we have analysed patients with and without dementia separately. There is merit in this approach, as it allows for different age effects and weightings. An alternative is to model the whole data set in a single analysis. We shall allow the weighting functions to be stratified by the dementia indicator dem: thus, separate weighting functions are allowed for patients with and without dementia. This is done by specifying covariates=factor(dem) in function eventdepenobs; the default is covariates=NULL.

In our first joint model, we shall assume common relative incidences for patients with and without dementia:

```
ageall <- floor(seq(45,95,5)*365.25)
ap.mod9 <- eventdepenobs(event~ap+age, indiv=case, astart=sta,
           aend=end, aevent=stro, adrug=ap, aedrug=endap,
           washout=c(1,92,182), agegrp=ageall, censor=cen,
           covariates=factor(dem), data=apdat,
           initval=rep(0.9,4))
```

This produces the following results.

```
> ap.mod9
......
               EWA         EWI         EGA         EGI
Loglik  -2410.021   -2502.625   -2516.036   -2562.558
AIC      4836.041    5021.250    5048.072    5141.116
......
      exp(coef) exp(-coef) lower .95 upper .95
ap1      1.3133     0.7614    1.13959     1.5136
ap2      1.0166     0.9837    0.86722     1.1917
ap3      0.8373     1.1943    0.65244     1.0745
```

The optimal weights are those from weighting model EWA, with $AIC = 4836.04$. The relative incidences, unsurprisingly, lie between those obtained separately for patients with and without dementia. In the next model, we include the interaction between the dementia indicator and the exposure variable:

```
ap.mod10 <- eventdepenobs(event~factor(dem)/ap+age, indiv=case,
             astart=sta, aend=end, aevent=stro, adrug=ap,
             aedrug=endap, washout=c(1,92,182), agegrp=ageall,
             censor=cen, covariates=factor(dem), data=apdat,
             initval=rep(0.9,4))
```

This model yields:

```
> ap.mod10
......
              EWA        EWI        EGA        EGI
Loglik  -2410.021  -2502.625  -2516.036  -2562.558
AIC      4836.041   5021.250   5048.072   5141.116
......
                  exp(coef) exp(-coef) lower .95 upper .95
......
factor(dem)0:ap1   1.0688     0.9356    0.90180    1.2668
factor(dem)1:ap1   2.3871     0.4189    1.81057    3.1471
factor(dem)0:ap2   0.8641     1.1573    0.71335    1.0467
factor(dem)1:ap2   1.7125     0.5839    1.26830    2.3123
factor(dem)0:ap3   0.7865     1.2715    0.58201    1.0627
factor(dem)1:ap3   1.1422     0.8755    0.72701    1.7944
```

The weight models are exactly the same as those for model ap.mod9, as expected, since inclusion of the interaction term only affects the SCCS model. The relative incidences are very similar to those obtained with models ap.mod7 and ap.mod8. The factor dem is coded 1 for patients with dementia, 0 for patients without dementia. For patients with dementia, the relative incidences are: 2.39, 95% CI $(1.81, 3.15)$ on drug; 1.71 $(1.27, 2.31)$ and 1.14 $(0.73, 1.79)$ for the first and second washout periods, respectively. For patients without dementia, the relative incidences are: 1.07, 95% CI $(0.90, 1.27)$ on drug; 0.86 $(0.71, 1.05)$ and 0.79, $(0.58, 1.06)$ for the washout periods.

One advantage of the combined modelling approach is that formal comparisons between nested models may be undertaken, provided the same weighting function is used for both models so that like is compared with like. This is the case for models ap.mod9 and ap.mod10. The likelihood ratio test may be undertaken with function lrtsccs, with the syntax adjusted to take account of the expanded model output.

```
> lrtsccs(ap.mod9$summary,ap.mod10$summary)
   test df     pvalue
   26.31  3 8.213e-06
```

The p-value is less than 0.0001, and so the interaction term is highly statistically significant. Thus the association differs significantly between patients with and without dementia.

We conclude that, after adjusting for the effect of event-dependent observation periods, there is evidence of a strong positive association between antipsychotics and stroke in patients with dementia, but little evidence of any association for patients without dementia.

7.2.5 Experimenting with initial values

In the applications in Sections 7.2.3 and 7.2.4, the weight models were obtained using special choices of initial values for the parameters, specified using the argument initval. In this section, the choice of initial parameter values is explored in greater detail.

The issue is important because the four weight models are mixtures of an exponential (E) component and either a gamma (G) or Weibull (W) component. Mixture models can be tricky to fit using maximum likelihood. This is because different combinations of parameter values may provide fits of similar quality: an issue of parameter identifiability. In addition, the likelihood may be multimodal, and the fitting algorithm may converge to a local rather than to the global maximum. In our case, however, the actual parameter values for the weight models are not of primary interest: we just need the weight models to provide a reasonable fit to the data on intervals from event to end of observation. Provided that this is the case, the results obtained from the SCCS model will not be overly sensitive to different weight models.

Further details of the weight models and their parameterisation are in Section 7.2.7. For all the weight models discussed in the applications in Sections 7.2.2 to 7.2.4 there are 4 initial values. More complex weight models, incorporating a regression component, may be fitted: these are described in Section 7.2.7. The default settings set all initial values to be equal to 0.1. Some experimentation is usually needed to choose reasonable initial values. This is done by changing the initial values specified in initval and refitting the model, to see if a lower AIC can be obtained. Extreme choices of initial values can cause the model fitting procedure to fail completely.

To illustrate the impact of using different initial values, we refit the models for nicotine replacement therapy and myocardial infarction with 100 randomly chosen sets of initial values, each being specified using the uniform distribution on $[-2, 0.5]$. The R code is as follows:

```
set.seed(1234)
svs <- matrix(rep(0,400), ncol=4)
aic <- rep(0,100)
par <- matrix(rep(0,400), ncol=4)
for (i in 1:100){
    pi <- runif(4,-2,0.5)
    modi <- eventdepenobs(event~nrt, indiv=case, astart=nrt,
            aend=act, aevent=mi, adrug=nrt, aedrug=nrt+28,
            censor=cen, expogrp=c(0,8,15,22), agegr=NULL,
            data=nrtdat, initval=pi)
    svs[i,] <- pi
```

```
aic[i] <- min(modi$modelfit[2,1:4])
par[i,] <- modi$summary$conf.int[,1]
}
```

These 100 sets of initial parameters produce 8 'best' AIC values (to 2 decimal places):

```
> table(round(aic,2))
```

58.82	59.3	61.22	61.4	61.73	64.21	65.16	65.18
65	3	3	23	2	1	2	1

The lowest of these values is the most common, and was obtained in Section 7.2.2 with model **nrt.mod6** using the default initial values. In spite of the variation in 'best' AICs according to initial values, the relative incidences estimated from the corresponding SCCS models are very similar, as shown in Figure 7.18. The conclusion from this figure is that the SCCS model results

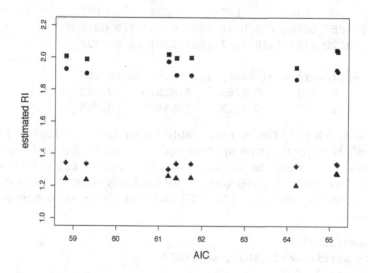

FIGURE 7.18
Relative incidences in successive periods after NRT initiation by AIC. Dots, 0–7 days; squares, 8–14 days; triangles, 15–21 days; diamonds, 22–28 days. Results obtained with 100 sets of randomly chosen initial values.

are not overly sensitive to the choice of initial values for the weight models. This figure was obtained using the following code.

```
par(mar=c(4.1,4.1,1,1), cex.lab=1.4)
plot(c(min(aic), max(aic)), c(1,2.2), type="n", xlab="AIC",
    ylab="estimated RI")
```

```
points(aic, par[,1], pch=19, cex=1.3)
points(aic, par[,2], pch=15, cex=1.3)
points(aic, par[,3], pch=17, cex=1.3)
points(aic, par[,4], pch=18, cex=1.6)
```

A similar conclusion may be drawn for the respiratory infections data of Section 7.2.3. Model mi.mod5 was specified using initval=rep(1.1,4) after a little experimentation. If we had used the same age groups but default initial values, the model would have been:

```
mi.mod6 <- eventdepenobs(event~rti+age, indiv=case, astart=sta,
           aend=end, aevent=mi, adrug=rti, aedrug=rti+14,
           expogrp=c(0,8), agegrp=ageq, censor=cen, data=midat)
```

This produces:

```
> mi.mod6
......
            EWA        EWI        EGA        EGI
Loglik -656.3878  -703.5649  -664.6195  -719.0211
AIC    1320.7757  1415.1297  1337.2391  1446.0421
......
       exp(coef) exp(-coef) lower .95 upper .95
rti1    6.3901     0.1565    4.8257     8.462
rti2    2.4223     0.4128    1.5460     3.795
```

The 'best' AIC is 1320.78, appreciably higher than the 1289.33 for model mi.mod5. However the exposure parameters of the SCCS model have changed only marginally from the previously obtained values rti1 = 6.45 and rti2 = 2.44. To obtain a broader picture, we randomly select 100 sets of starting values from the interval $[-1.25, 1.25]$ and refit the model for each of these selections:

```
set.seed(1234)
svs <- matrix(rep(0,400), ncol=4)
aic <- rep(0,100)
par <- matrix(rep(0,200), ncol=2)
for (i in 1:100){
    pi <- runif(4,-1.25,1.25)
    modi <- eventdepenobs(event~rti+age, indiv=case, astart=sta,
                aend=end, aevent=mi, adrug=rti, aedrug=rti+14,
                expogrp=c(0,8), agegr=ageq, censor=cen,
                data=midat, initval=pi)
    svs[i,] <- pi
    aic[i] <- min(modi$modelfit[2,1:4])
    par[i,] <- modi$summary$conf.int[1:2,1]
    }
```

This takes some time to run, eventually producing the following 'best' AIC values (rounded to integers):

```
> table(round(aic))

1289 1295 1306 1318 1321 1322 1415
  59   14    3   17    5    1    1
```

The lowest value is that obtained with model mi.mod5. However, the estimated exposure-related relative incidences vary very little, as shown in Figure 7.19. The implication of this figure is that results of the SCCS analysis are robust to the choice of initial values for the weight models.

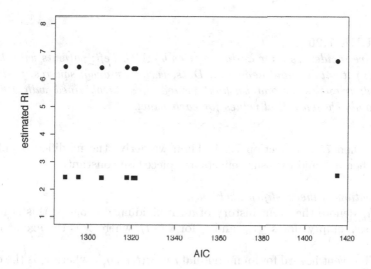

FIGURE 7.19

Relative incidences in successive periods after respiratory tract infections by AIC. Dots, 0–7 days; squares, 8–14 days. Results obtained with 100 sets of randomly chosen initial values.

Similar observations apply to the antipsychotics data, though the code to fit models with 100 random starting values, selected uniformly from $[-0.75, 1.75]$, takes appreciably longer to run. Figure 7.20 shows the parameter values for the 'best' AIC values obtained in this way. Again, there is little variation in parameter estimates for these models.

7.2.6   Adjusting for event-dependent observation periods*

In this section we first derive the modified SCCS likelihood contribution in

---

* This section may be skipped.

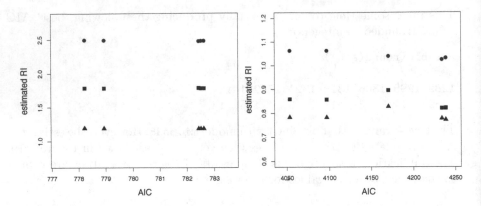

FIGURE 7.20

Relative incidences after antipsychotics by AIC. Left: patients with dementia. Right: patients without dementia. Dots, period on drug; squares, first washout period; triangles, second washout period. Results obtained with 100 sets of randomly chosen initial values for each panel.

Expression 7.12 of Section 7.2.1. Then we derive the modified likelihood for use when age and exposure effects are piecewise constant.

Derivation of the modified likelihood

Let h_i^s denote the event history of an individual i at age s; this is null (that is to say, empty) for $s \leq t_i$, and t_i for $s > t_i$, where t_i is the age at event for case i.

The event hazard for an individual i is $\lambda_i(t|x_i, \boldsymbol{y}_i)$, where x_i is the exposure history over $(a_i, b_i]$ (exposures are assumed not to be event-dependent up to the end of observation), and $\boldsymbol{y}_i$ is a vector of time-invariant covariates.

The censoring hazard function for an individual i is denoted $\mu_i(s|h_i^s, \boldsymbol{y}_i)$. This depends on the event history, and possibly also on the time-invariant covariates $\boldsymbol{y}_i$ which, without loss of generality, are the same as those for the event hazard. For a case i, if $s \leq t_i$, then since the event history h_i^s is null we write $\mu_i(s|h_i^s, \boldsymbol{y}_i) = \mu_i(s|\boldsymbol{y}_i)$. The censoring hazard is assumed not to depend on the exposure history x_i for individual i.

For ages s and t let $s \wedge t$ denote the minimum of s and t. Thus, we have $b_i = c_i \wedge b_i^*$.

We begin with an individual i within the underlying cohort. Let E_i denote the event indicator, equal to 1 if individual i experiences an event within the observation period $(a_i, b_i]$ and 0 otherwise; if $E_i = 0$ we nominally assume that the event age $t_i > b_i$. I_i is the censoring indicator defined in Equation 7.11 of

Section 7.2.1. The cohort likelihood contribution for individual i is

$$L_{ci}(t_i, b_i) = \lambda_i(t_i|x_i, \boldsymbol{y}_i)^{E_i} \exp\left(-\int_{a_i}^{t_i \wedge b_i} \lambda_i(s|x_i, \boldsymbol{y}_i)ds\right)$$

$$\times \mu_i(b_i|h_i^{b_i}, \boldsymbol{y}_i)^{I_i} \exp\left(-\int_{a_i}^{b_i} \mu_i(s|h_i^s, \boldsymbol{y}_i)ds\right).$$

We now condition on the actual observation period $(a_i, b_i]$ and the number of events n_i (0 or 1) within it. The conditional likelihood contribution for individual i is

$$L_i = \frac{L_{ci}(t_i, b_i)}{\int_{a_i}^{b_i} L_{ci}(t, b_i)dt}.$$

If $E_i = 0$, the conditional likelihood is the constant $(b_i - a_i)^{-1}$. Thus, as with the standard SCCS method, non-cases contribute no information and need not be sampled. If $E_i = 1$, the conditional likelihood contribution L_i is

$$\frac{\lambda_i(t_i|x_i, \boldsymbol{y}_i)\mu_i(b_i|t_i, \boldsymbol{y}_i)^{I_i} \exp\left(-\int_{a_i}^{t_i} \lambda_i(s|x_i, \boldsymbol{y}_i)ds - \int_{a_i}^{b_i} \mu_i(s|t_i, \boldsymbol{y}_i)ds\right)}{\int_{a_i}^{b_i} \lambda_i(t|x_i, \boldsymbol{y}_i)\mu_i(b_i|t, \boldsymbol{y}_i)^{I_i} \exp\left(-\int_{a_i}^{t} \lambda_i(s|x_i, \boldsymbol{y}_i)ds - \int_{a_i}^{b_i} \mu_i(s|t, \boldsymbol{y}_i)ds\right)dt}. \tag{7.13}$$

Since events are rare, we have

$$\exp\left(-\int_{a_i}^{t} \lambda_i(s|x_i, \boldsymbol{y}_i)ds\right) \simeq 1. \tag{7.14}$$

Also, if the age at event is t we may write

$$\int_{a_i}^{b_i} \mu_i(s|t, \boldsymbol{y}_i)ds = \int_{a_i}^{t} \mu_i(s|\boldsymbol{y}_i)ds + \int_{t}^{b_i} \mu_i(s|t, \boldsymbol{y}_i)ds. \tag{7.15}$$

Now define

$$\lambda_i^*(t|x_i, \boldsymbol{y}_i) = \lambda_i(t|x_i, \boldsymbol{y}_i) \exp\left(-\int_0^t \mu_i(s|\boldsymbol{y}_i)ds\right), \tag{7.16}$$

and

$$w_i(b_i|t, I_i, \boldsymbol{y}_i) = \mu_i(b_i|t, \boldsymbol{y}_i)^{I_i} \exp\left(-\int_t^{b_i} \mu_i(s|t, \boldsymbol{y}_i)ds\right). \tag{7.17}$$

Substituting Expressions 7.14 to 7.17 in Expression 7.13, noting that the constant terms $\exp(-\int_0^{a_i} \mu_i(s|\boldsymbol{y}_i)ds)$ cancel out, we obtain

$$L_i = \frac{\lambda_i^*(t_i|x_i, \boldsymbol{y}_i) \times w_i(b_i|t_i, I_i, \boldsymbol{y}_i)}{\int_{a_i}^{b_i} \lambda_i^*(t|x_i, \boldsymbol{y}_i) \times w_i(b_i|t, I_i, \boldsymbol{y}_i)dt}.$$

This is Expression 7.12, incorporating the time-invariant covariates $\boldsymbol{y}_i$. The weight function $w_i(b|t, I_i, \boldsymbol{y}_i)$ is the density of the censoring time b for individual i conditional on an event at t, defined on the truncated support $(t, b_i^*]$, with I_i the indicator for the event $b = b_i^*$.

Modified likelihood for piecewise constant effects

Assume now that the event hazard is piecewise constant on $J+1$ age periods indexed by $j = 0, \ldots, J$ and $K+1$ exposure periods indexed by $k = 0, \ldots, K$. Suppose that case i experiences n_{ijk} events in age period j, $j = 0, 1, \ldots, J$ and exposure period k, $k = 0, \ldots, K$. This is always 0 or 1 as $\sum_{j,k} n_{ijk} = 1$. The extended piecewise constant SCCS model is parameterised by J age-related parameters α_j^*, $j = 1, \ldots, J$ and K exposure-related parameters β_k, $k = 1, \ldots, K$. The α_j^* are starred solely to emphasise that they represent log relative age effects that take into account the thinning effect of censoring.

As for the standard SCCS model described in Chapter 4, Section 4.1, time-invariant multiplicative factors in $\lambda_i^*(t|x_i, \boldsymbol{y}_i)$ drop out of the likelihood, leaving the incidence kernel that depends on age and exposure parameters:

$$\nu_{ijk}^* = \exp(\alpha_j^* + \beta_k).$$

Let A_{ijk} denote the set of ages t for which case i is in age group j and exposure group k. Define

$$W_{ijk} = \int_{t \in A_{ijk}} w_i(b_i|t, I_i, \boldsymbol{y}_i)dt. \tag{7.18}$$

The W_{ijk} are constants that do not depend on the parameters to be estimated. The modified likelihood contribution for case i is then

$$L_i = \text{constant} \times \prod_{j,k} \left(\frac{\nu_{ijk}^* \times W_{ijk}}{\sum_{r,s} \nu_{irs}^* W_{irs}} \right)^{n_{ijk}}.$$

This is of exactly the same form as the standard SCCS likelihood, with $e_{ijk} = \text{length}(A_{ijk})$ replaced by W_{ijk}. Thus, once the weights W_{ijk} have been obtained, the model is fitted in the same was as the standard SCCS model, with the W_{ijk} in place of the e_{ijk}. These are accommodated using the offset terms $\log(W_{ijk})$.

7.2.7　Estimating the weights*

In this section we provide more detail on the method used for obtaining the weight functions $w_i(b_i|t_i, I_i, \boldsymbol{y_i})$. We shall assume that the functions are the same for all individuals, that is, $w_i \equiv w$ for all i. The case subscripts on b_i, t_i, I_i and $\boldsymbol{y}_i$ may occasionally be dropped, for greater clarity. The four parametric weight models for the censoring process used in the R function

---

* This section may be skipped.

eventdepenobs are described. Finally, we outline the procedure used for fitting these extended SCCS models.

Weight functions
The weight functions $w(b|t, I, \boldsymbol{y})$ may be obtained by maximum likelihood estimation of parametric densities $f(b|t, \boldsymbol{y}; \boldsymbol{\theta})$ on (t, ∞) for parameters $\boldsymbol{\theta}$. Here t is the age at event and $\boldsymbol{y}$ is a vector of time-invariant covariates. Given data $(b_i, t_i, I_i, \boldsymbol{y}_i)$ and a parametric model f, the likelihood contribution is

$$L_i^w(\theta) = f(b_i|t_i, \boldsymbol{y}_i; \boldsymbol{\theta})^{I_i} \times P(b > b_i|t_i, \boldsymbol{y}_i; \boldsymbol{\theta})^{1-I_i},$$

where

$$P(b > b_i|t_i, \boldsymbol{y}_i; \boldsymbol{\theta}) = 1 - \int_{t_i}^{b_i} f(x|t_i, \boldsymbol{y}_i; \boldsymbol{\theta})dx.$$

Maximisation of the likelihood $L^w = \prod_i L_i^w(\theta)$ yields maximum likelihood estimates $\hat{\theta}$. The estimated weight function for case i, as a function of t, is:

$$w(b_i|t, I_i, \boldsymbol{y}_i) = f(b_i|t, \boldsymbol{y}_i; \hat{\boldsymbol{\theta}})^{I_i} \times P(b > b_i|t, \boldsymbol{y}_i; \hat{\boldsymbol{\theta}})^{1-I_i}.$$

Weight models for the censoring process
The R function **eventdepenobs**, by default, fits four parametric weight models and selects the best fitting. We now describe these four models.

It is natural to think of the density of age at censoring c, given an event at age t, as the mixture of two components. The first component corresponds to the acute, short-term impact of the event at age t, and is formulated as a density for $c - t$. The second component reflects the underlying censoring process which may not depend on age at event t, or the longer term impact of an event at age t. Thus, a natural model for $f(c|t, \boldsymbol{y}; \boldsymbol{\theta})$ is

$$f(c|t, \boldsymbol{y}; \boldsymbol{\theta}) = \pi(t|\boldsymbol{y}; \boldsymbol{\theta})g(c - t|\boldsymbol{y}; \boldsymbol{\theta}) + \{1 - \pi(t|\boldsymbol{y}; \boldsymbol{\theta})\}h(c|t, \boldsymbol{y}; \boldsymbol{\theta}). \quad (7.19)$$

Here, π is a probability; g is a density on $(0, \infty)$, and h is a density on (t, ∞). We consider two versions of this model. In the age version, the second component models the absolute age at censoring c, and age at start of observation a is included among the time-independent covariates. In the interval version, the second component models the interval $c - t$. In the age version of the model, we have

$$h(c|t, \boldsymbol{y}) = \frac{h'(c|\boldsymbol{y})}{\int_t^\infty h'(u|\boldsymbol{y})du},$$

and in the interval version, we have

$$h(c|t, \boldsymbol{y}) = h'(c - t|\boldsymbol{y}),$$

for some density h' on $(0, \infty)$.

We now describe specific choices for the densities g and h' (and hence the age and interval versions of density h). The density g for the first component is exponential with (small) mean ρ. Thus,

$$g(x) = \rho^{-1} \exp(-x/\rho).$$

The densities h' for the second component are either gamma or Weibull, with location parameter θ and shape parameter η:

Gamma: $\quad h'(x) = \dfrac{\eta^\eta}{\Gamma(\eta)} \left(\dfrac{x}{\theta}\right)^{\eta-1} \exp(-\eta x/\theta),$

Weibull: $\quad h'(x) = \dfrac{\eta}{\theta} \left(\dfrac{x}{\theta}\right)^{\eta-1} \exp\left\{-(x/\theta)^\eta\right\}.$

These define four mixture models: the exponential–gamma (age) mixture model EGA, the exponential–gamma (interval) mixture model EGI, the exponential–Weibull (age) model EWA, and the exponential–Weibull (interval) model EWI.

Finally, we define regression models for the mixture probabilities π and the model parameters ρ, θ and η. We assume that the time-invariant covariate vector $\boldsymbol{y}$ includes a, the age at start of observation, and categorical covariates $\boldsymbol{z}$ specified in the `covariates` argument. As before, t is age at event. The analysis is thus stratified by the levels of the covariates $\boldsymbol{z}$.

For the age models EGA and EWA, the regression models are:

$$
\begin{aligned}
\text{logit}\{\pi(t, \boldsymbol{z})\} &= \pi_z + \gamma_z t, \\
\rho(\boldsymbol{z}) &= \rho_z, \\
\log\{\theta(a, \boldsymbol{z})\} &= \theta_z + \zeta_z a, \\
\log\{\eta(a, \boldsymbol{z})\} &= \eta_z + \xi_z a.
\end{aligned}
$$

For the interval models EGI and EWI, the regression models are:

$$
\begin{aligned}
\text{logit}\{\pi(t, \boldsymbol{z})\} &= \pi_z + \gamma_z t, \\
\rho(\boldsymbol{z}) &= \rho_z, \\
\log\{\theta(t, \boldsymbol{z})\} &= \theta_z + \zeta_z t, \\
\log\{\eta(t, \boldsymbol{z})\} &= \eta_z + \xi_z t.
\end{aligned}
$$

Fitting procedure

The default procedure used by R function `eventdepenobs` is as follows. In the first stage, the four weight models EGA, EGI, EWA and EWI are fitted, for user-specified covariates $\boldsymbol{z}$. The model with the smallest value of the AIC (Akaike information criterion) $-2 \log \hat{L}^w + 2p$, where $\hat{L}^w$ is the maximised likelihood and p is the number of estimated parameters, is chosen to estimate the weight functions. The weights W_{ijk} are obtained from Expression 7.18 by numerical integration. In the second stage, the SCCS model with piecewise constant age and exposure effects is fitted in much the same way as the standard SCCS model, with offsets $\log(W_{ijk})$.

Confidence intervals are obtained as for the standard SCCS model. Thus, no adjustment is made for the fact that the weights are estimated from the data. It turns out that the confidence intervals obtained in this manner are slightly conservative (that is, too wide), though the loss in efficiency is typically small. Further details are provided in Farrington et al. (2011).

Fitting mixture models by the method of maximum likelihood can be tricky owing to lack of identifiability of the parameters and convergence to local maxima. In consequence, results are often sensitive to the choice of initial parameter values for the weight models. In the present context, these difficulties are mitigated by the fact that our primary interest lies in the SCCS models based on weights obtained from the mixture models rather than in the mixture models themselves. Generally, an approximate fit is likely to be sufficient.

By default, the weight models in R function eventdepenobs do not include the regression terms: the regression parameters γ_z, ζ_z and ξ_z are set equal to zero. The regressions can be included by specifying regress=T. Unless the data are extensive, including the regressions is likely to compound any problems with parameter identifiability or convergence. The examples described in Sections 7.2.2 to 7.2.4 all used the default setting regress=F.

It is advisable to experiment with different initial parameter values. These are specified with initval. The default is initval=rep(0.1,4) when regress=F and initval=rep(0.1,7) when regress=T. The initial values are for the vector of parameters $(\log(\rho), \theta, \eta, \pi, \zeta, \xi, \gamma)$, in that order. When covariates are present, common initial values are used for the parameters corresponding to all covariates. The four weight models EGA, EGI, EWA and EWI use the same initial values. For the purpose of fitting the weight models, all times (and hence the dimensions of the location parameters) are in years (that is, days/365.25).

7.3 Deaths in SCCS studies

In this final section we discuss how to handle deaths in SCCS studies. Most of the section is devoted to SCCS studies in which death is the outcome event of interest. Before turning to this, we briefly recapitulate earlier material on how to handle censorship due to death.

When observation periods are censored at random (Kalbfleisch and Prentice, 2002, page 53) by death, then the SCCS method is valid without modification. This applies, for example, when deaths arise in a process unconnected with the outcome event of interest: observation periods are not event-dependent.

If, on the other hand, deaths are influenced by (but distinct from) the event of interest, then observation periods are event-dependent and the extension described in Section 7.2 may be required.

We now turn to the most extreme situation of all, in which deaths are the outcomes of interest.

7.3.1   Death as the outcome event

Death as the outcome event is tricky to handle in self-controlled case series analyses. The reason is that two key assumptions of the method are violated: deaths censor both exposure and observation, so that both exposures and observation periods are event-dependent. (There are exceptions, an example of which is described in Section 7.3.4.)

Nevertheless, in some circumstances it is possible to undertake a valid SCCS analysis when the outcome event of interest is death. However, three requirements need to be met. First, the deaths of interest must be rare in the study population over the observation period of interest, in the sense described in Chapter 5, Section 5.1. Second, the duration of the risk periods must be known once they begin, and must not be indefinite. And third, it must be possible to define a nominal end of observation for each case.

Suppose that the observation period for case i starts at a_i. By a nominal end of observation, we mean a pre-specified age b_i for case i such that, if the event (in our case, death due to the cause of interest) had arisen at any time in $(a_i, b_i]$, then that event would have been observed and thus case i would feature in our data set. Typically, nominal observation periods are defined using the age and calendar time boundaries specified for ascertaining cases, but there are other possibilities – for example, $b_i = a_i + \tau$ for some pre-specified value of τ.

The reason a nominal observation period must be specified is that the methods of Section 7.2 cannot be used to account for event-dependence of the observation period. This is because observation is censored at the event: conditioning on the actual observation period determines the event time. It follows that neither the standard SCCS likelihood nor the extension described in Section 7.2 can be used.

Instead, the SCCS analysis proceeds with observation period $(a_i, b_i]$ for each case i, where b_i is the nominal end of observation. This gets round the problem of event-dependence of the observation period, but not event-dependence of exposures. Thus, the methods of Section 7.1 must be used. In some cases, when there is at most a single exposure and observation starts at the age of exposure, a standard SCCS model may be applied. This latter model is in fact a special case of the extension described in Section 7.1. The two models will yield the same parameter estimates, though the standard errors and confidence intervals will generally differ, as the extension uses robust rather than likelihood-based standard errors.

Summary

- When the outcome event of interest is death, a SCCS analysis may be undertaken provided that a nominal end of observation can be defined for each case.

- A nominal end of observation for a case i observed from age a_i is a pre-specified age b_i such that, if death were to occur at any time in $(a_i, b_i]$, then that death would be ascertained and so case i would be included in the data set.

- Additional requirements are that deaths are rare in the population studied, and that risk period durations are known once they begin and are not indefinite.

- The analysis proceeds with the extension to the SCCS method for event-dependent exposures, applied with the nominal observation periods.

7.3.2   Bupropion and sudden death

Bupropion is a smoking cessation therapy which was launched in 2000 in the United Kingdom. In 2001, anecdotal press reports suggested that bupropion may be associated with an increase in the risk of sudden death. A SCCS study was undertaken using data from The Health Improvement Network. The observation period was specified to stretch from age at first bupropion prescription to age on 11th November 2003, the last day of data collection. There were 121 sudden deaths, including two in the risk period which was chosen to be 0–28 days after first bupropion prescription (the recommended duration of bupropion treatment). Note the use of a nominal age at end of observation, since for the 121 cases actual observation ended at event.

We illustrate the analysis using 121 cases simulated based on Hubbard et al. (2005b). These data are in data frame `bupdat`. Calendar time is expressed in days, with day 0 corresponding to 1st October 2000. Calendar time at first bupropion prescription is in variable `date`. Age at first bupropion prescription is in variable `bup`.

We begin by defining the start and end of observation. The start of observation is the age at first bupropion precription. The nominal end of the observation period is age on 11th November 2003, which is day 1136 counted from 1st October 2000 (day 0). Thus, we define:

```
bupdat$sta <- bupdat$bup
bupdat$end <- bupdat$sta + (1136 - bupdat$date)
```

The distribution of the dates at first bupropion prescription are obtained as follows.

```
par(mar=c(4.1,4.1,1,1), cex.lab=1.4)
hist(bupdat$date/365, breaks=seq(0.0833,2.9988,0.0833), xlab=
    "date at bupropion (years from 1 Oct 2000)", main=NULL)
```

This histogram is displayed in Figure 7.21. The drop in the number of bupro-

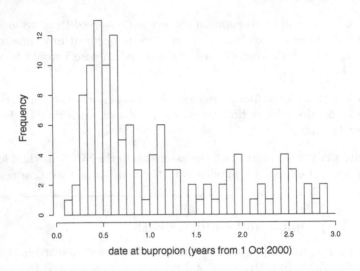

FIGURE 7.21
Date of first bupropion prescription (years from 1st October 2000).

pion prescriptions from mid-2001 reflects the impact of media reports of a
possible link between bupropion and sudden death.

Since we are using a nominal end of observation, the end of observation
is not event-dependent. And since the exposure of interest relates to the first
prescription of bupropion, and the observation period starts at the age of first
prescription, there are no subsequent exposures. Thus, exposure is not event-
dependent either. Finally, sudden deaths are uncommon. Thus, we may apply
the standard SCCS model, with risk period $[0, 28]$ days after first bupropion
prescription.

Before applying the model, we first check that exposure periods, which
coincide with the start of the observation period, are not clustered by age,
which would make it difficult to separate age and exposure effects. The nominal observation periods, and ages at death, are shown in Figure 7.22. The
starts of observation are spread across the age range, so it should be possible
to separate age and exposure effects. Figure 7.22 was obtained as follows:

```
par(mar=c(4.1,4.1,1,1), cex.lab=1.4)
os <- order(bupdat$sta)
plot(c(min(bupdat$sta/365.25),max(bupdat$end/365.25)), c(1,
```

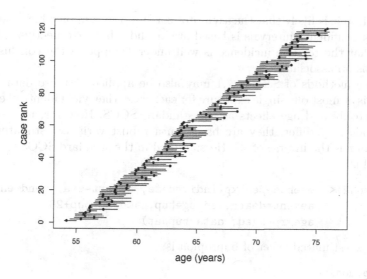

FIGURE 7.22
Nominal observation periods (line segments) and age at death (points) for bupropion data.

```
       length(bupdat$case)), type="n", xlab="age (years)",
       ylab="case rank")
segments(bupdat$sta[os]/365.25, bupdat$case,
         bupdat$end[os]/365.25, bupdat$case)
points(bupdat$death[os]/365.25, bupdat$case, pch=20)
```

We shall use 10 age groups determined by the 0.1-quantiles of age at death. The standard SCCS model is specified as follows:

```
ageq <- floor(quantile(bupdat$death,seq(0.1,0.9,0.1),names=F))
bup.mod1 <- standardsccs(event~bup+age, indiv=case, astart=sta,
            aend=end, aevent=death, adrug=bup, aedrug=bup+28,
            agegr=ageq, data=bupdat)
```

This yields the following results:

```
> bup.mod1
.....
      exp(coef) exp(-coef) lower .95 upper .95
bup1    0.2972    3.3652    0.07167     1.232
```

The relative incidence of sudden death in the 28-day period after first bupropion prescription is 0.30, with 95% CI (0.072, 1.23). Thus there is very little evidence of any positive association. There are only two events within the risk period, so it is likely that the asymptotic assumptions upon which the calculation of confidence intervals is based are invalid – but, irrespective of this, the fact that the relative incidence is well under 1 supports the conclusion that there is no association.

The methods of Section 7.1 may also be applied to these data. Because there is at most one single exposure for each case, they yield identical estimates of exposure and age effects as the standard SCCS. However, the confidence intervals may differ: they are based on a robust variance estimator, rather than minus the inverse of the Hessian used in the standard SCCS model. The model is

```
bup.mod2 <- eventdepenexp(indiv=case, astart=sta, aend=end,
             aevent=death, adrug=bup, aedrug=bup+28,
             agegrp=ageq, data=bupdat)
```

and the estimated effect of bupropion is

```
> bup.mod2
......
      exp(coef) exp(-coef) lower .95 upper .95
bup1    0.2972     3.3652   0.07370     1.198
```

As expected, the estimated relative incidence is the same as that obtained with the standard SCCS model, but the confidence interval differs slightly.

If unexposed cases had been included, the methods of Section 7.1 could be applied to all cases, including those with no bupropion prescription. Including unexposed cases in this way is recommended when age at event and age at exposure are highly correlated, which as shown in Figure 7.22 is not the case in the bupropion data set.

7.3.3   Hexavalent vaccines and sudden infant deaths

In 2000, two hexavalent vaccines were introduced in Germany, for administration at 2, 3 and 4 months of age with a booster dose after 11 months. The question soon arose as to whether these vaccines were associated with sudden deaths (von Kries et al., 2005). A case-control study was undertaken; the cases were also analysed using SCCS (Kuhnert et al., 2011, 2012). The data for the present example have been simulated based on this study.

The data, in data frame `siddat`, comprise 300 cases of sudden infant death syndrome (SIDS) occurring between the ages of 28 and 365 days of age. Age at death is in variable `sids`. Only the first three doses of hexavalent vaccine are included in the analysis; the ages at vaccination are in variables `hex`, `hexd2` and `hexd3`. Of the 300 SIDS cases, 180 received the first dose, 98 the second and 53 the third. The data are in format `multi`. The distribution of ages at hexavalent vaccination and SIDS are shown in Figure 7.23.

The age distribution of SIDS peaks around the age at which the first doses of hexavalent vaccine are administered. Because the events are deaths,

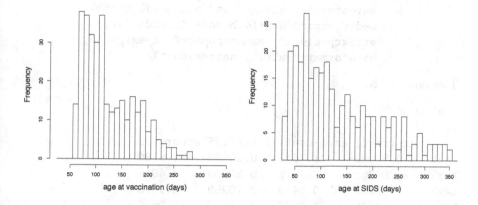

FIGURE 7.23
Left: age at hexavalent vaccination (three doses combined). Right: age at SIDS.

both observation and exposures are censored at the event. However, since all
cases under 365 days of age were sought, we may define the nominal end of
observation to be 365 days of age for each case. This gets round the problem
of event-dependent observation periods. We then apply the SCCS extension
for event-dependent exposures. We shall use 28-day age groups and the risk
periods 0–3 days and 4–14 days post-vaccination, at each dose.

First, we specify the model with a common parameter at each dose:

```
age <- seq(42,350,28)
sid.mod1 <- eventdepenexp(indiv=case, astart=sta, aend=end,
            aevent=sids, adrug=cbind(hex,hexd2,hexd3),
            aedrug=cbind(hex+14,hexd2+14,hexd3+14),
            expogrp=c(0,4), sameexpopar=T, agegrp=age,
            dataformat="multi", data=siddat)
```

This yields the following exposure parameters:

```
> sid.mod1
......
     exp(coef) exp(-coef) lower .95 upper .95
hex1   0.87387    1.1443    0.46890    1.6286
hex2   1.02598    0.9747    0.70022    1.5033
```

In the $[0, 3]$-day risk period, $RI = 0.87$ with 95% CI $(0.47, 1.63)$; in the $[4, 14]$-
day risk period, $RI = 1.03$, 95% CI $(0.70, 1.50)$. These results do not indicate
any evidence of association. In case they conceal a dose effect, we fit the model
with separate parameters at each dose using `sameexpopar=F`. This model is
specified as follows.

```
sid.mod2 <- eventdepenexp(indiv=case, astart=sta, aend=end,
```

```
        aevent=sids, adrug=cbind(hex,hexd2,hexd3),
        aedrug=cbind(hex+14,hexd2+14,hexd3+14),
        expogrp=c(0,4), sameexpopar=F, agegrp=age,
        dataformat="multi", data=siddat)
```

This now yields:

```
> sid.mod2
......
        exp(coef) exp(-coef) lower .95 upper .95
hex1     0.57089    1.7517    0.20646    1.5786
hex2     0.86363    1.1579    0.50006    1.4915
hex3     1.82228    0.5488    0.79258    4.1898
hex4     1.17572    0.8505    0.60907    2.2696
hex5     0.40665    2.4591    0.05544    2.9828
hex6     1.23234    0.8115    0.58215    2.6087
```

Parameters hex1 and hex2 are the relative incidences at dose 1, hex3 and hex4 are the RIs at dose 2, and hex5 and hex6 are those at dose 3. None are statistically significant: thus there is little evidence of a dose effect.

We conclude that the temporal association observed simply reflects the fact that SIDS tends to occur at the age at which hexavalent vaccines are administered; the data provide little evidence in support of a causal association.

7.3.4   Partner bereavement and death

In all the examples so far considered, exposure can only meaningfully be defined when the case is alive. In this elegant application of SCCS methodology, the event of interest is death, and the exposure is death of a partner (King et al., 2017). Thus, exposure is observed even after the case has died. Consequently, a standard SCCS analysis may be used, using nominal observation periods for each case. For this reason, we focus on the design of the study, rather than the analysis.

The study was undertaken within The Health Improvement Network database. Cases included persons who died aged 50 to 99 years during the period 2003 to 2014; these age and time boundaries, and dates on which GP practice data were available, were used to define nominal observation periods. Only cases living with a single adult of the opposite sex aged within 15 years of the case were included. Exposure was defined as death of the partner. The risk period included the 24 months after the death of the partner, subdivided in eight 3-month periods.

A pre-exposure risk interval of 24 months was also included, to mitigate the likely event-dependence of exposures. Note that, if the death of the case precipitates the death of the partner, the resulting bias will be to reduce the relative incidence.

Two separate SCCS analyses were undertaken: in male cases (death of the female partner being the exposure), and in female cases (death of the male partner being the exposure). The design is represented in Figure 7.24.

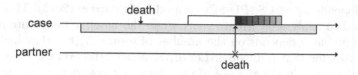

FIGURE 7.24
Definition of risk periods for study of death and partner bereavement.

Age was adjusted for in eight age groups. Supplementary analyses were undertaken by cause of death of the partner. The results indicated a positive association, highest in the first three months after death of the partner, and declining thereafter. For males (exposure being death of the female partner), the relative incidence was 1.63, 95% CI $(1.45, 1.83)$. For females (exposure being death of the male partner), the relative incidence was 1.70, 95% CI $(1.52, 1.90)$.

A key and unusual feature of this analysis is that the exposure is observed even after the case has died, though it might still be influenced by the death of the case. The benefit of the SCCS approach in this context is that fixed multiplicative confounders are automatically controlled, and hence the issues surrounding choice of suitable controls arising in other epidemiological designs are circumvented.

7.4 Bibliographical notes and further material

The extension of the SCCS method to event-dependent exposures was developed by Farrington et al. (2009). Further evaluation of the method is described in Hua et al. (2013). The extension is based on the theory of estimating equations, further details of which may be found in Jesus and Chandler (2011). The estimating equations were developed using counterfactuals. The use of counterfactuals in statistical inference is reviewed in Höfler (2005).

The SCCS method for event-dependent observation periods was proposed by Farrington et al. (2011). A related model, in a different context, was developed by Roy et al. (2006). Further details of the efficiency issues relating to the estimation of the weights is discussed in Rathouz (2004).

Analysis of deaths with SCCS for a single exposure using nominal end of observation was first used by Hubbard et al. (2005b). Kuhnert et al. (2011) extended this approach to multiple exposures, when there is a minimum known separation between successive exposures, as is the case with some multi-dose vaccines.

Other extensions of the SCCS model have been proposed. One is the positive dependence SCCS (PD-SCCS) model of Simpson (2013). This model can be used to analyse recurrent events when the baseline event rate at age t for an individual i depends on the number of events $N_i(t^-)$ that have occurred prior to t for that individual. Let $E_i(t)$ denote the event and exposure history at time t. In the absence of time-invariant covariates, the event rate for individual i is

$$\lambda_i(t|E_i(t)) = \{\phi_i + \delta N_i(t^-)\}\psi(t)\rho(t|x_i).$$

The parameter $\delta \geq 0$ controls the degree of positive dependence between successive events; the SCCS model is retrieved when $\delta = 0$. In this extension, events are no longer assumed to arise in a non-homogeneous Poisson process, but in a non-homogeneous pure birth process with immigration. The model may apply when occurrence of one event increases the chance of another, as with myocardial infarction.

A further extension to the SCCS model is the measurement error SCCS (MECS) model proposed by Mohammed et al. (2012). This model was developed in the context of a study of infection-associated cardiovascular events, in which the exact times of the infections (which in this application are the exposures) cannot accurately be ascertained, and are therefore subject to measurement error. The authors propose a bias-corrected estimation procedure. In Mohammed et al. (2013b) the same authors investigate the impact of measurement errors on hypothesis tests. They conclude that, when there is a single risk period, hypothesis tests that ignore the impact of measurement error are valid.

8

Design and presentation of SCCS studies

This final chapter is devoted to aspects of the design, efficiency, presentation and contextualisation of SCCS studies.

We begin in Section 8.1 by discussing some of the key choices that need to be made when designing a SCCS study. These include the primary time line, risk periods, observation periods, and age groups. Some of these choices are illustrated by examples in Section 8.1.5. In Section 8.1.6 we discuss a special SCCS design sometimes called the self-controlled risk interval design.

Section 8.2 is devoted to sample size and power calculations. The R package SCCS may be used to obtain nominal sample sizes with and without age effects, and to undertake simulations in more realistic scenarios. Sample size formulas are provided in Section 8.2.5 which is starred, and may be skipped.

In Section 8.3, we discuss the asymptotic efficiency and identifiability of the SCCS design. We compare the efficiencies of the SCCS method, the cohort method and the 1:1 matched case-control method. We also discuss how SCCS design features may impact upon its efficiency. The focus is practical; the theory is covered in Section 8.3.4 which is starred, and may be skipped.

In Section 8.4, we touch upon the presentation of SCCS studies. We show how to use the R package SCCS to obtain event counts and person-time, and discuss the presentation of results tables. We also review some of the graphs introduced in earlier chapters, which help to illustrate aspects of SCCS studies.

The final Section 8.5 is devoted to the wider contextualisation of SCCS studies. We discuss when, and how, measures of attribution including the attributable fraction, population attributable fraction, and attributable risk may validly be obtained in SCCS studies.

8.1 Choice of design

The very first step in designing a SCCS study is to choose the primary time line: the choice is usually age or calendar time. Next, the observation period and the risk periods must be specified. These choices should be motivated primarily by subject matter considerations relating to the scientific question of interest. However, they also have implications in terms of the efficiency of the SCCS design relative to other designs, which will be explored further in

Section 8.3. In most SCCS study designs it is also necessary to specify age groups or time periods, unless semiparametric or spline-based methods are to be used.

The requirement to specify the observation and risk periods is, of course, not unique to SCCS studies. Similar choices must be made when designing a cohort or case-control study, for example. However, because the SCCS method bases inference exclusively on the timings of events within individual observation periods, rather than marginal information (which is conditioned upon, and therefore is not used for estimation), it is particularly important to specify observation and risk periods appropriately.

8.1.1   The primary time line

The primary time line should generally be that most relevant to variation in event rates and exposures within individuals over the time scale of interest. In the majority of SCCS studies in pharmacoepidemiology, it is likely to be age rather than calendar time, since events and treatments within individuals are often strongly age-related. This is particularly relevant for childhood vaccines that are routinely administered according to an age-dependent schedule.

There are exceptions, in which calendar time is the most natural time line. In pharmacoepidemiology, these exceptions usually relate to events or exposures that arise seasonally. Examples, both relating to influenza vaccination, were described in Chapter 2, Section 2.3.2 and Chapter 4, Section 4.9.1. The environmental epidemiology applications of Chapter 6, Section 6.6, also used calendar time as the primary time line. In some circumstances, time dimensions other than age or calendar time, such as time since exposure, might be relevant.

Whichever primary time line is chosen, it is possible to adjust for variation on other time lines. Adjustment for seasonality in SCCS analyses in which age is the primary time line was discussed in Chapter 4, Section 4.9. Note also that SCCS analyses by age are insensitive to exponential calendar time trends, as was pointed out in Chapter 6, Section 6.1.1. Finally, cohort effects are time and age invariant, as they depend solely on the date of birth of each case. In consequence, they cannot be estimated within a SCCS proportional incidence model, as they factor out of the likelihood like other time-invariant multiplicative covariates.

Finally, the unit of time must be chosen. For the functions in R package SCCS, all times must be expressed as integers in these units. In virtually all the examples in this book, the time unit is one day, as events and exposures are usually recorded to the nearest day. However, there is no reason why, in other contexts (as in Chapter 6, Section 6.5.2), other units of time should not be chosen, provided that all times are expressed as integers in these units.

8.1.2 Risk periods

The choice of risk period, or periods, is usually based on a prior hypothesis relating to a potential association between the exposure and the event of interest, on prior data from other studies, or on an understanding of the underlying biological process. For applications in pharmacoepidemiology, such an understanding may relate to the pharmacodynamics of the pharmaceutical drug of interest.

If a point exposure is involved, as is the case with vaccination or initiation of therapy with a pharmaceutical drug, then risk periods are specified using time intervals from this point exposure. For some pharmaceutical drugs, the risk period may be defined as the time or times on drug. Several risk periods may be used, for example to capture the effects of initiation of treatment, followed by the longer term effect of the drug. Washout periods after the end of treatment may also be specified. If the event of interest is not acute, or if its onset is difficult to pinpoint, longer (possibly indefinite) risk periods should be used.

In specifying risk periods, it is important to distinguish between studies designed to test a specific hypothesis, and hypothesis-generating studies. In studies undertaken to test a specific hypothesis, for example to confirm results obtained elsewhere, it is important, if applying the methods described in this book, to choose the risk period a priori, rather than using the data to identify the most strongly associated interval. The reason is that basing the risk period on the data inflates the type I error probability, namely the probability that a statistically significant effect is found when in reality there is none, unless this effect is corrected using special statistical methods (see Section 8.6).

This is illustrated in Figure 8.1, which summarises the results of a simulation study in which there is no association between a point exposure and an event. In this simulation, all possible risk periods of durations 7 to 14 days wholly contained within a 30-day post-exposure period are investigated. Each point plotted is based on 500 runs of 500 cases.

The lower points (circles) represent the proportions of runs that yielded a statistically significant effect (that is, the 95% confidence interval for the relative incidence did not include 1) for the earliest post-exposure risk period $[0, r]$ for $r = 6, \ldots, 13$. The proportions vary between 3.2% and 6%, in line with the nominal type I error probability of 5%. The upper points (black dots) represent the proportion of runs in which a significant effect was found for at least one interval, when all possible intervals of that length were investigated. For example, when $r = 6$, the interval length is 7, and the 25 intervals $[0, 6], [1, 7], \ldots, [24, 30]$ are investigated. These proportions are much greater than 5%. The decline in these proportions as the risk period duration increases simply reflects the drop in the number of intervals investigated.

Figure 8.1 illustrates the perils of basing the choice of risk period on the data: even if there is no effect, a short interval close to the exposure can often be found in which there appears to be a statistically significant effect.

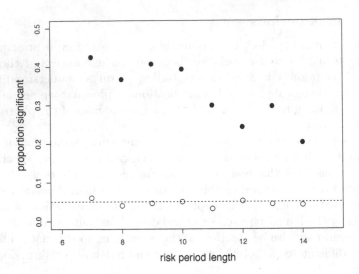

FIGURE 8.1
Proportion significant by length of risk period. Full dots: all intervals of that length investigated. Circles: first interval only. The dashed line is at 0.05.

In hypothesis-generating studies, on the other hand, a more relaxed approach to choosing the risk period may be taken, since the purpose is to develop a hypothesis relating to the presence or absence of an association, to be confirmed in other studies. Even so, it is seldom sensible to try all possible intervals. One approach is to use several contiguous risk periods, with the aim of exploring the shape of the relative incidence function. An alternative is to use the spline-based methods of Chapter 6, Section 6.3.

The choice of pre-exposure risk period, if one is required, is less of an issue as it is not the focus of inference. However, the choice can sometimes be guided by expert advice. For example, if the exposure of interest is vaccination and the event involves hospitalisation, the vaccination is unlikely to happen while the individual is in hospital. Thus, the pre-exposure risk period should be related to the typical duration of a hospital stay.

In the case of studies undertaken within databases of administrative or clinical records, account should be taken of the idiosyncracies of these databases. For example, in some databases, past events may be recorded when a patient's history is taken on the day of consultation, rather than attributed to times past. This can create entirely spurious associations if risk periods begin on the day of consultation. This particular problem can be handled by including a day of consultation effect in the SCCS model, or by excluding the day of consultation from the risk period.

8.1.3   Case ascertainment and observation periods

The specification of the observation period to be used in a SCCS study is governed by case ascertainment. In turn, this depends, first, on the substantive scientific question of interest (namely, the potential association between an exposure and an event, perhaps in a specific population) and, second, on the source of the data (for example, hospital or general practitioner records).

Typically, cases are ascertained subject to constraints on age and time within a specific database or other sampling frame. Assuming that the primary time line is age, the observation period for each case ascertained (with at least one event) is the age interval $(a_i, b_i]$ such that, if an event had occurred at any time in $(a_i, b_i]$, that event would have been captured by the case ascertainment process.

In the next few paragraphs we shall describe in more detail the three time lines (calendar time, age, and follow-up) that typically constrain case ascertainment and, in consequence, define individual observation periods. The Lexis diagram in Figure 8.2 shows the three time lines, to be discussed in the next paragraphs.

Calendar time constraints

Calendar time constraints are always present insofar as all events ascertained must have occurred prior to the time at which case ascertainment takes place – call this time P (for present). Other calendar time constraints may also be necessary or sensible.

For example, if the drug of interest comes into use at calendar time T_1, then in a study of that drug it may make sense to select only events occurring after time T_1. On the other hand, if it is required to include unexposed cases, because age and exposure effects are likely to be confounded (see the discussion in Chapter 4, Section 4.8.2, and Chapter 6, Section 6.2.4), then it may make sense to include events occurring before T_1. If it takes some time for events to be recorded on the database, it might be wise to halt ascertainment at some calendar time T_2 before P, the interval $P - T_2$ being chosen to ensure that most events targeted are recorded. Using a cut-off time $T_2 < P$ might also be sensible if events are ascertained at diagnosis, but retrospectively dated to the earlier appearance of first symptoms.

Even if there are no such constraints, for operational reasons it might make sense to restrict case ascertainment to some calendar time interval T_1 to T_2, where $T_1 < T_2 \leq P$. In Figure 8.2 calendar time is on the horizontal axis. The point P denotes the present time; events occurring outside the calendar time interval $[T_1, T_2]$ are excluded.

If the primary time line is age, then calendar times T_1 and T_2 must be converted to ages for the purpose of defining observation periods. If an individual was born at calendar time B_i, the calendar time constraints for this individual translate into ages $T_1 - B_i$ and $T_2 - B_i$.

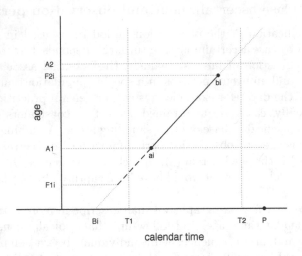

FIGURE 8.2
Lexis diagram showing calendar time, age and follow-up constraints on case
ascertainment for a case i with observation period $(a_i, b_i]$ (see text).

Age constraints
Age constraints on case ascertainment may be determined by the exposure of
interest, the event of interest, the population of interest, and the risk period
– and very likely a combination of all four.

For example, if the exposure is primary MMR vaccination and the event
of interest is convulsion, then the vaccine is administered in the second year
of life, the event is acute, and the post-vaccination risk period is relatively
short, so it makes sense to restrict the observation period to the second year
of life. To take another example, if the event of interest is hip fracture in
the elderly, one might restrict case ascertainment to hip fractures in persons
above a certain age, but with no upper limit. For some events, for example
Guillain–Barré syndrome, no age restriction might be imposed.

In general, age constraints are of the form A_1 to A_2, where A_1 is the lower
age and A_2 the upper age of case ascertainment (and A_2 might be left unspecified). In Figure 8.2, age is on the vertical axis. Events occurring at ages
outside the age interval $[A_1, A_2]$ are excluded.

Follow-up constraints
Follow-up constraints, as the name suggests, are constraints on the follow-
up time for each individual. These vary according to circumstance; several
may apply. Trivially, follow-up is constrained to include time between birth
and death (though in some SCCS analyses a nominal end of observation after
death is used – this is described in Chapter 7, Section 7.3).

However, there may be more meaningful constraints. If cases are ascertained within a particular database, then follow-up is constrained by the duration of each subject's record in the database. Thus, if an event is ascertained for a case i, the follow-up constraint for that case is the age interval F_{1i} to F_{2i}, where F_{1i} is the age at which the database record begins for case i and F_{2i} is the age at which the record ends (this may be the current age). In some instances, further restrictions might be imposed: for example, it might be required that a case has at least a year's event-free follow-up in the database before the first event; then F_{1i} corresponds to the start of the record plus one year. Finally, in some applications, cases are only ascertained from exposed subjects, with follow-up determined by age at exposure or start of exposure. Let E_i be the age at exposure for case i, and τ_1, τ_2 some pre-determined positive time intervals. The exposure-dependent follow-up is then F_{1i} to F_{2i} with $F_{1i} = E_i - \tau_1$ and $F_{2i} = E_i + \tau_2$.

In Figure 8.2, follow-up for case i is represented as the diagonal line starting at B_i (the date of birth). Events occurring outside the interval $[F_{1i}, F_{2i}]$ are excluded; the interval includes the thick dashed and full segments of the diagonal line.

Combining constraints

The calendar time, and age follow-up constraints are then combined to determine the observation period $(a_i, b_i]$ for each case i:

$$a_i = \max\{T_1 - B_i, A_1, F_{1i}\}, \quad b_i = \min\{T_2 - B_i, A_2, F_{2i}\}.$$

Thus, the observation period for case i comprises:

> *all times between calendar times T_1 and T_2*
> *that lie between ages A_1 and A_2*
> *and between follow-up age limits F_{1i} and F_{2i}.*

In Figure 8.2, the observation period for case i is represented by the full line segment on the diagonal follow-up time line; the endpoints at ages a_i and b_i are indicated by dots. For case i with this configuration, $a_i = A_1$ and $b_i = F_{2i}$.

The definition of the observation period ensures that, if an event for case i had arisen at any time within it, then the event would have been ascertained as it falls within all the time constraints used for ascertaining cases. In consequence, case i would have been ascertained whatever the timing of the event or events within the observation period.

It is worth reiterating that while it is acceptable for observation periods to be determined by age at exposure, they must not be determined by age at event, as this violates the assumptions of the method (see Chapter 3, Sections 3.7.3 and 3.7.4). Finally, while in mathematical terms we use the interval $(a_i, b_i]$ (which includes b_i but not a_i), in practice time and age are measured in discrete units, typically one day, and the first and last day of the observation period for each case are specified.

8.1.4 Age groups

For the standard SCCS model, age groups must be specified. This specification depends on the age profile of the event incidence function: typically, narrower intervals are required where the age-related incidence varies most. When possible, age groups can be determined a priori based on knowledge of the likely variation in incidence. Alternatively, they may be selected after the data have been assembled, using quantiles (rounded to integer values) of the ages at event. Such a data-dependent choice is acceptable since age effects are not usually the primary target of estimation.

Age effects may also reflect features of the case ascertainment process – for example, delays in ascertaining cases, or retrospective dating of events to the appearance of first symptoms. Such age-related effects will not introduce bias in the exposure-related relative incidence provided that the case ascertainment process is independent of exposure status. If any adjustment to event onset dates is to be made, this should ideally be undertaken blind to information on exposure.

When observation periods are short relative to the age range of the events, choosing a large number of age groups can produce unreliable or undefined age effects: this may occur, for example, when there are cases with disjoint – that is, non-overlapping – observation periods. Some of the age parameters may then not be identifiable. This does not usually affect the estimation of the exposure effect, but if required can usually be remedied by reducing the number of age groups.

8.1.5 Some examples of design choices

We illustrate contrasting SCCS designs with four examples from the literature.

Point exposures in a laboratory-based study: MMR vaccination and CSF-confirmed aseptic meningitis
This is the application that motivated the development of the SCCS method, described in Section 2.1 of Chapter 2. Prior to this study, cases of aseptic meningitis in temporal association with some MMR vaccines had been observed, albeit at a much lower rate than surveillance reports suggested in the United Kingdom.

Cases of aseptic meningitis confirmed by investigation of cerebrospinal fluid samples were obtained from five public health laboratories. Age at event was taken to be age at hospital admission. Based on earlier studies, such as Fujinaga et al. (1991), the risk period for aseptic meningitis was chosen to be 15 to 35 days after MMR vaccination, day 0 corresponding to the day of vaccination.

Each participating laboratory retrospectively ascertained all cases aged between 366 and 730 days of age inclusive arising between two calendar dates. These dates differed between laboratories: for example, for the Preston laboratory, admissions were sought between 1st April 1989 and 31st June 1992. The age range was chosen so as to capture most primary MMR vaccinations, for which the recommended age was 12 to 15 months, with some variation in practice.

MMR vaccination histories for the cases were obtained from local authority and general practitioner records. Note that, in view of the 15–35 day risk period, information on MMR vaccination was required from age $366-35 = 331$ days of age, to $730 - 15 = 715$ days of age, in order that each day within the second year of life could be classified as lying within the risk period or not.

The observation period for each case from a given laboratory began at the latest of age 366 days and age at the first day of case ascertainment for that laboratory, and ended on the earliest of age 730 days and age at the last day of case ascertainment for the laboratory. Thus, in this study, $A_1 = 366$ days and $A_2 = 730$ days; the calendar times T_1 and T_2 varied between laboratories; and no follow-up constraints were used.

The data are described in Miller et al. (1993). The SCCS analysis is reported in Farrington (1995), and used 4 quarterly age groups.

Drug initiation, time on drug and washout periods in a database study: antidepressants and hip fracture
This study, which was published in Hubbard et al. (2003), was undertaken to investigate an association between antidepressants and hip fractures that had been reported in several earlier studies. One of these, a case-control study, found that the association was strongest for new users of antidepressants, suggesting an increased risk associated with therapy initiation (Liu et al., 1998). The present study also contrasted tricyclic antidepressants and selective serotonin reuptake inhibitors, but noted the potential for bias due to channelling – a form of indication bias. This study was referred to in Section 2.3.2 of Chapter 2 and Section 4.3.3 of Chapter 4.

The SCCS study was designed in conjunction with a case-control study, both undertaken within the Clinical Practice Research Datalink (CPRD). Age was chosen as the primary time line, since the incidence of hip fracture varies substantially with age. The risk period was chosen to include all time on an antidepressant, starting at the first prescription and ending 31 days after the last prescription, this interval being chosen based on the median interval between successive prescriptions. To study the effect associated with initiation of antidepressants, the risk period was split into three intervals: the period 0–14 days after the first prescription (day 0 being the day of prescription), the period 15–42 days after first prescription, and the rest of the time on antidepressants. Since the end of treatment was estimated (based on durations of individual prescriptions) rather than known precisely, and to capture any residual effect after coming off treatment, two washout periods were used: 1–91 and 92–182 days after the end of treatment.

The observation period was defined as follows. There were no age restrictions: first recorded diagnoses of hip fractures or fractured neck of femur at any age were included. Thus, in this study, $A_1 = 0$ and $A_2 = \infty$. There were time restrictions: events were ascertained between specified dates in 1987 and 1999, which define the calendar time limits T_1 and T_2. Finally, the follow-up constraint was available time within the CPRD database, so for a case i, $F_{1i} =$ age at start of CPRD record, and $F_{2i} =$ age at end of CPRD record. Ages were grouped in 1-year bands.

Multiple exposures in a database study: NSAIDs, antidepressants and gastro-intestinal bleeds

The Health Improvement Network (THIN) is a database of computerised medical records from general practices (GPs) across England and Wales. In the present study, data from THIN were used to investigate the association between antidepressants and gastro-intestinal bleeds, and their possible interaction with non-steroidal anti-inflammatory drugs (NSAIDs). The data from Chapter 4, Section 4.5.2 were based on this study. The authors used a case-control design, supplemented by a SCCS study based on the same cases.

Age is the most relevant time line in this context. As the primary interest lay in the possible interaction between antidepressants and NSAIDs, risk periods were defined as treatment episodes with either drug. (Where the end of treatment was not specified explicitly, it was imputed as 30 days from the last prescription.) Thus, each case could have several risk periods for each drug, and the risk periods typically varied in duration.

Case ascertainment, and hence the observation period for each case, was determined as follows. All instances of first gastro-intestinal bleed were identified between 1st January 1990 and 1st November 2003, which define the calendar time limits T_1 and T_2. Only events occurring at age 18 years or later were included: thus $A_1 = 6575$ days of age (this is 18×365.25, rounded up); there was no upper age limit, so $A_2 = \infty$. In order to ensure that events were indeed first bleeds, and to obtain full information on exposures (the start of which may have predated the start of observation), each case was required to have been registered with the participating GP for at least 6 months. Thus the follow-up constraints were as follows for each case i: $F_{1i} =$ age at start of THIN record plus 183 days, and $F_{2i} =$ age at end of THIN record.

Observation periods completely determined by the exposure: antibiotics and pregnancy

Two of the examples so far described have used follow-up constraints based on database records. It is perfectly valid to define observation periods using follow-up constraints determined by exposures. Nor is it strictly necessary for the observation period to be an interval of age or time: it could comprise several disjoint intervals.

An example with both these features is the study of antibiotics and pregnancy by Petersen et al. (2010). In this study, a woman is regarded as exposed during pregnancy, and the events of interest are antibiotic prescriptions. The observation period is defined to include, as well as the period of pregnancy, two control periods of the same duration, starting exactly one year before and one year after the start of the pregnancy. Figure 8.3 illustrates the design.

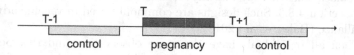

FIGURE 8.3
Observation and risk periods for the antibiotics and pregnancy study. The pregnancy risk period begins at calendar time T years. The two control periods begin 1 year before and 1 year after T. All three periods last 9 months.

The observation period thus comprises three disjoint intervals of approximately 9 months. The reason for choosing control periods starting exactly one year before and one year after the start of the pregnancy is to control for any seasonal effects that might be associated with the prescription of antibiotics: such effects have thus been designed out. The alternative would have been to adjust for them explicitly in the SCCS model using seasonal factors.

In this study, the events are antibiotic prescription episodes (of different types), ascertained in the THIN database described in the previous example. If a woman had several pregnancies, one was chosen at random. Every pregnant woman with at least one antibiotic prescription during her observation period was included in the study. The only further constraints on ascertainment were to include only women who were not pregnant at any time within the two control periods, and who were registered with their GP for their entire observation period. Thus, in this design, effective age and calendar time constraints are not used (so $A_1 = 0$, $A_2 = \infty$, $T_1 = -\infty$, $T_2 = P$) and the observation periods are determined solely by constraints on follow-up determined by pregnancy and duration of registration with the GP in the THIN database.

Calendar time is perhaps the most relevant primary time line, though the fact that seasonal effects are controlled for by design removes the need to allow for them explicitly. Secular changes in prescribing practice could be adjusted for, though they are perhaps unlikely to be detectable on a 3-year timescale (similarly with age effects). It is also sensible to distinguish between pre-exposure and post-exposure control periods in the analysis. Designs of this type have sometimes been called self-controlled risk interval studies. These are discussed further in Section 8.1.6.

8.1.6 Self-controlled risk interval designs

SCCS designs with short observation periods determined by a point exposure, in which all cases share the same risk and control periods, have also been called self-controlled risk interval designs. In such studies, age effects are usually assumed to be ignorable. The study of antibiotics and pregnancy described in Section 8.1.5 is of this type. Another example is the study of nicotine replacement therapy and myocardial infarction first described in Chapter 4, Section 4.8.3. Such designs are commonly used in vaccine adverse event surveillance (Baker et al., 2015).

When all individuals have the same observation and risk periods, and age effects are ignored, then the maximum likelihood estimator of the relative incidence is the same whether or not the analysis is conditional on the number of events experienced by each case. It follows that, as far as inference on the log relative incidence β is concerned, it matters not whether the study is restricted to cases: in this respect, cohort and self-controlled designs yield the same inferences, though of course cohort designs also allow absolute rates to be estimated.

This is because, in these circumstances, the cohort and SCCS (or self-controlled risk interval) designs share the same estimator of the relative incidence. Provided that events arise in a Poisson process and that the exposure effect is multiplicative, these designs are all self-matched in the sense that time-invariant confounders do not affect the relative incidence.

The reason is as follows. Suppose each individual in a cohort of M exposed subjects has a control period of duration e_0 and a single risk period of duration e_1. The total Poisson event rate in the control period is λe_0, where

$$\lambda = \sum_{i=1}^{M} \lambda_i$$

is the sum of the individual event rates λ_i in the absence of exposure. In the risk period, the total event rate is $e^{\beta} \lambda e_1$, where e_1 is the duration of the risk period.

If N events arise in the cohort, of which N_0 are in the control period and N_1 in the risk period, the maximum likelihood estimator of the relative incidence, obtained from the Poisson cohort likelihood, is

$$e^{\hat{\beta}} = \frac{N_1 \times e_0}{N_0 \times e_1}$$

which only involves the N events. This is identical to the maximum likelihood estimator obtained from the SCCS analysis based only on cases.

Furthermore, the cohort variance of $\hat{\beta}$ is

$$\text{var}_{\text{cohort}}(\hat{\beta}) = \frac{e_0 + e^{\beta} e_1}{\lambda e_0 e^{\beta} e_1},$$

and the SCCS variance of $\hat{\beta}$ is

$$\text{var}_{\text{SCCS}}(\hat{\beta}) = \frac{(e_0 + e^{\beta} e_1)^2}{N e_0 e^{\beta} e_1}.$$

But since, in the cohort model, the mle $\hat{\lambda} = N(e_0 + e^{\hat{\beta}}e_1)^{-1}$, the estimated cohort variance reduces to that of the SCCS method:

$$\text{vâr}_{\text{cohort}}(\hat{\beta}) = \text{vâr}_{\text{SCCS}}(\hat{\beta}).$$

Thus, the cohort and SCCS designs result in exactly the same inference on β. The same conclusion holds (with different expressions for the variance from those in the above equations) if there are several risk periods.

The assumption that exposures must not be event-dependent remains relevant to these designs. For this reason it might be sensible to exclude times immediately preceding the exposure from the control period. Note also that using a short control period adjacent to the risk period may be more prone to misclassification bias resulting from an incorrect specification of the risk period than would arise with longer control periods. This can be mitigated by inserting a washout interval between the risk and control periods.

Although age is assumed not to affect the incidence over the short observation periods used, age homogeneity of the relative incidence may still be investigated. This is achieved by including in the model an interaction between the exposure effect and age at exposure, and testing this interaction using a likelihood ratio test. Some further issues relating to the interpretation of relative incidences estimated in self-controlled risk interval studies in which the control period always follows the risk period are discussed in Section 8.3.3.

Summary

- Designing a SCCS study requires the primary time line of analysis, the risk periods, and the observation periods to be defined.

- In hypothesis-testing studies, data-dependent choice of the risk period should be avoided.

- Defining observation periods will in general depend on a combination of calendar time, age, and follow-up constraints.

- Age categories should reflect the age distribution of events.

- Self-controlled risk interval designs are SCCS studies with observation periods defined in relation to exposure, in which cases share the same risk and control periods. Typically, observation periods are brief and age effects are ignored.

8.2 Sample size and power

Self-controlled case series studies are usually observational, and consequently formal sample size and power calculations are not as central to the study design as for controlled clinical trials. However, such calculations can be useful when several design options are contemplated, especially when dealing with uncommon events for which the number of cases available for study is likely to be small.

In the context of SCCS studies, the sample size is the number of events. This may or may not be the same as the number of cases, depending on whether cases experience more than one event. The sample size calculation aims to estimate the sample size required to detect a specified design value of the relative incidence associated with exposure, for a given significance level and power. These quantities are defined in terms of the null hypothesis that there is no effect associated with exposure, that is, that the relative incidence is 1. The significance level is the probability that the null hypothesis is rejected when it is true; the power is the probability that the null hypothesis is rejected when the relative incidence equals the design value.

In a SCCS study, the sample size required depends on the significance level, the design value of the relative incidence, and the power required for that design value. It also depends on the relative durations of the risk period and the observation period, and on the proportion of individuals exposed in the population. Finally, it is influenced by the distribution of the risk periods within the observation period, and by the age effects. The formula used to obtain the sample size is approximate: in particular it relies on asymptotic approximations that ignore the fact that event counts in risk and other periods are discrete.

The R package SCCS contains two functions relevant to sample size and power calculations. Function samplesize calculates the sample size for given design parameters. Examples of the use of this function, and the assumptions required, are described in Sections 8.2.1 and 8.2.3. The sample size formula underpinning this function is based on the likelihood ratio test. Further details of this formula and its derivation are given in Section 8.2.5, which is starred and may be skipped.

The second function is simulatesccsdata. This function creates a simulated SCCS data set with given design parameters, and can be used to generate cases with observation and risk periods of different durations, multiple risk periods, repeated exposures, and washout periods. This facility is useful for investigating more realistic scenarios. In Sections 8.2.2 and 8.2.4, simulations are used to obtain the empirical power for a given design.

Summary

- In a SCCS study, the sample size is the number of events rather than the number of cases.

- The sample size required for a given design value of the relative incidence depends on the significance level, the design value of the relative incidence, and the power sought for this design value.

- The sample size also depends on the relative durations of the risk and observation periods, and on the proportion of individuals exposed in the population. It is influenced by the distribution of the risk periods and the age effects.

- An approximate value of the sample size required may be obtained using a sample size formula. Specific designs may be evaluated by simulation.

8.2.1 Estimating the sample size: no age effects

In this section we consider sample size calculations ignoring any age effects that may affect the distributions of exposures or events. We illustrate the use of R function `samplesize` in such a setting.

In this example, it is required to estimate the sample size for a study of MMR vaccine, with observation period nominally including the second year of life, that is, days 366 to 730 of age inclusive. The risk period is 15–35 days after MMR vaccination: a duration of 21 days. The significance level is the conventional value $\alpha = 0.05$.

We seek 80% power for a design value of the relative incidence of 2.5. Suppose first that only vaccinated cases are to be sampled, so that the proportion exposed in the target population is 1. The required sample size is computed as follows:

```
ss1 <- samplesize(eexpo=2.5, risk=21, astart=366, aend=730,
    p=1, alpha=0.05, power=0.8)
```

Here, `eexpo` is the design value of the relative incidence; `risk` is the duration of the risk period, `p` is the proportion vaccinated in the target population, `alpha` is the significance level, and `power` is the power required. This yields:

```
> ss1
[1] 110
```

Thus, the sample of vaccinated cases must include 110 events. To estimate how many events are required when their vaccination status is not known in advance, we need information about MMR vaccine coverage in the second year of life. Suppose that it is 75%. The sample size required is then obtained by specifying `p = 0.75`:

```
ss2 <- samplesize(eexpo=2.5, risk=21, astart=366, aend=730,
       p=0.75, alpha=0.05, power=0.8)
```

This yields:

```
> ss2
[1] 143
```

Thus, the sample of cases (vaccinated or unvaccinated) should include 143 events. Note that $110/143 \simeq 0.77$ rather than 0.75: vaccinees are slightly over-represented among cases, owing to the positive association between vaccination and the event.

When the proportion exposed in the population is not known with any degree of accuracy, it is usually best to plan the study based on the sample size of events in exposed cases, and take steps to recruit the appropriate number of exposed cases.

It is good practice to estimate sample sizes for a range of design parameters, to assess the sensitivity of the design to variation in these parameters. For illustration, suppose that, in the MMR vaccine example, sample sizes are sought for design values of the relative incidence in the range 1.5(0.5)3.5, and for powers in the range 75(5)95%. Rather than calculating the 25 sample sizes individually, a rudimentary sample size table may be obtained as follows (with $p = 1$).

```
ri <- c(1.5,2.0,2.5,3.0,3.5)
po <- c(0.75,0.8,0.85,0.9,0.95)
m <- cbind(rep(ri,length(po)), rep(po,each=length(ri)))
ssfun1 <- function(x){
          samplesize(eexpo=x[1], risk=21, astart=366, aend=730,
          p=1, alpha=0.05, power=x[2])}
ssm1 <- matrix(apply(m,MARGIN=1,FUN=ssfun1), nrow=length(po),
          byrow=T, dimnames=list(po,ri))
```

This yields:

```
> ssm1
       1.5    2 2.5    3 3.5
0.75   633  187  96   61  44
0.8    719  213 110   70  50
0.85   826  246 127   81  58
0.9    972  291 150   96  69
0.95  1211  363 188  120  87
```

The top row gives the five design values of the relative incidence; the first column the five powers. Thus, if the design value of the relative incidence is 2, a sample size of 213 events in vaccinated cases is required for 80% power, rather than the 110 required with design value 2.5.

8.2.2 Power assessment by simulation

The power associated with a given study design may be assessed by simulation using the R function `simulatesccsdata`. This function creates a simulated data frame from specified inputs. For example, continuing the MMR vaccine example of Section 8.2.1, suppose we wish to simulate a data set comprising 110 events in 110 cases who have received MMR vaccine, with risk period duration 21 days and design value `eexpo=2.5`. In the following example, the observation period for each case is $[366, 730]$ days and the start of the risk period is uniformly distributed within the observation periods. There are no age effects; simulations including age effects are discussed in Section 8.2.4.

```
set.seed(1234)
arisk <- round(runif(110,366,730))
simdata <- simulatesccsdata(nindivs=110, astart=366, aend=730,
             adrug=arisk, aedrug=arisk+20, eexpo=2.5)
```

This creates a simulated data frame `simdata` with 110 rows (one event per row) and the following columns:

```
> simdata
  indiv astart adrug1 aedrug1 aend aevent
1     1    366    407     427  730    553
2     2    366    593     613  730    725
3     3    366    588     608  730    419
4     4    366    593     613  730    605
5     5    366    679     699  730    603
6     6    366    599     619  730    527
......
```

The function `simulatesccsdata` also accepts vectors as inputs for `astart` and `aend`, thus allowing observation periods of different durations.

This simulation facility can be used to evaluate the power of a design. This is done by simulating a large number of data sets with this design, analysing each one with the SCCS method, and counting the proportion of data sets that yield a statistically significant result.

For illustration, we evaluate the power of the proposed study of MMR vaccine with design value `eexpo=2.5`. The estimated sample size is 110, there are no age effects, and the risk period duration is 21 days for each case. For definiteness we assume each case has the same risk period $[457, 477]$ days (as there are no age effects, this choice makes no difference to the results). Statistical significance is assessed using the 95% confidence interval for the relative incidence from the SCCS model, fitted without any age effects. For 1000 simulations, the required code is as follows.

```
set.seed(1234)
rilim <- rep(0,1000)
for (i in 1:1000){
```

```
simdati <- simulatesccsdata(nindivs=110, astart=366, aend=730,
          adrug=457, aedrug=477, eexpo=2.5)
sim.modi <- standardsccs(event~adrug1, indiv=indiv,
            astart=astart, aend=aend, adrug=adrug1,
            aedrug=aedrug1, aevent=aevent, data=simdati)
rilim[i] <- sim.modi$conf.int[1,3]
}
```

The vector `rilim` contains the lower 95% confidence limits for the relative incidences obtained from the SCCS model (without age adjustment) fitted to each of 1000 simulated data sets. The empirical power is then obtained as follows:

```
> sum(rilim>1)/1000
[1] 0.793
```

The simulated power is thus 79.3%, only marginally lower than the value of 80% specified in the sample size calculation. This power estimate is subject to Monte Carlo variation. The Monte Carlo (MC) standard error for a simulated probability p based on R replicates is $\sqrt{p*(1-p)/R}$. Thus, in this case the MC standard error is

$$\sqrt{\frac{0.793 \times (1 - 0.793)}{1000}} = 0.013.$$

The simulated power should be quoted as 79.3% (MC error 1.3%). The MC standard error reduces as the number of replicates increases; with 10 000, the simulated power is 79.8% (MC error 0.4%).

Using the lower 95% confidence limit of the relative incidence to calculate the power is, in effect, to use a 1-tailed hypothesis test. The corresponding 2-tailed test would also consider the proportion of 95% confidence intervals with upper limit less than 1. However, when the true relative incidence is 2.5 this proportion is close to zero, so ignoring it does not materially affect the power. We shall briefly return to the issue of 1-tailed and 2-tailed hypothesis tests in Section 8.2.4.

Sample size calculations are only ever approximate, especially when the sample sizes produced are not large. This is because the sample size formula relies on asymptotic approximations. In particular, the formula makes no allowance for the fact that the numbers of events occurring in and outside the risk period are discrete. Figure 8.4 shows the true relationship between sample size and power, assessed by simulation, and the relationship obtained using the sample size formula. The stepped line obtained using the sample size formula is non-decreasing: as the sample size increases, so does the power. In reality, however, the power to sample size relationship is one of steady increases interrupted by sudden drops. This is revealed by the sawtooth pattern of the points in Figure 8.4. Each point was obtained by simulation with 10 000 replicates using the code previously described, with values of `nindivs` ranging from 85 to 135.

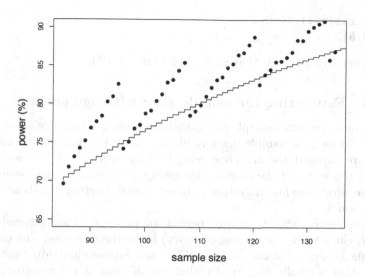

FIGURE 8.4
Power to sample size relationships for MMR study. Stepped line: obtained using sample size formula. Points: obtained by simulation.

It is sometimes possible to incorporate a continuity correction in sample size formulas to mitigate this effect. The alternative (espoused here) is to use the sample size formula as a guide, to be refined by simulation. An advantage of simulations is that greater realism can be introduced. Thus, for the MMR example, we can allow the risk period to start at any time in the interval [366, 730], and also fit the SCCS model with an adjustment for age. In the following code, quarterly age groups are used.

```
set.seed(1234)
ageg <- c(457,548,639)
rilim <- rep(0,1000)
for (i in 1:1000){
arisk <- round(runif(110,366,730))
simdati <- simulatesccsdata(nindivs=110, astart=366, aend=730,
            adrug=arisk, aedrug=arisk+20, eexpo=2.5)
sim.modi <- standardsccs(event~adrug1+age, indiv=indiv,
            astart=astart, aend=aend, adrug=adrug1,
            aedrug=aedrug1, aevent=aevent, agegrp=ageg,
            data=simdati)
rilim[i] <- sim.modi$conf.int[1,3]
}
```

Note that the simulations do not incorporate any age effects, even though the fitted SCCS models do. This now yields:

```
> sum(rilim>1)/1000
[1] 0.812
```

The simulated power is thus 81.2% (MC error 1.3%).

8.2.3 Estimating the sample size: with age effects

To be more realistic, sample size calculations should take age effects into account. To keep the sample size formula manageable, some restrictive assumptions are imposed, the main one being that the risk period duration must not exceed the width of the shortest age group. Furthermore, it is assumed that the age effects are known, rather than estimated. Further details are provided in Section 8.2.5.

Suppose that the observation period comprises $J+1$ age intervals labelled 0 to J, category 0 (the earliest category) being the reference. The sample size formula assumes that the risk period for each exposed individual in the target population is wholly contained within one of these $J + 1$ age groups. Let p_j denote the proportion of the target population exposed in age group j. Then

$$p = \sum_{j=0}^{J} p_j$$

is the proportion of the target population who are exposed. Also, let $\exp(\alpha_j)$ denote the age-specific relative incidence in age group j, relative to age group 0, with $\exp(\alpha_0) = 1$.

The sample size formula requires the age groups, the p_j, and the $\exp(\alpha_j)$ (for $j = 1, \ldots, J$) to be specified.

We illustrate the calculation of sample sizes with age effects using the example on MMR vaccine. To begin with, we assume that the target population comprises only vaccinated individuals whose risk period is in the second year of life. We shall use quarterly age groups specified by the cutpoints 457, 548, 639 days using `agegrp=c(457,548,639)`.

Next, we specify the proportions exposed in each age group within the target population. Most children are vaccinated in the first quarter; we shall use the distribution specified as follows: `p=c(0.50,0.35,0.1,0.05)`. This means that 50% of the target population are vaccinated in the first quarter, 35% in the second, 10% in the third, and 5% in the fourth. These proportions sum to 100%, in line with our assumption that the target population comprises individuals vaccinated in the second year of life.

Finally, we specify the effects of age on the event incidence. The first age group is taken as reference, with relative incidence 1. Suppose that the incidence increases with age; we enter `eage=c(1.2,1.6,2.0)`. This means that the age-specific relative incidence, relative to the first age group, is 1.2 for the second age group, 1.6 for the third and 2.0 for the fourth. The code required is as follows.

```
ss3 <- samplesize(eexpo=2.5, risk=21, astart=366, aend=730,
       p=c(0.50,0.35,0.1,0.05), alpha=0.05, power=0.8,
       eage=c(1.2,1.6,2.0), agegrp=c(457,548,639))
```

This yields the following sample size:

```
> ss3
[1] 132
```

The sample size required is 132 events among exposed cases. This is greater than the sample size 110 required when there were no age effects. The increase is due to the negative correlation between age at vaccination and age at event.

Different age distributions will have different impacts on the sample size. For example, suppose that the incidence of the event of interest declines during the second year of life, with `eage=c(0.8,0.6,0.5)`. The sample size is then specified as follows:

```
ss4 <- samplesize(eexpo=2.5, risk=21, astart=366, aend=730,
       p=c(0.50,0.35,0.1,0.05), alpha=0.05, power=0.8,
       eage=c(0.8,0.6,0.5), agegrp=c(457,548,639))
```

This yields:

```
> ss4
[1] 95
```

The required sample size is now 95, which is less than the sample size 110 required without age effects.

The sample sizes so far calculated in this section have been obtained for a target population including only individuals exposed in the second year of life. Suppose now that we wish to sample from the entire population, in which the proportion vaccinated within the second year of life is 0.75. We now specify `p=0.75*c(0.50,0.35,0.1,0.05)`:

```
ss5 <- samplesize(eexpo=2.5, risk=21, astart=366, aend=730,
       p=0.75*c(0.50,0.35,0.1,0.05), alpha=0.05, power=0.8,
       eage=c(1.2,1.6,2.0), agegrp=c(457,548,639))
```

This yields the following sample size:

```
> ss5
[1] 172
```

This is the number of events required among cases sampled from a target population including both vaccinated and unvaccinated individuals. It contrasts with the sample size 143 required without age effects, for a target population in which 75% of individuals are vaccinated in the second year of life.

8.2.4   Simulated power with age effects present

The R function `simulatesccsdata` can readily incorporate age effects, affecting both the distribution of exposures and the distribution of events. We illustrate these features again using the MMR vaccination example. Specifically, we base the simulations on the sample size 132 events obtained in Section 8.2.3 with quarterly age groups, `p=c(0.50,0.35,0.1,0.05)` and `eage=c(1.2,1.6,2.0)`.

One purpose of using a simulation is to achieve greater realism, so we shall use more realistic distributions than those used to obtain the sample size. We shall base the distribution of risk periods on a scaled and shifted beta density with parameters $\alpha = 2, \beta = 4$. One realisation is shown in the left panel of Figure 8.5. The panel on the right shows two choices for the age effect,

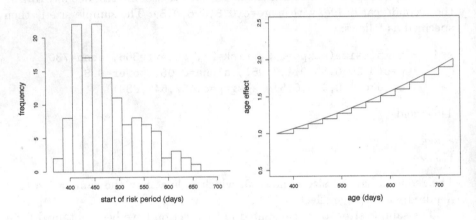

FIGURE 8.5
Left: a sample of 132 risk interval starts simulated using a scaled and shifted beta density. Right: continuous curve and step function representing the age effect.

which increase from 1 to 2 over the observation period. The step function uses roughly monthly age groups; the continuous curve is exponential. Figure 8.5 was obtained as follows.

```
age <- 366:730
agegp <- c(366, seq(401,731,30))
eagec <- exp((age-366)*log(2)/(730-366))
eageg <- exp((agegp-366)*log(2)/(731-366))
set.seed(1234)
arisk <- round(366+364*rbeta(132,2,4))
par(mfrow=c(1,2), mar=c(4.1,4.1,1,1), cex.lab=1.4)
hist(arisk, main=NULL, xlab="start of risk period (days)",
    ylab="frequency", breaks=seq(366,730,20))
```

```
plot(age, eagec, type="l", xlim=c(366,730), ylim=c(0.5,2.5),
    xlab="age (days)", ylab="age effect")
lines(agegp, eageg, type="s")
```

The following simulation code is used to obtain 1000 replicates each with a sample size of 132, with age effects as a monthly step function. The SCCS model fitted still uses quarterly age groups, however. This is not a problem: indeed it is more realistic to use a simpler model to analyse the simulated data than was used in generating those data.

```
eage <- exp((seq(401,701,30)-366)*log(2)/(731-366))
set.seed(1234)
rilim <-rep(0,1000)
for (i in 1:1000){
arisk <- round(366+364*rbeta(132,2,4))
simdati <- simulatesccsdata(nindivs=132, astart=366, aend=730,
            adrug=arisk, aedrug=arisk+20, eexpo=2.5,
            agegrp=seq(401,701,30), eage=eage)
sim.modi <- standardsccs(event~adrug1+age, indiv=indiv,
            astart=astart, aend=aend, adrug=adrug1,
            aedrug=aedrug1, aevent=aevent, agegrp=
            c(457,548,639), data=simdati)
rilim[i] <- sim.modi$conf.int[1,3]
}
```

The estimated power is as follows:

```
> sum(rilim>1)/1000
[1] 0.832
```

The power is thus 83.2% (MC standard error 1.2%). This compares with the nominal 80% power specified in the sample size calculation.

Using a continuous age effect in the simulation would be more realistic than the monthly step function, but takes much longer as a cutpoint is used for each day of observation. To enter the age effects as a continuous exponential curve, use the following code.

```
eage <- exp((seq(366,730,1)-366)*log(2)/(730-366))
eage <- eage[-1]
```

The second line removes the reference value 1 at age 366 days. The simulation then proceeds as follows.

```
set.seed(1234)
rilim <-rep(0,1000)
for (i in 1:1000){
arisk <- round(366+364*rbeta(132,2,4))
simdati <- simulatesccsdata(nindivs=132, astart=366, aend=730,
```

```
                 adrug=arisk, aedrug=arisk+20, eexpo=2.5, eage=eage)
sim.modi <- standardsccs(event~adrug1+age, indiv=indiv,
             astart=astart, aend=aend, adrug=adrug1,
             aedrug=aedrug1, aevent=aevent, agegrp=
             c(457,548,639), data=simdati)
rilim[i] <- sim.modi$conf.int[1,3]
}
```

This yields:

```
> sum(rilim>1)/1000
[1] 0.84
```

Thus the power is 84.0% (MC standard error 1.2%).

One important practical use of simulations is to obtain empirical power curves for a proposed study design. A power curve shows the power for a range of values of the design parameter, and can thus be used to assess the sensitivity of the design to the value of the design parameter. With the design parameter equal to 1, the curve also indicates the actual significance level.

So far we have used the lower 95% confidence limit on the relative incidence to assess statistical significance. This corresponds to a 1-tailed test, with significance level 2.5%. The following code (using age effects represented by a monthly step function) also incorporates a 2-tailed test based on the likelihood ratio test statistic:

```
eage <- exp((seq(401,701,30)-366)*log(2)/(731-366))
set.seed(1234)
rilim <- plrt <- rep(0,1000)
for (i in 1:1000){
arisk <- round(366+364*rbeta(132,2,4))
simdati <- simulatesccsdata(nindivs=132, astart=366, aend=730,
             adrug=arisk, aedrug=arisk+20, eexpo=1,
             agegrp=seq(401,701,30), eage=eage)
sim.modi <- standardsccs(event~adrug1+age, indiv=indiv, astart=
             astart, aend=aend, adrug=adrug1, aedrug=aedrug1,
             aevent=aevent, agegrp=c(457,548,639), data=simdati)
sim.mod0 <- standardsccs(event~age, indiv=indiv, astart=astart,
             aend=aend, adrug=adrug1, aedrug=aedrug1, aevent=
             aevent, agegrp=c(457,548,639), data=simdati)
rilim[i] <- sim.modi$conf.int[1,3]
plrt[i] <- lrtsccs(sim.modi,sim.mod0)[1,3]
}
```

The vector plrt contains the *p*-values of the likelihood ratio test for the exposure effect. The 1-tailed and 2-tailed empirical significance levels are obtained as follows:

```
> sum(rilim>1)/1000
[1] 0.032
> sum(plrt<0.05)/1000
[1] 0.044
```

The 1-tailed significance level from the lower 95% confidence limit is 3.2% (MC standard error 0.56%); the 2-tailed significance level from the likelihood ratio test is 4.4% (MC standard error 0.65%). The nominal values are 2.5% and 5%, respectively. The MC standard errors in this case are perhaps a little too large in relation to the target parameter values; increasing the number of simulation replicates to 10 000 yields 2.95% (MC standard error 0.17%) for the 1-tailed test and 5.00% (MC error 0.22%) for the 2-tailed test, but takes a lot longer.

Figure 8.6 shows the power curves for values of the design parameter between 1 and 3.5. Each point was obtained using the code above with 10 000 replicates. The power curve provides an indication of the sensitivity of the

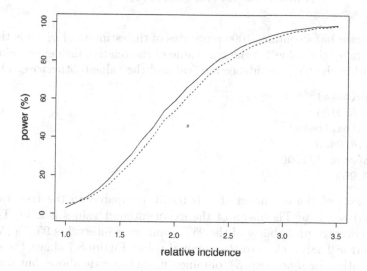

FIGURE 8.6
Power curves for the MMR study design. Full line: 1-tailed test based on lower 95% confidence limit. Dashed line: 2-tailed test based on likelihood ratio.

design, which in this instance is based on a sample size of 132 events, to the value of the design parameter. For example, the power for a relative incidence of 2 is only 54 to 59% depending on which test is applied.

Simulations may be used to assess many other aspects of a study design, notably the validity of asymptotic assumptions for the sample size used. In our MMR vaccine example, the sampling distribution of the maximum likelihood estimator of β, the log relative incidence, and the coverage probability of the 95% confidence interval when $\exp(\beta) = 2.5$ may be obtained using the following code, for the sample size 132.

```
eage <- exp((seq(401,701,30)-366)*log(2)/(731-366))
set.seed(1234)
beta <- cover <- rep(0,1000)
for (i in 1:1000){
arisk <- round(366+364*rbeta(132,2,4))
simdati <- simulatesccsdata(nindivs=132, astart=366, aend=730,
            adrug=arisk, aedrug=arisk+20, eexpo=2.5, agegrp=
            seq(401,701,30), eage=eage)
sim.modi <- standardsccs(event~adrug1+age, indiv=indiv, astart=
            astart, aend=aend, adrug=adrug1, aedrug=aedrug1,
            aevent=aevent, agegrp=c(457,548,639), data=simdati)
beta[i] <- sim.modi$coef[1,1]
cover[i] <- (sim.modi$conf.int[1,3]<2.5)*
            (2.5<sim.modi$conf.int[1,4])
}
```

The vector `beta` contains 1000 replicates of the estimate of β, while the vector `cover` takes the value 1 if the true value of the relative incidence (namely 2.5) lies within the 95% confidence interval and the value 0 otherwise. Then

```
> mean(beta)
[1] 0.873134
> mean(exp(beta))
[1] 2.490439
> sum(cover)/1000
[1] 0.952
```

The mean of the estimates of β is 0.873, compared to the true value $\beta = \log(2.5) = 0.916$. The mean of the exponentiated values is 2.49. The simulated coverage probability of the 95% confidence interval is 95.2% (MC standard error 0.68%), close to the nominal value. Figure 8.7 shows the sampling distribution for β and $\exp(\beta)$, obtained using the code above, but with 10 000 replications. The sampling distributions of $\hat{\beta}$ and $\exp(\hat{\beta})$ are roughly normal in appearance, suggesting that the asymptotic assumptions underpinning the estimation method are acceptable.

In this simulation we have used the mean of the estimates of β to summarise its location. With smaller sample sizes, we might have obtained large negative estimated values (in effect, $-\infty$), corresponding to 0 events in the risk period. Similarly, when risk periods are long, we might obtain large positive estimated values (in effect, $+\infty$), when all events occur within the risk period. If such values arise, the median or trimmed mean provide more relevant measures of location than the mean. From a theoretical perspective, the maximum likelihood estimator $\hat{\beta}$, in finite samples, can take the values $\pm\infty$ with positive probability, so its central moments do not exist.

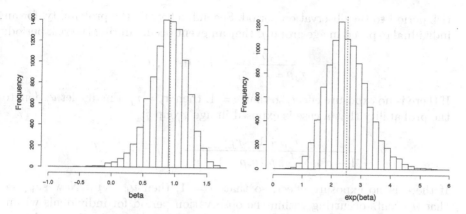

FIGURE 8.7

Simulated sampling distribution. Left: log relative incidence. Right: relative incidence. The dashed lines indicate the true values.

8.2.5 A formula for the sample size*

In this section the sample size formula behind the R function `samplesize` is presented. The calculation is based on the likelihood ratio test statistic, in the following simplified scenario.

We assume all individuals share the same observation period, covering $J+1$ age groups of duration $e_0, e_1, \ldots, e_J$. The age-specific relative incidence is assumed to vary as a step function with log values $\alpha_j, j = 1, \ldots, J$ relative to the first age group, so that $\alpha_0 = 0$.

We also assume that individuals in the target population (the population from which the cases are to be sampled), if exposed, have a single risk period of duration e^*, which is entirely contained within a single age group. This implies that $e^* \leq e_j$ for all $j = 0, \ldots, J$. The relative incidence associated with exposure is $\rho = e^\beta$. The probability that an individual randomly sampled from the target population is exposed in age group j is $p_j, j = 0, \ldots, J$. The probability that an individual is exposed at any time during the observation period is $p = \sum_{j=0}^{J} p_j$.

We make the further assumption that the values of the α_j are known, so that only β is to be estimated. We define the following intermediate quantities. First, let r_j be the weighted ratio of time at risk to the whole observation period for a risk period contained within age group j:

$$r_j = \frac{e^{\alpha_j} e^*}{\sum_{s=0}^{J} e^{\alpha_s} e_s}, \quad j = 0, \ldots, J.$$

If there are no age effects, so that $\alpha_j = 0$ for all j, then r_j is the ratio of the

---

* This section may be skipped.

risk period to the observation period. Second, let π_j be the probability, for an individual exposed in age group j, that an event occurs during the risk period:

$$\pi_j = \frac{r_j\rho}{r_j\rho + 1 - r_j}, \quad j = 0, \dots, J.$$

If there is no exposure effect, so that $\rho = 1$, then $\pi_j = r_j$. Finally, let ν_j denote the probability that a case is exposed in age group j:

$$\nu_j = \frac{p_j(r_j\rho + 1 - r_j)}{1 - p + \sum_{s=0}^{J} p_s(r_s\rho + 1 - r_s)}, \quad j = 0, \dots, J.$$

If there is no exposure effect, so that $\rho = 1$, then $\nu_j = p_j$. Now suppose that n events occurring within the observation period for individuals within the target population are randomly sampled. Let x denote the number of events occurring within a risk period, and m_j the number of events occurring for individuals exposed at age j. The log likelihood ratio test statistic for β obtained from the standard SCCS log likelihood (which is conditional on the m_j) may be written

$$D(\beta; x) = 2\left\{ x\beta - \sum_{j=0}^{J} m_j \log(r_j e^{\beta} + 1 - r_j) \right\}.$$

The maximum likelihood estimate $\hat{\beta}$ of β maximises $D(\beta; x)$ and satisfies the identity

$$x = \sum_{j=0}^{J} m_j \hat{\pi}_j.$$

Let x_j denote the number of events occurring in the risk period, among the m_j events in individuals exposed in age group j. The x_j are independent binomial $B(m_j, \pi_j)$ variates, and $x = \sum_j x_j$. The mean and variance of x, conditional on the m_j, are thus:

$$E(x|m) = \sum_{j=0}^{J} m_j \pi_j,$$

$$\mathrm{var}(x|m) = \sum_{j=0}^{J} m_j \pi_j (1 - \pi_j). \tag{8.1}$$

We shall base the sample size calculation on the signed root likelihood ratio statistic

$$T(\hat{\beta}; x) = \mathrm{sgn}(\hat{\beta})\sqrt{D(\hat{\beta}; x)}.$$

Under the null hypothesis $\beta = 0$, $T(\hat{\beta}; x)$ is approximately distributed as a standard normal variate $N(0,1)$. To obtain an approximate distribution for a design value $\beta \neq 0$, we first expand $T(\beta; x)$ in a Taylor series around $\hat{\beta}$. Since $\hat{\beta}$ optimises $T(\beta; x)$, this yields:

$$T(\beta; x) = T(\hat{\beta}; x) + O_p(n^{-1/2}),$$

where n is the number of events. A second Taylor expansion, of $T(\beta; x)$ around $E(x|\boldsymbol{m})$, together with Expressions 8.1, gives to first order:

$$E\{T(\hat{\beta}; x)\} \simeq \text{sgn}(\beta)\left[2\sum_{j=0}^{J} m_j\{\beta\pi_j - \log(r_j e^\beta + 1 - r_j)\}\right]^{1/2},$$

$$V\{T(\hat{\beta}; x)\} \simeq \frac{\beta^2}{[E\{T(\hat{\beta} : x)\}]^2}\sum_{j=0}^{J} m_j\pi_j(1 - \pi_j).$$

Now replace m_j by $n\nu_j$ in these expressions. Thus,

$$T(\hat{\beta}; x) \approx N\big(\text{sgn}(\beta)\sqrt{nA}, B\big),$$

where

$$A = 2\sum_{j=0}^{J} \nu_j\{\pi_j\beta - \log(r_j e^\beta + 1 - r_j)\},$$

$$B = \frac{\beta^2}{A}\sum_{j=0}^{J} \nu_j\pi_j(1 - \pi_j).$$

The required sample size formula for 100γ percent power at the 100α percent significance level (two-sided) is then

$$n = \frac{1}{A}\left(z_{1-\alpha/2} + z_\gamma\sqrt{B}\right)^2,$$

where $z_{1-\alpha/2}$ is the $1 - \alpha/2$-quantile of the standard normal distribution and z_γ is its γ-quantile.

8.3   Efficiency and identifiability

The SCCS method is based on a conditional likelihood, derived from a Poisson model for the underlying cohort from which cases are sampled. Conditioning in this way incurs a cost in efficiency (that is, the variance of the relative incidence estimator is increased). The question then arises: how much efficiency is lost in this way? A related question is: how does the performance of the SCCS method depend on the choice of design parameters? Finally, under what circumstances are the parameters of the SCCS model identifiable?

These are the issues addressed in this section. It is fair to say that they will seldom prove decisive in the choice of design, which is usually, and quite correctly, determined primarily by the practical application at hand. But an understanding of these issues can help to guide the implementation of the method more generally, and to anticipate or explain features of the results.

In Section 8.3.1 we discuss the relative efficiency of the SCCS method, compared to cohort and case-control studies with the same cases. Then in Section 8.3.2 we describe how the performance of the SCCS method depends on its design, in an asymptotic sense. In Section 8.3.3 we briefly discuss some identifiability issues, and how to tackle them. In these three sections, mathematical details are kept to a minimum. A more elaborate treatment is provided in Section 8.3.4, which is starred and may be skipped.

8.3.1 Relative efficiency of the SCCS method

The maximum likelihood estimator of the relative incidence from a SCCS study is asymptotically efficient, which implies that, in large samples, no estimator with lower variance can be derived from a SCCS study. This fact follows from the theory of maximum likelihood estimation. However, it is of interest to compare the efficiency of the relative incidence estimator from a SCCS study with that from a cohort or case-control study with the same cases as the SCCS study.

Recall from Chapter 3, Section 3.8, that the SCCS likelihood is obtained from an underlying Poisson cohort model by conditioning on the number of events experienced by each individual in the cohort. This means that any information about the relative incidence that is contained in these marginal counts is not used in the SCCS method. Accordingly, the SCCS method will generally be less efficient than the underlying Poisson cohort model.

Efficiencies are most readily compared using the asymptotic relative efficiency or ARE. In our case, this is the ratio of the variances of the log relative incidence estimators $\hat{\beta}$ for a single risk period obtained from a SCCS model and from the underlying cohort model with the same cases, as the number of events n grows large. Thus, in mathematical notation,

$$ARE = \lim_{n \to \infty} \frac{\text{var}(\hat{\beta}_{\text{cohort}})}{\text{var}(\hat{\beta}_{\text{SCCS}})}.$$

A general expression for the ARE is derived and discussed in Section 8.3.4. However, the salient points are conveniently illuminated in a special case, in which all individuals in the underlying cohort have an observation period of equal duration $b - a$, a proportion p are exposed and experience a single risk period of duration d, and in which there are no age effects. In this scenario,

$$ARE = \frac{1 + pre^{\beta}/(1 - pr)}{1 + re^{\beta}/(1 - r)} \tag{8.2}$$

where $r = d/(b - a)$ is the ratio of the risk period to observation period durations.

Note from Equation 8.2 that when $p = 1$, $ARE = 1$. Thus, when all individuals in the underlying cohort are exposed, then the asymptotic efficiency of the SCCS method is identical to that of the cohort method based on the same exposed cases. The practical implication is that, when an exposure is widespread, or when only exposed individuals are included, then a SCCS study is virtually as efficient as a cohort study based on the same exposed cases.

Figure 8.8 illustrates how the asymptotic relative efficiency ARE varies with r, the ratio of the risk period to the observation period, for a range of values of the relative incidence $\rho = e^\beta$, in two scenarios: $p = 0.3$ (moderate exposure probability) and $p = 0.7$ (high but not universal exposure probability).

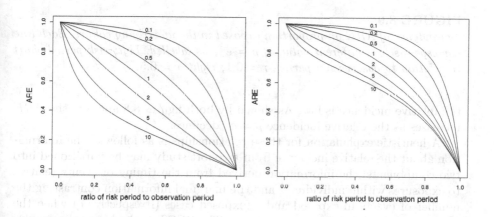

FIGURE 8.8

Dependence of ARE on ratio of risk to observation periods. Each line corresponds to a different value of $\rho = e^\beta$, as labelled. Left: proportion exposed in the underlying cohort $p = 0.3$; right: $p = 0.7$.

Figure 8.8 shows that ARE is high when r is small, but declines as r increases. The decline is slow when the relative incidence is less than 1, more rapid when the relative incidence is greater than 1. In other words, the SCCS design is most efficient, compared to a cohort analysis based on the same cases, when the risk period is short compared to the observation period.

Figure 8.9 shows how the ARE varies with p, the proportion of individuals exposed in the underlying cohort, in two scenarios: $r = 0.1$ (risk periods short relative to observation periods) and $r = 0.5$ (risk periods longer relative to observation periods). As shown in Figure 8.9, the ARE increases with the proportion exposed. When the proportion exposed is high, the ARE is high in all scenarios. When the proportion exposed is low, the ARE is high when

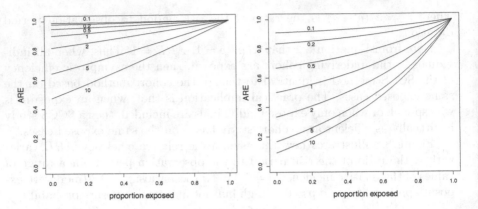

FIGURE 8.9

Dependence of ARE on proportion exposed in the underlying cohort. Each line corresponds to a different value of $\rho = e^\beta$, as labelled. Left: risk period short in relation to observation period, $r = 0.1$; right: $r = 0.5$.

the relative incidence is low. As shown by both figures 8.8 and 8.9, the *ARE* increases as the relative incidence $\rho = e^\beta$ declines.

A heuristic explanation for these relationships is as follows. The information about the relative incidence from a cohort study may be partitioned into two components: the information derived from the timing of events relative to exposures within individuals, and the marginal information contrasting the number of events in exposed and unexposed cases (irrespective of when the event occurred in relation to exposure). The SCCS method uses the within-individual information, but not the marginal information. In circumstances where there is little or no marginal information, the SCCS method will be virtually as efficient as the cohort method. This occurs, for example, when all or nearly all individuals are exposed (p close to 1). When $p < 1$, the contribution of marginal information increases when the duration of the risk period relative to the observation period increases, and also when the relative incidence increases, and so the SCCS method becomes less efficient compared to the cohort method.

The asymptotic relative efficiency of the SCCS method compared to designs other than cohort methods may also be obtained. Of particular interest is to compare the efficiency of a 1:1 matched case-control study with that of a SCCS study with the same cases; when the event rate is low the odds ratio and the relative incidence are virtually identical. Denoting both by $\rho = e^\beta$, the asymptotic relative efficiency is defined as follows:

$$ARE = \lim_{n \to \infty} \frac{\mathrm{var}(\hat{\beta}_{1:1 \text{ casecon}})}{\mathrm{var}(\hat{\beta}_{\text{SCCS}})}$$

Consider rare events in the following simple scenario: all individuals in the target population (from which both cases and controls are drawn) have an observation period of equal duration, a proportion p are exposed and experience a single risk period, the ratio of the risk period to the observation period durations being r, and there are no age effects. The relative efficiency is then:

$$ARE = \frac{(1-r)(1+\rho)}{(1-pr)(\rho r + 1 - r)}.$$

Note that when $p = 1$, so that all individuals in the target population are exposed, then $ARE > 1$. Thus, in this setting the SCCS design is more efficient than the 1:1 matched case-control design with the same cases. This also applies when r is less than or equal to 0.5. Figure 8.10 shows the relationship between ARE and r for the same scenarios as in Figure 8.8. This shows that the ARE

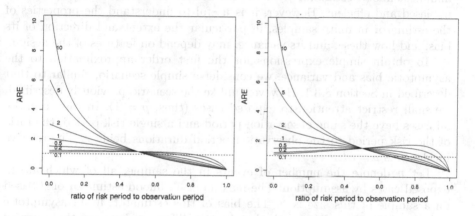

FIGURE 8.10
Dependence of ARE (1:1 matched case-control vs SCCS) on ratio of risk to observation periods. Each line corresponds to a different value of $\rho = e^\beta$, as labelled. Left: proportion exposed in the target population $p = 0.3$; right: $p = 0.7$. The horizontal dashed line indicates $ARE = 1$.

drops below 1 only when r is large. When the relative incidence is large and the risk period duration is small compared to the observation period, the ARE can be very much greater than 1.

These relationships may be explained heuristically as follows. The 1:1 matched case-control study only uses discordant case-control pairs, excluding cases whose matched control has the same exposure as the case. When r is small, the proportion of discordant case-control pairs drops and so the SCCS method becomes more efficient. On the other hand, when r is close to 1, the proportion of discordant pairs can remain substantial provided that $p < 1$, and so in some circumstances the SCCS method becomes less efficient.

Summary

- The efficiency of the SCCS design may be compared to that of others with the same cases using the asymptotic relative efficiency, or *ARE*.

- The SCCS method has good efficiency compared to cohort and case-control designs when the proportion exposed is high and when the risk period is short relative to the observation period.

8.3.2 Impact of design on parameter estimates

It follows from the theory of maximum likelihood estimation that the maximum likelihood estimator $\hat{\beta}$ of the log relative incidence is asymptotically unbiased and efficient. However, it is useful to understand the properties of the estimator in finite samples, in particular the extent and direction of its bias, and how these, and its variance, may depend on features of the design.

To obtain simple expressions for the first order approximation to the asymptotic bias and variance, we consider a simple scenario, similar to that described in Section 8.3.1. However, unlike the scenario previously described, we shall restrict attention to exposed cases (thus, $p = 1$). In this scenario, all cases have the same observation period and a single risk period, the ratio of the risk period to the observation period durations being r. The relative incidence is $\rho = e^{\beta}$.

Let n denote the number of events in the sample, all of which are in exposed cases by assumption. The maximum likelihood estimator of β based on a sample of this size is $\hat{\beta}$. The bias of this estimator, in an asymptotic sense, is $\text{bias}(\hat{\beta}) = E(\hat{\beta}) - \beta$, that is, the difference between the mean of the estimator (more precisely, its asymptotic limit) and the true value of the parameter. While both the bias and the variance $\text{var}(\hat{\beta})$ of the estimator tend to zero as n grows large, the rate at which they do so provides some indication as to how the estimator behaves in finite samples.

The first order expressions for the asymptotic (as n grows large) bias and variance of $\hat{\beta}$ are as follows.

$$\text{bias}(\hat{\beta}) \simeq \frac{1}{2n}\{re^{\beta} - (1-r)\}\left(\frac{1}{re^{\beta}} + \frac{1}{1-r}\right), \qquad (8.3)$$

$$\text{var}(\hat{\beta}) \simeq \frac{1}{n}\frac{\{re^{\beta} + (1-r)\}^2}{re^{\beta}(1-r)}. \qquad (8.4)$$

Bias and variance are often combined into a single measure of estimator performance, the mean squared error:

$$MSE = \text{bias}(\hat{\beta})^2 + \text{var}(\hat{\beta})$$

When the asymptotic quantities in Equations 8.3 and 8.4 are substituted in the expression for the MSE, we obtain the asymptotic mean squared error. To first order in n, this is the same as the asymptotic variance.

Note that the bias is zero (asymptotically, to first order in n) when $re^\beta = 1 - r$, that is, when the expected number of events in the risk period equals the expected number of events outside the risk period. The variance and MSE are lowest in this situation as well. More generally, the dependence of the bias and variance on r and e^β specified by Equations 8.3 and 8.4 is illustrated in Figure 8.11. In this figure, the bias and variance have both been multiplied by n, the number of events, to remove the dependence on n. The curves in

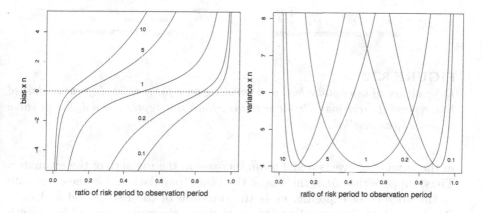

FIGURE 8.11

Dependence of asymptotic scaled bias and variance on r. Left: bias $\times n$; dashed line represents zero bias. Right: variance $\times n$. Each line represents a different value of $\rho = e^\beta$, as labelled.

Figure 8.11 indicate that estimators can potentially be badly behaved for values of r close to 0 or 1. These curves, however, are scaled by the sample size. The actual bias and variance expected in a sample of size $n = 20$ is shown in Figure 8.12.

Even with a sample size as low as $n = 20$, the bias is generally close to zero except for extreme combinations of r and ρ. To summarise, problems may arise in small samples, especially when the risk period is very short or very long in relation to the observation period. This is particularly so for short risk periods when the the relative incidence is well below 1, and for long risk periods when the relative incidence is well above 1. Most importantly, when the risk period is very short, the bias is likely to be negative, so that the estimated value of the relative incidence may be lower than the true value.

If the risk period is short, the best way to reduce an anticipated small-sample bias at the design stage of the study is to increase the number of events to be sampled among exposed cases. Reducing the duration of the observation period with the aim of increasing r will not help: it would lead to a reduction

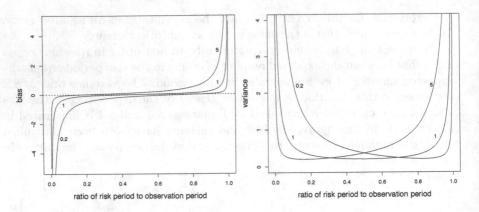

FIGURE 8.12
Dependence of asymptotic bias and variance on r for n = 20. Left: bias; dashed line represents zero bias. Right: variance. Each line represents a different value of $\rho = e^\beta$, as labelled.

in the number of events n and to an increase in the variance of the estimator. Thus, suppose that M is the size of the target population, λ is the event rate in the absence of exposure, e_1 is the duration of the risk period and e_0 is the duration of the control period, so that the observation period has length $e_0 + e_1$. Then the expected number of events is

$$E(n) = M\lambda(e_1\rho + e_0).$$

Substituting this expression for n in Equation 8.4, we obtain (to first order in M),

$$\text{var}(\hat{\beta}) = \frac{1}{M\lambda}\left(\frac{1}{e_0} + \frac{1}{e_1 e^\beta}\right).$$

Thus the variance of $\hat{\beta}$ decreases as the control period length e_0 increases, for a fixed risk period duration e_1. The asymptotic relative efficiency associated with a control period of duration e_0 relative to $e_0 = \infty$ is:

$$ARE_\infty = \left(1 + \frac{e_1 e^\beta}{e_0}\right)^{-1}.$$

This function is plotted in Figure 8.13. When $e_0 = e_1 \times \rho$, the bias is zero, but ARE_∞ is only 0.5. Thereafter, as e_0 increases, the relative efficiency increases towards 1.

As stated above, if the issue of bias is potentially of concern, efforts should be made at the design stage to increase the sample size. In some circumstances, it may be possible to maximise the number of exposed cases by choosing the

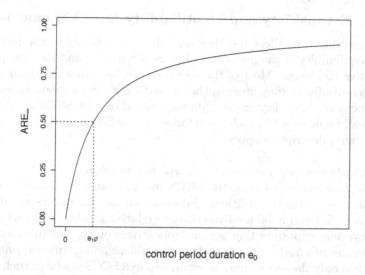

FIGURE 8.13
Asymptotic relative efficiency ARE_∞ by control period duration e_0.

observation period so as to capture the age range at which most exposures occur. Increasing the number of exposed cases will reduce both the finite sample bias and the asymptotic mean squared error.

Summary

- In simple scenarios, the asymptotic bias and variance of the estimator of the log relative incidence may be obtained in terms of the number of events in exposed cases, the ratio of the risk period to the observation period, and the relative incidence.

- In such scenarios, the bias is zero, and the variance is lowest, when the expected number of events in the risk period equals the expected number of events outside the risk period.

- Extreme combinations of relative incidence and risk period can produce biased estimates with large variances in small samples.

- SCCS analyses in small samples with very short risk periods are likely to produce estimates with negative bias, that is, an estimated relative incidence lower than the true value.

- The observation period should be chosen in such a way as to maximise the number of exposed cases.

8.3.3 Estimability and identifiability in SCCS models

In this section, we collect together several topics relating to the estimability and identifiability of the parameters in a SCCS model, and the interpretation of relative incidences. Most of these issues have been touched upon in earlier chapters, insofar as they arose in the context of SCCS analyses. Our aim here is to focus on how they might influence the choice of SCCS design. These issues can be dealt with much more formally (see Section 8.3.4). Here we take an informal, descriptive approach.

Estimability and interpretation of the relative incidence

As it is based on cases only, the SCCS method cannot be used to estimate absolute risks without additional information, as will be described in Section 8.5.1. Nor can it be used to estimate relative incidences associated with time-invariant exposures that act multiplicatively on the baseline incidence. If an exposure has both a time-invariant component and a time-varying component, then only the second may be estimated in a SCCS study. In such settings, some care is needed in interpreting a relative incidence obtained from a SCCS study.

In Chapter 1, Section 1.2, we gave the example of physical exercise: regular exercise may be beneficial in reducing the risk of cardiovascular disease, but episodes of physical exertion may increase the short-term risk. The long-term benefit associated with taking regular exercise cannot realistically be estimated in a SCCS study, as it is essentially time-invariant. Estimation of this effect requires a comparison between individuals taking and not taking regular exercise. On the other hand, the relative incidence associated with episodes of physical exertion can be estimated in a SCCS study, as the exposure varies within individuals. The two exposures – taking regular exercise, and episodic exertion – should thus be regarded as distinct. Effect modification of the episodic risk by regular exercise may, however, be estimated in a SCCS study, provided that covariate information on taking regular exercise is collected on the cases.

Note that the SCCS method does not require the exposure to be transient: however the exposure cannot be time-invariant. Examples of SCCS analyses with exposures that are time-varying but not transient were presented in Chapter 4, Sections 4.8.1 and 4.8.2.

Care in interpretation is also required with SCCS studies in which the observation period starts at exposure, especially when the control period, which follows the risk period, is of short duration. Such studies may certainly be used to identify a risk gradient after exposure. However, estimating the relative incidence relative to an unexposed baseline level requires that the incidence should return to this level in the control period. This assumption will often be reasonable, but it cannot be tested in a SCCS study in which the observation periods start at exposure. The issue arises, in particular, in self-controlled risk interval studies, described in Section 8.1.6, in which the control period is typically brief.

An example was described in Chapter 4, Section 4.8.3: the exposure was nicotine replacement therapy (NRT), and the event was myocardial infarction (MI). The question of interest was whether MI is associated with the initiation of NRT therapy. The observation periods were relatively short: one year from first NRT prescription. Thus, the relative incidence is based on a contrast between the ratio of incidences in the period immediately following the initiation of NRT therapy, and the incidence in the remaining period up to one year later. Such a SCCS study can certainly identify or rule out a risk gradient, but cannot necessarily determine, without further information, whether the exposure is associated with an elevated or reduced relative incidence.

Aside from the efficiency considerations discussed in Section 8.3.2, it is advisable when possible to use longer observation periods, not necessarily starting at exposure, as these offer more opportunities to test the assumptions of the model, and to contextualise the risk profile.

Identifiability of parameters
The parameters of a SCCS model may be unidentifiable if exposure and age effects are confounded. To take an extreme example, if an exposure were universal, and always occurred at exactly the same age or time for all individuals, then it would not be possible to separate the effects associated with exposure from the effects associated with age or time. This is true whatever the study design, including the SCCS design.

We encountered such a situation, in which exposure and temporal effects are confounded, in Chapter 6, Section 6.6. The exposure was environmental, and affected everyone in the population studied at the same time. Thus, it was not possible to identify separately the effect of the exposure from the effect associated with temporal variation.

The solution in this case was to choose the observation periods so that temporal variation within observation periods could be ignored. By removing the temporal confounder from the model, the exposure effect can then be identified. Such an approach usually – and exceptionally – requires observation periods to be of short duration.

More generally, it is not uncommon for age and exposure effects to be confounded to some degree. For example, childhood vaccinations are typically administered according to a strict age-related schedule. In practice, there is variation in age at vaccination, so this is not a problem provided that the risk period is short. However, if the post-vaccination risk period is long or indefinite, as was the case for the MMR vaccine and autism example discussed in Chapter 4, Section 4.8.2, then there may be little between-individual variation in exposure history among vaccine recipients. As a result, the long-term effects of vaccination are to some degree confounded with age effects.

In this example, there happened to be more variation in age at vaccination owing to the MMR catch-up programme (in which older unvaccinated children were offered MMR vaccination). And in addition, confounding was reduced by the inclusion of cases who did not receive MMR vaccine.

To get round the problem of lack of variability in exposure between exposed individuals, unexposed cases should be included in the SCCS analysis. Such cases enable the effects of age and exposure to be separately identified.

A further instance of non-identifiability relates to the inclusion of temporal as well as age effects within a SCCS model. Multiplicative cohort effects are not estimable in a SCCS model, as they are time-invariant. Multiplicative age and time effects may or may not be identifiable when included together in a SCCS model. As noted in Chapter 6, Section 6.1.1, an exponential time effect is not separately identifiable within a semiparametric SCCS model. Thus, if a temporal effect $\eta(u)$ (u representing calendar time) is exponential, with $\eta(u) = \exp(\delta u)$, and u_i denotes the calendar time of birth of an individual i, so that $u = t + u_i$, (t being age) then

$$\eta(u) = \exp(\delta t) \times \exp(\delta u_i).$$

The term $\exp(\delta u_i)$ is a cohort effect. This drops out of the SCCS likelihood, and the term $\exp(\delta t)$ is incorporated into the age effect. In standard SCCS models, exponential time trends, with times grouped in distinct categories, are only partially identifiable when the model also includes an age effect.

The practical implication is that estimated age effects encompass exponential calendar time trends. When the calendar time effect is cyclical, as is the case with seasonality, then age and calendar time effects may be separately identified. If the temporal effect includes both an exponential trend and a cyclical seasonal component, the exponential trend will be absorbed into the age effect, and only the seasonal component need be specified explicitly.

Summary

- Only time-varying effects can be estimated in a SCCS study. Effect modification by time-invariant factors can also be estimated.

- In SCCS studies with initial risk periods and short observation periods, only the presence or absence of a risk gradient can reliably be identified without further assumptions.

- If there is little variation in the timing of exposures within exposed cases, the exposure and age effects may be confounded.

- In such circumstances, including unexposed cases, or choosing observation periods so that age effects may be ignored, enables exposure effects to be identified.

- In a SCCS model, exponential calendar time trends are largely confounded with age effects. Non-exponential calendar time effects, such as cyclical seasonal variation, may be identified.

8.3.4 More on identifiability and relative efficiency*

In this section we discuss identifiability and efficiency issues from a more theoretical perspective, in an asymptotic setting. In particular we derive an expression for the asymptotic relative efficiency of the cohort method and the SCCS method with the same cases, in the presence of age effects.

To simplify the calculations, we consider a target population of individuals with the same observation period $(a, b]$. Let X denote the exposure history of a randomly selected individual from this population; the observation history is not represented explicitly. We assume that X has a well-defined density. As in Chapter 4, Section 4.10, we assume that the age-specific relative incidence $\psi(t)$ may be written $\psi(t) = \exp\{u(t)^T\alpha\}$ and that the relative incidence function associated with an exposure history $X = x$ is $\rho(t|x) = \exp\{v(t; x)^T\beta\}$. This parameterisation applies to the standard SCCS model. Furthermore, we assume that there are no time-invariant covariates, though these could readily be incorporated. A cohort of M individuals is randomly sampled from this population, including $N \le M$ cases. The N cases $i = 1, \ldots, N$ are listed first, followed by the $M - N$ non-cases. Individual i experiences n_i events, with $n_i > 0$ for $i = 1, \ldots, N$, and $n_i = 0$ for $i = M - N + 1, \ldots, M$. For case i, t_{ij} is the time of the jth event.

The event rate for an individual i with exposure history x_i from this cohort may be written

$$\lambda(t|x_i) = \exp\{\gamma + u(t)^T\alpha + v(t; x_i)^T\beta\}.$$

The cohort model involves the parameters γ, α and β, whereas the SCCS model involves just α and β. The likelihood for the SCCS model is as follows:

$$L_{\text{SCCS}} = \prod_{i=1}^{N} \prod_{j=1}^{n_i} \left(\frac{\exp\{u(t_{ij})^T\alpha + v(t_{ij}; x_i)^T\beta\}}{\int_a^b \exp\{u(t)^T\alpha + v(t; x_i)^T\beta\}dt} \right). \tag{8.5}$$

The cohort likelihood is:

$$L_{\text{cohort}} = \prod_{i=1}^{N} \prod_{j=1}^{n_i} \exp\{\gamma + u(t_{ij})^T\alpha + v(t_{ij}; x_i)^T\beta\}$$

$$\times \prod_{i=1}^{M} \exp\left(-\int_a^b \exp\{\gamma + u(t)^T\alpha + v(t; x_i)^T\beta\}dt \right). \tag{8.6}$$

At its heart, the relative efficiency of the SCCS and cohort methods derives from the interplay of within and between-individual variability in exposure and age effects. We begin by defining suitable measures of within-individual and between-individual variability. For an individual with exposure history x, define the density

$$f_x(t) = \frac{\exp\{u(t)^T\alpha + v(t; x)^T\beta\}}{\int_a^b \exp\{u(s)^T\alpha + v(s; x)^T\beta\}ds}.$$

---

* This section may be skipped.

Now define the within-individual mean $\boldsymbol{\mu}_x$ and variance $\boldsymbol{\nu}_x$ of the exposure vector $\boldsymbol{v}(t;x)$ with respect to this density:

$$\boldsymbol{\mu}_x = \int_a^b \boldsymbol{v}(t;x) f_x(t) dt,$$

$$\boldsymbol{\nu}_x = \int_a^b \boldsymbol{v}(t;x)\boldsymbol{v}(t;x)^T f_x(t) dt - \boldsymbol{\mu}_x\boldsymbol{\mu}_x^T,$$

the integrations being undertaken component-wise. Also define the following within-individual mean and variance of the age vector $\boldsymbol{u}(t)$ and its within-individual covariance with the exposure vector:

$$\boldsymbol{\theta}_x = \int_a^b \boldsymbol{u}(t) f_x(t) dt,$$

$$\boldsymbol{\delta}_x = \int_a^b \boldsymbol{u}(t)\boldsymbol{u}(t)^T f_x(t) dt - \boldsymbol{\theta}_x\boldsymbol{\theta}_x^T,$$

$$\boldsymbol{\kappa}_x = \int_a^b \boldsymbol{v}(t;x)\boldsymbol{u}(t)^T f_x(t) dt - \boldsymbol{\mu}_x\boldsymbol{\theta}_x^T.$$

We will need to average these within-individual quantities across individuals in the cohort. Define the mean intensity Λ and weights ω_x as follows:

$$\Lambda = E\left[\int_a^b \exp\{\gamma + \boldsymbol{u}(t)^T\boldsymbol{\alpha} + \boldsymbol{v}(t;X)^T\boldsymbol{\beta}\} dt\right],$$

$$\omega_x = \frac{1}{\Lambda}\int_a^b \exp\{\gamma + \boldsymbol{u}(t)^T\boldsymbol{\alpha} + \boldsymbol{v}(t;x)^T\boldsymbol{\beta}\} dt,$$

where the expectation E is with respect to the distribution of exposure histories X of the individuals within the target population from which the cohort is drawn. The ω_x give greater weight to individuals that are more likely to experience greater numbers of events. We define the average within-individual variances and covariances as follows:

$$\mathrm{var_w}(\boldsymbol{v}) = E(\omega_X \boldsymbol{\nu}_X),$$

$$\mathrm{var_w}(\boldsymbol{u}) = E(\omega_X \boldsymbol{\delta}_X),$$

$$\mathrm{cov_w}(\boldsymbol{v}, \boldsymbol{u}) = E(\omega_X \boldsymbol{\kappa}_X).$$

The subscripts w indicate that these refer to (average) within-individual quantities. We also define between-individual variances and covariances, subscripted by the letter b, as follows, with $\boldsymbol{\mu} = E(\omega_X \boldsymbol{\mu}_X)$ and $\boldsymbol{\theta} = E(\omega_X \boldsymbol{\theta}_X)$.

$$\mathrm{var_b}(\boldsymbol{v}) = E(\omega_X \boldsymbol{\mu}_X \boldsymbol{\mu}_X^T) - \boldsymbol{\mu}\boldsymbol{\mu}^T,$$

$$\mathrm{var_b}(\boldsymbol{u}) = E(\omega_X \boldsymbol{\theta}_X \boldsymbol{\theta}_X^T) - \boldsymbol{\theta}\boldsymbol{\theta}^T,$$

$$\mathrm{cov_b}(\boldsymbol{v}, \boldsymbol{u}) = E(\omega_X \boldsymbol{\mu}_X \boldsymbol{\theta}_X^T) - \boldsymbol{\mu}\boldsymbol{\theta}^T.$$

Also define the total variances and covariances as the sum of the within and between quantities, that is, $\mathrm{var}_t \equiv \mathrm{var}_w + \mathrm{var}_b$ and $\mathrm{cov}_t \equiv \mathrm{cov}_w + \mathrm{cov}_b$.

The matrix of second derivatives of the SCCS log likelihood from Expression 8.5, times -1, may be written

$$\sum_{i=1}^{M} n_i \begin{pmatrix} \nu_{x_i} & \kappa_{x_i} \\ \kappa_{x_i}^T & \delta_{x_i} \end{pmatrix}, \tag{8.7}$$

since $n_i = 0$ for $i > N$. The expectation of n_i is $M\Lambda\omega_{x_i}$. As the cohort size M, and hence the number of cases N, increases, Expression 8.7 is asymptotically equivalent to

$$I_{\mathrm{SCCS}} = n \begin{pmatrix} \mathrm{var}_w(v) & \mathrm{cov}_w(v, u) \\ \mathrm{cov}_w(v, u)^T & \mathrm{var}_w(u) \end{pmatrix},$$

where n is the number of events, which has expectation $M\Lambda$ in a cohort of size M. For the cohort model, the matrix of second derivatives of the likelihood from Expression 8.6, times -1, may be written

$$\sum_{i=1}^{M} \Lambda\omega_{x_i} \begin{pmatrix} \nu_{x_i} + \mu_{x_i}\mu_{x_i}^T & \kappa_{x_i} + \mu_{x_i}\theta_{x_i}^T & \mu_{x_i} \\ \kappa_{x_i}^T + \theta_{x_i}\mu_{x_i}^T & \delta_{x_i} + \theta_{x_i}\theta_{x_i}^T & \theta_{x_i} \\ \mu_{x_i}^T & \theta_{x_i}^T & 1 \end{pmatrix}.$$

As the cohort size M increases, this is asymptotically equivalent to

$$I_{\mathrm{cohort}} = n \begin{pmatrix} \mathrm{var}_t(v) + \mu\mu^T & \mathrm{cov}_t(v, u) + \mu\theta^T & \mu \\ \mathrm{cov}_t(v, u)^T + \theta\mu & \mathrm{var}_t(u) + \theta\theta^T & \theta \\ \mu^T & \theta^T & 1 \end{pmatrix}.$$

The asymptotic variances of $\hat{\beta}$, the maximum likelihood estimator of β, for the SCCS and cohort models, are obtained by inverting the matrices I_{SCCS} and I_{cohort}. We use a standard identity for partitioned matrices: if

$$D = \begin{pmatrix} A & B \\ B^T & C \end{pmatrix},$$

then the upper left corner of D^{-1} is $(A - BC^{-1}B^T)^{-1}$, provided all inverses exist. In the case of the cohort model, this identity is applied twice.

The asymptotic variances of $\hat{\beta}$ are as follows:

$$\mathrm{var}_{\mathrm{SCCS}}(\hat{\beta}) = \frac{1}{n}\{\mathrm{var}_w(v) - \mathrm{cov}_w(v, u)\mathrm{var}_w(u)^{-1}\mathrm{cov}_w(v, u)^T\}^{-1}, \tag{8.8}$$

$$\mathrm{var}_{\mathrm{cohort}}(\hat{\beta}) = \frac{1}{n}\{\mathrm{var}_t(v) - \mathrm{cov}_t(v, u)\mathrm{var}_t(u)^{-1}\mathrm{cov}_t(v, u)^T\}^{-1}. \tag{8.9}$$

In the SCCS model, the variance of $\hat{\beta}$ is undefined if $v(t, X)$ is of the form $Au(t) + c_X$, where A is a time-invariant matrix and c_X is a time-invariant vector that may vary between individuals. This corresponds to the situation in which the exposure and the age profiles are collinear within individuals. In this case, exposure and age effects are wholly confounded, and so β is unidentifiable and hence cannot be estimated with the SCCS method.

In the cohort model, on the other hand, the exposure and age effects are wholly confounded when $v(t, X) = Au(t) + c$, where c is a constant vector that does not vary between individuals – a more stringent condition than for the SCCS method. Thus, when exposure and age profiles are collinear within individuals, the exposure effect β may still be estimable within the cohort model, provided there is sufficient between-individual variation.

Now suppose that there is a single log relative incidence parameter β to be estimated, so $v(t, x)$ is a time-varying indicator function taking the values 0 in control periods and 1 in risk periods. The asymptotic relative efficiency of $\hat{\beta}$ in the SCCS design compared with the cohort design is obtained from the ratio of the variances, that is, Expression 8.9 divided by Expression 8.8. This ratio may be written:

$$ARE = \frac{\mathrm{var_w}(v)}{\mathrm{var_t}(v)} \times \frac{1 - R_w^2}{1 - R_t^2},$$

where R_w^2 and R_t^2 are akin to multiple squared correlations (Mardia et al., 1979, page 168).

Thus, the asymptotic relative efficiency of the SCCS method is high when the average within-individual variation in exposure accounts for a large proportion of the total variation in exposure, and when there is little collinearity between exposure and age profiles within individuals.

For the special case described in Section 8.3.1, there are no age effects so $ARE = \mathrm{var_w}(v)/\mathrm{var_t}(v)$. The exposure histories are binary:

$$v(t; X) = \begin{cases} I_{(a, a+d]}(t) & \text{if } X = 1, \\ 0 & \text{if } X = 0, \end{cases}$$

with $X = 1$ occurring with probability p. Then $\Lambda = e^\gamma \{p(re^\beta + 1 - r) + (1 - p)\}$, and

$$\mathrm{var_w}(v) = \frac{pre^\beta(1 - r)}{\{p(re^\beta + 1 - r) + 1 - p\}(re^\beta + 1 - r)},$$

$$\mathrm{var_t}(v) = \frac{pre^\beta(1 - rp)}{\{p(re^\beta + 1 - r) + 1 - p\}^2}.$$

Thus we have

$$\mathrm{var_{SCCS}}(\hat{\beta}) = \left(\frac{1}{Mpe^\alpha}\right)\frac{re^\beta + 1 - r}{re^\beta(1 - r)},$$

$$\mathrm{var_{cohort}}(\hat{\beta}) = \left(\frac{1}{Mpe^\alpha}\right)\frac{p(re^\beta + 1 - r) + 1 - p}{re^\beta(1 - rp)},$$

from which the ARE in Equation 8.2 may be derived.

8.4 Presentation of SCCS studies

The presentation of a SCCS study should follow the same principles that apply to any other type of epidemiological investigation: the conduct of the study should be described in sufficient detail to enable readers, in principle, to reproduce it. It should include precise information on how observation periods and risk periods are specified, how events and exposures are defined, and how cases are sampled. It should also include details of what sensitivity analyses were undertaken and other steps to verify the assumptions when these are in doubt.

Rather than expanding further on these broad principles, in this section we focus on some very much more practical issues. We begin by describing how to obtain event counts and person-time totals, and how to use them in results tables. Then we briefly review some of the graphs that can be displayed to present SCCS data and results.

8.4.1 Results tables for SCCS studies

When reporting the results of a SCCS study, notably in results tables, it is good practice to state not just the relative incidences, with 95% confidence limits, but also the number of events within each risk period. Presenting event counts is particularly important for assessing the strength of evidence, as well as the validity of asymptotic assumptions. It may also be useful to present data summaries on the total or average person-time within each risk period for the cases in the study, though care is needed in interpreting such information: owing to the self-matching involved, they are not denominators in the usual sense.

Obtaining such descriptive statistics is readily achieved using the R package SCCS with the function `formatdata`, which reshapes the data in a form suitable for SCCS analysis using the standard SCCS model. This function, which was described in Chapter 4, Section 4.3.2, may be used to obtain event counts and person-time totals in the various exposure and age groups.

8.4.2 MMR vaccine and ITP: relative incidence table

We return in this example to the data on ITP and MMR vaccine first discussed in Chapter 4, Section 4.3.1. The data, in data frame `itpdat`, comprise 44 events in 35 cases. The risk period included days 0 to 42 after MMR vaccine; an analysis was also done with three 2-week risk periods, $[0, 14]$, $[15, 28]$ and $[29, 42]$ days after MMR vaccine. In these analyses, the observation periods, which were all comprised within the second year of life from 366 to 730 days of age, were partitioned into six roughly 2-month age groups with cutpoints at 427, 488, 549, 610 and 671 days of age.

The estimated relative incidences were 1.31, 95% CI (0.30, 5.73) in the [0, 14]-day risk period; 5.95, 95% CI (2.52, 14.1) in the [15, 28]-day risk period, and 2.60, 95% CI (0.75, 9.07) in the [29, 42]-day risk period. Over the whole 6-week risk period, $RI = 3.23$, 95% CI (1.53, 6.79).

To better contextualise these results, we shall obtain event counts using the R function formatdata. Thus:

```
itp.dat1 <- formatdata(indiv=case, astart=sta, aend=end,
                aevent=itp, adrug=mmr, aedrug=mmr+42,
                expogrp=c(0,15,29), agegrp=c(427,488,549,610,671),
                data=itpdat)
```

Obtaining the event counts by exposure group is readily achieved as follows:

```
> tapply(itp.dat1$event, itp.dat1$mmr, sum)
 0  1  2  3
31  2  8  3
```

Thus, there are 31 events in control (unexposed) periods, 2 in the first 2-week risk period, 8 in the second 2-week risk period, and 3 in the third 2-week risk period. Event counts in each age group are obtained in a similar fashion:

```
> tapply(itp.dat1$event, itp.dat1$age, sum)
 1  2  3  4  5  6
16 11  3  4  5  5
```

Table 8.1 shows the results as they might be presented in a report of the study. When reading this table, it is apparent that the relative incidences for

TABLE 8.1
Relative incidences (RI) for MMR and ITP.

Risk period	No. events	RI	95% CI
Unexposed	31	1.00	–
0 - 14 days	2	1.31	(0.30, 5.73)
15 - 28 days	8	5.95	(2.52, 14.1)
29 - 42 days	3	2.60	(0.75, 9.07)
0 - 42 days	13	3.23	(1.53, 6.79)

the first and third 2-week periods are based on very small numbers of events (2 and 3 events, respectively). Thus, the estimate obtained for the 0–42 day risk period may be more robust.

Person-time within each risk or age category for the cases in the study may also be obtained using the R function formatdata. However, some care is needed: when reshaping the data, individuals with multiple events are replicated and a new individual counter, indivL, is created. For these data, indivL takes values 1 to 44 (the number of events) rather than 1 to 35 (the number of cases). To obtain person time for the 35 cases, we need to de-duplicate the cases. This is achieved by subsetting the data:

```
itp.dat2 <- formatdata(indiv=case, astart=sta, aend=end,
                aevent=itp, adrug=mmr, aedrug=mmr+42,
                expogrp=c(0,15,29), agegrp=c(427,488,549,610,671),
                data=subset(itpdat,duplicated(case)==0))
```

The total person-time for the exposure groups is then obtained as follows:

```
> tapply(itp.dat2$interval, itp.dat2$mmr, sum)
     0     1     2     3
11147   464   426   408
```

Thus, for the 35 cases, there are 11147 person-days in control periods, and 464, 426 and 408 in the three risk periods, respectively. Similarly for the age groups:

```
> tapply(itp.dat2$interval, itp.dat2$age, sum)
   1    2    3    4    5    6
2013 2096 2135 2135 2135 1931
```

The interpretation of person-time in a SCCS study requires some caution. It is important to remember that person-time does not represent a denominator, as in a cohort study, since it is calculated from cases alone. The relative incidence estimator in a SCCS study is not a simple age-adjusted ratio of absolute rates (a rate being a count divided by person-time), except in very particular circumstances such as those described in Section 8.1.6.

8.4.3 Multiple exposures: NSAIDs and antidepressants

The presentation of results is complicated when there are several distinct exposure types to be included in the same model. In this case, it may be best to provide a separate table giving the cross-classification of event counts and person-time totals by exposure type and level.

In Chapter 4, Section 4.5.2, data on 1000 gastro-intestinal bleeds were presented. Of particular interest was the possible interaction between non-steroidal anti-inflammatory drugs (NSAIDs) and antidepressants (ADs), in Section 4.7.2 of the same chapter. The data are in data frame addat, and include only first bleeds.

First, we reshape the data using formatdata, using the age groups previously specified for these data:

```
ageq <- floor(quantile(addat$bleed[duplicated(addat$case)==0],
         seq(0.025,0.975,0.025),names=F))
ad.dat1 <- formatdata(indiv=case, astart=sta, aend=end,
             aevent=bleed, adrug=cbind(ns,ad),
             aedrug=cbind(endns,endad), agegrp=ageq, data=addat)
```

The cross-classification of event counts by exposure type is obtained by entering the exposures as a list as follows.

```
> tapply(ad.dat1$event, list(ad.dat1$ns,ad.dat1$ad), sum)
    0   1
0 710  78
1 184  28
```

In this table, the rows correspond to NSAIDs (specified first in the list), and the columns to ADs. Thus, 710 GI bleeds occurred when not exposed to either NSAIDs or ADs, 78 occurred when exposed to ADs but not NSAIDs, 184 occurred when exposed to NSAIDs but not to ADs, and 28 occurred when exposed to both NSAIDs and ADs. Similarly, person-time, expressed as person-years, is obtained as follows; as the data comprise only first events, there are no recurrent events, so we do not need to subset the data.

```
> tapply(ad.dat1$interval, list(ad.dat1$ns,ad.dat1$ad),
         sum)/365.25
        0         1
0 7540.7721 527.4743
1  994.2478 172.7009
```

So the 1000 cases experienced 7540.77 person-years of observation with no exposure, 994.25 years of exposure to NSAIDs alone, 527.47 person-years of exposure to ADs alone, and 172.70 years of exposure to both NSAIDs and ADs. These summaries are presented together in Table 8.2.

TABLE 8.2
Person time and GI bleeds by exposure type.

Exposure	Person-years	GI bleeds
Neither	7540.77	710
NSAID only	994.25	184
AD only	527.47	78
NSAID + AD	172.70	28

Unlike the MMR vaccine and ITP example in Section 8.4.2, the risk period durations vary from case to case. The person-time in Table 8.2 may be used to obtain the average times at risk. There are 1000 cases in this study. Thus, cases spent on average 7.54 years unexposed to NSAIDs or ADs, 0.99 years exposed to NSAIDs alone, 0.53 years exposed to ADs alone, and 0.17 years exposed to both NSAIDs and ADs.

In SCCS models with both the effects of NSAIDs and ADs, there may be no one-to-one correspondence between event counts and relative incidence estimates. For example, the relative incidence for NSAIDs in the model with no interaction is based on the number of events in the NSAID only and the NSAID + AD categories. Thus, rather than attempt to construct a table like Table 8.1, it is preferable to present the person-time and event counts in a table such as Table 8.2, and the relative incidences in a separate table.

8.4.4 Graphical displays for SCCS studies

In earlier chapters we have used several different types of graphs to present SCCS data and results from SCCS studies. In this subsection we review these different graphs, and comment briefly on their use.

Observation periods
Graphs displaying the observation periods are useful primarily for large data sets in which there is substantial variation in the ages at which the observation periods start and end. Such graphs provide a visual impression of the structure and spread of the data. For example, Figure 4.3 in Chapter 4, Section 4.3.3 shows that there is considerable overlap of observation periods between cases; in contrast the left panel of Figure 4.4 in Section 4.4.1 from the same chapter shows that observation periods are short in relation to their spread over the age range. An even more extreme case is Figure 4.18, in Section 4.8.3, which shows that there is very little overlap between observation periods. This carries implications for the modelling of age effects.

Graphs of observation periods are not likely to be very useful when most observation periods share the same endpoints.

Risk periods
Diagrams showing risk periods readily convey key information about the SCCS model. For example, Figure 4.2 in Chapter 4, Section 4.3.3 illustrates a complex succession of risk and washout periods. Such graphs can also display risk periods in relation to observation periods, as in Figure 4.13 in Chapter 4, Section 4.8.1.

Exposure and event distributions
Descriptive information about age at event and age at exposure is most readily presented in the form of histograms, as in Figure 4.6 from Chapter 4, Section 4.4.2. In this example each case experiences up to three doses of vaccine, which have been combined in one histogram: they could be plotted separately if preferred.

The shape of the histogram for age at event needs to be interpreted with some care, as it may reflect changes in durations of observation periods at different ages. When there is little variation in observation periods between cases, the shape of the histogram can help to inform the choice of age categories in the SCCS model.

A histogram of exposures and events by season can similarly be used to explore the desirability of including seasonal effects in the SCCS model, as in Figure 4.21 from Chapter 4, Section 4.9.2.

The histogram of age at exposure is perhaps most relevant for point exposures, such as vaccines, and risk periods of fixed duration. When risk period durations vary substantially between cases, a representation such as that used in the right panel of Figure 4.4 in Chapter 4, Section 4.4.1 may be more useful.

Centred plots

Centred event plots, in which the time intervals between exposures and events are plotted, were discussed in Chapter 5, Sections 5.4.1 and 5.5.1. These plots, which may be supplemented by centred observation plots, can be used for two different purposes.

First, they provide a useful representation of the data which can help to illustrate the presence or absence of an association, and can therefore supplement the numerical results obtained from a SCCS model. This can be particularly useful for risk communication. An example is Figure 5.12 from Section 5.5.2 of Chapter 5. Figure 2.1 in Section 2.1 of Chapter 2 is also a centred plot. However, an important proviso surrounds the use of such plots: they should not be used to choose the risk period when applying the methods described in this book. To do so would invalidate the inferences drawn from the model, as the risk period would then be data-dependent. For this reason, we avoided them entirely in Chapter 4 which focused on model fitting.

Second, centred plots may be used to investigate short-term event dependence of exposures, as described in Section 5.4.1 of Chapter 5. Examples from Chapter 5 include Figure 5.7 in Section 5.4.2, Figure 5.9 in Section 5.4.3 and Figure 5.10 in Section 5.4.4.

Fitted models

For most SCCS models, graphical representations of the exposure effect are unenlightening, as there are only a small number of parameters: tabular presentation of the results, discussed in Section 8.4.1, is usually preferable. Spline models for the exposure effect are the exception: indeed for such models, only a graphical representation makes sense. An example of such a graph is Figure 6.9 from Section 6.3.2 of Chapter 6.

While age effects are not usually the focus of inference, it may sometimes be appropriate to display the fitted relative age effect. It may be preferable to do so using a graph rather than a list of parameter estimates. Examples include Figure 4.11 of Section 4.7.1 and Figure 4.15 in Section 4.8.1 of Chapter 4. For the semiparametric SCCS model, the cumulative relative age effect is plotted, as in Figure 6.1 of Section 6.1.2, Chapter 6. Age effects for spline-based SCCS models may also be plotted, as in Figure 6.4 from Section 6.2.2 of Chapter 6.

Sensitivity analyses

Several special plots were described in Chapter 5 relating to testing assumptions and sensitivity analyses. These include the cumulative hazard plot for gap times, such as Figure 5.1 in Section 5.2.2; histograms of the interval from event to end of observation in censored and uncensored cases, such as Figure 5.6 in Section 5.3.3; plots of relative incidences by duration of pre-exposure risk interval such as Figure 5.8 in Section 5.4.2. The use of these and other such plots should be governed by the specific application under consideration.

Summary

- Event counts in risk and control periods are required to interpret relative incidences, and should be quoted or included in results tables.

- It may also be appropriate to present person-time totals or averages. Person-time totals should not be interpreted as denominators as they relate only to cases.

- A wide range of graphs may be used to display key features of the data to guide model choice, to illustrate the findings of a SCCS analysis, or to summarise sensitivity analyses.

8.5 Measures of attribution in SCCS studies

If a relative incidence is found to be statistically significantly different from 1, the issue arises as to whether the association is causal or artefactual. This issue cannot be decided on statistical grounds alone, though a detailed investigation of the assumptions, as described in Chapter 5, and other types of bias is a necessary part of such an assessment.

If a statistically significant positive association is believed to be causal, it may be relevant, for the purpose of contextualising the results and risk communication, to present further estimates of the burden of disease attributable to the exposure. Two such measures are the attributable fraction, or AF, and the population attributable fraction, or PAF. Although SCCS studies do not provide direct estimates of absolute effects, in certain circumstances an estimate of the absolute risk, or AR, may also be obtained indirectly using additional information.

In Section 8.5.1 we discuss measures of attribution, including the attributable fraction, population attributable fraction, attributable risk and number needed to harm, and when and how these can be obtained from a SCCS study. Sections 8.5.2 and 8.5.3 give examples of such calculations.

8.5.1 Attributable fraction and attributable risk

Suppose first that just one relative incidence ρ is involved, which might relate to unique or repeated exposures. We shall consider multiple relative incidences later. In the context of SCCS studies, the attributable fraction is the proportion of events arising within a risk period that may be attributed to the exposure. This is obtained as follows from the relative incidence ρ:

$$AF = \frac{\rho - 1}{\rho}. \tag{8.10}$$

It is estimated by substituting the RI estimate $\hat{\rho}$ for ρ in Expression 8.10. Since AF is a monotone function of ρ, a confidence interval for AF may be obtained by substituting the confidence limits for ρ in Expression 8.10. The description of the attributable fraction should always mention the risk period to which it relates. This also applies to other measures of attribution, to be described below.

In some circumstances, an estimate of the population attributable fraction PAF may also be obtained from a SCCS study. The PAF is the proportion of events arising in a defined population that are attributable to the exposure. Estimating the PAF from SCCS data requires one key condition to be fulfilled: the SCCS study must be based on a simple random sample or a census of all events arising in the population. If n denotes the total number of events in the SCCS study and n_1 denotes the number of events in risk periods, then

$$PAF = \frac{\rho - 1}{\rho} \times \frac{n_1}{n}. \tag{8.11}$$

This is estimated by substituting $\hat{\rho}$ for ρ in Expression 8.11.

In yet more restricted circumstances, a rough estimate of the attributable risk AR may be obtained from a SCCS study. This is the probability that an exposed individual from the population studied will experience an event caused by the exposure. Estimating the AR from a SCCS study requires two key conditions to be met. First, the SCCS study must include all events arising in exposed subjects (subjects with at least one exposure) within the population of interest; second, the number of exposed subjects within the relevant population must be known. Let E be this number. Then:

$$AR = \frac{\rho - 1}{\rho} \times \frac{n_1}{E}, \tag{8.12}$$

where n_1 is the total number of events arising within the risk period in this population. AR is estimated by substituting $\hat{\rho}$ for ρ in (8.12). Often, only a rough estimate of E is available, and hence only a rough estimate of AR can be obtained. Nevertheless, AR can still usefully convey the order of magnitude of the attributable risk. Sometimes the reciprocal of AR is more readily interpretable; this is called the number needed to harm, or NNH.

Suppose now that K distinct relative incidences $\rho_1, \ldots, \rho_K$ are found to be statistically significantly greater than 1, and that the corresponding associations are believed to be causal. For each k, ρ_k may relate to one or several risk periods at exposure level k. The different exposure levels k typically relate to distinct risk periods for the same exposure.

The attributable fraction AF_k is then calculated for each k, and applies specifically to risk periods at exposure level k:

$$AF_k = \frac{\rho_k - 1}{\rho_k}.$$

Let n_{1k} denote the number of events in risk periods at exposure level k. Then the population attributable fraction is:

$$PAR = \frac{1}{n} \sum_{k=1}^{K} \left(\frac{\rho_k - 1}{\rho_k} \right) \times n_{1k}.$$

The attributable risk is obtained as PAR with E in place of n:

$$AR = \frac{1}{E} \sum_{k=1}^{K} \left(\frac{\rho_k - 1}{\rho_k} \right) \times n_{1k}.$$

As before, estimates of AF_k, PAR and AR are obtained by substituting the estimated relative incidences $\hat{\rho}_k$ for ρ_k.

Obtaining confidence intervals for PAR and AR should take into account the fact that $\hat{\rho}$ and n_1 are correlated; one approach is to use bootstrapping. However, in view of the additional assumptions required, the values of PAR and AR obtained from a SCCS study are best thought of as providing rough orders of magnitude, especially if E is known only approximately.

8.5.2 Attributable risk: MMR and ITP

We derive measures of attribution for the study of ITP and MMR vaccine, using the results reported in Section 8.4.2. Using a 0–42 day risk period post-MMR, the relative incidence reported in Table 8.1 was found to be 3.23, with 95% CI $(1.53, 6.79)$.

This estimate is significantly greater than 1. Assuming that the association is causal, the attributable fraction for the 0–42 day risk period may then be obtained as follows:

$$AF = \frac{3.23 - 1}{3.23} = 0.690.$$

A 95% confidence interval for AR may be obtained by substituting the confidence limits 1.53 and 6.79 in the same expression, yielding 0.346 and 0.853. Thus the attributable fraction, expressed as a percentage, is 69.0%, with 95% CI $(34.6\%, 85.3\%)$. Of the 13 events in the 0–42 day risk period, about

$0.69 \times 13 = 9.0$ may reasonably be attributed to MMR vaccine, if the association is deemed to be causal.

The cases obtained in this SCCS study included all hospital admissions for ITP within two health regions, which arose in children aged between 1 and 2 years who could be matched to immunisation records. The number of MMR vaccine doses administered in the underlying cohort from which the cases in this SCCS study were drawn was estimated to be about 193 000 (Miller et al., 2001). Thus, a rough estimate of the attributable risk in the 0–42 day risk period may be obtained:

$$AR = \frac{3.23 - 1}{3.23} \times \frac{13}{193000} = 0.0000465.$$

A more readily interpretable measure is provided by number needed to harm, which is the reciprocal of AR:

$$NNH = \frac{1}{AR} = \frac{1}{0.0000465} = 21504.$$

Thus, the number needed to harm is about 21 500. In conclusion, the attributable risk for the 0–42 day post-vaccination risk period in this population is about 1 episode of ITP per 21 500 MMR doses. Such information on the order of magnitude of the attributable risk can usefully help to contextualise the relative incidence estimate.

8.5.3   Attributable risk: intussusception and rotavirus vaccine

In Chapter 7, Section 7.1.3 we presented jittered data on rotavirus vaccine and intussusception from the United Kingdom. The vaccine is administered in two doses, and the risk periods of interest comprised the intervals 1–7 days and 8–21 days after each dose.

The results obtained suggest elevated relative incidences of intussusception in the 1–7 day risk period after dose 1 and in the 8–21 day period after dose 2, the RIs being statistically non-significant in the other two risk periods. As it makes little sense to calculate measures of attribution for relative incidences that are not statistically significant, our first step is to re-run the analyses using a single combined 1–21 day risk period for each dose.

This is done as follows:

```
age <- seq(56,168,14)
rot.mod4 <- eventdepenexp(indiv=case, astart=sta, aend=end,
            aevent=intus, adrug=cbind(rv,rvd2),
            aedrug=cbind(rv+21,rvd2+21), sameexpopar=F,
            agegrp=age, dataformat="multi", data=rotdat)
```

This yields:

```
> rot.mod4
......
        exp(coef) exp(-coef) lower .95 upper .95
rv1       4.426      0.2259   2.4161     8.108
rv2       2.556      0.3913   1.4052     4.648
```

The relative incidences are statistically significantly elevated for both doses over the 1–21 day risk period. As recommended in Section 8.4.1, we next obtain the event counts in the two risk periods.

```
rot.dat1 <- formatdata(indiv=case, astart=sta, aend=end,
              aevent=intus, adrug=cbind(rv,rvd2),
              aedrug=cbind(rv+21,rvd2+21), sameexpopar=F,
              agegrp=age, dataformat="multi", data=rotdat)
```

We may then obtain the event counts by exposure level at each dose:

```
> tapply(rot.dat1$event, rot.dat1$rv, sum)
  0   1   2
527  20  19
```

Thus there are 20 events in the 1–21 day risk period after dose 1, and 19 after dose 2. There are 527 events outside the risk period. Of these, 471 arose in a historical cohort prior to the introduction of rotavirus vaccination, and 56 arose after the introduction of the vaccine (Stowe et al., 2016); the historical cases contribute to the estimation of the age effects, but not directly to the exposure effects. These data are collected in Table 8.3.

TABLE 8.3
Relative incidences (RI) for rotavirus vaccine and intussusception.

Exposure	No. events	RI	95% CI
Pre-vaccination cohort	471	1.00	-
Post-vaccination, unexposed	56	1.00	-
Dose 1, 1–21 day risk period	20	4.43	(2.42, 8.11)
Dose 2, 1–21 day risk period	19	2.56	(1.41, 4.65)

The attributable fractions for the 1–21 day risk periods may be calculated separately for each dose. For dose 1, it is $(4.43 - 1)/4.43 = 0.774$, with 95% CI $(0.587, 0.877)$, and for dose 2, $(2.56 - 1)/2.56 = 0.609$, with 95% CI $(0.291, 0.785)$.

The data were obtained using Hospital Episode Statistics for England. The $56 + 20 + 19 = 95$ cases ascertained after rotavirus vaccination was introduced include all intussusceptions in infants aged 42–183 days arising between the introduction of the rotavirus vaccination programme and 31st October 2014, which met the Brighton levels 1 and 2 criteria of diagnostic certainty. For these cases, it therefore makes sense to calculate the population attributable fraction for the 1–21 day risk periods:

$$PAR = \frac{1}{95} \times \left(\frac{4.43 - 1}{4.43} \times 20 + \frac{2.56 - 1}{2.56} \times 19 \right)$$
$$= 0.285.$$

Thus, about 28.5% of intussusceptions in the target population were attributable to rotavirus vaccine within a 1–21 day risk period after either dose.

However, the PAR depends on the level of vaccine coverage and other defining characteristics of the target population. More informative, perhaps, is the attributable risk, the order of magnitude of which may be calculated based on rough estimates of the numbers of vaccine doses administered within the target population during the period of the study. These were estimated in Stowe et al. (2016) as 827 000 first doses and 782 000 second doses. The attributable risks in the 1–21 day risk periods after the first and second vaccine doses are as follows:

$$AR_{\text{dose 1}} = \frac{20}{827000} \times \frac{4.43 - 1}{4.43} = 0.000019,$$
$$AR_{\text{dose 2}} = \frac{19}{782000} \times \frac{2.56 - 1}{2.56} = 0.000015.$$

Thus, the attributable risks for the 1–21 day risk periods are about 1.9 per 100 000 first doses and 1.5 per 100 000 second doses. These can alternatively be expressed in terms of numbers needed to harm as 1 intussusception per 53 000 first doses and 1 intussusception per 68 000 second doses. These orders of magnitude usefully complement the more precise estimates of relative incidences, and can help to inform public health policy.

Summary

- If an association is found to be statistically significant and is believed to be causal, then measures of attribution may be presented.

- The attributable fraction may be estimated directly from the relative incidence. If the events in the SCCS study are a random sample, or a census, of all events arising in the population of interest, then the population attributable fraction may also be estimated.

- If the SCCS study includes all events in exposed individuals within the population of interest, and the number of exposed individuals in that population is known, then an estimate of the attributable risk, or its order of magnitude, may be obtained.

8.6   Bibliographical notes and further material

We have emphasised the need to specify the risk period a priori, to avoid making data-dependent choices that would invalidate the inferences drawn using the methods we have described. Alternative methods of analysis, including some in which prior specification of the risk period is not required, are described in Hunsberger and Proschan (2017).

Sample size formulas for the SCCS method are discussed by Musonda et al. (2006). The saw-tooth relationship between power and sample size occurs more generally, see Chernick and Liu (2002). Sample size and power calculations for the SCCS model with exposure measurement error proposed by Mohammed et al. (2012) are provided in Mohammed et al. (2013a).

The efficiency of the SCCS design relative to cohort and case-control designs in the simple scenarios described in Section 8.3.1 is discussed in Farrington et al. (1996) and Whitaker et al. (2009). The more general results on efficiency and identifiability of the SCCS model in Section 8.3.4 are derived in Farrington and Whitaker (2006).

The self-controlled risk interval design is described in Baker et al. (2015). Generally, control periods are chosen so that age effects may be ignored; Li et al. (2015) discuss various adjustments when temporal effects need to be included. The efficiency and power of the self-controlled risk interval design compared to SCCS is discussed in Li et al. (2016). These authors derive results on asymptotic relative efficiency which are related to those of Section 8.3.2.

Measures of attribution, including attributable risks, were first used in connection with the SCCS method in Farrington et al. (1995).

A further issue relevant to SCCS studies, but not covered here, is the impact of misclassification of events. Low specificity of the case definition will bias the relative incidence towards 1. However, low specificity may increase the sensitivity of the case definition, and hence power. These trade-offs are discussed in Quantin et al. (2013). Misclassification of outcome events is also discussed in Xu et al. (2014), in the context of signal detection.

Bibliography

Aalen, O. O., Borgan, Ø., and Gjessing, H. K. (2008). *Survival and Event History Analysis*. New York: Springer.

Aalen, O. O., Borgan, Ø., Keiding, N., and Thormann, J. (1980). Interaction between life history events. Nonparametric analysis for prospective and retrospective data in the presence of censoring. *Scandinavian Journal of Statistics*, 7:161–171.

Andersen, E. B. (1970). Asymptotic properties of conditional maximum-likelihood estimators. *Journal of the Royal Statistical Society, Series B*, 32(2):283–301.

Andersen, P. K. (2006). Discussion of the paper "Semiparametric analysis of case series data". *Journal of the Royal Statistical Society, Series C*, 55(5):587–589.

Andrews, N., Miller, E., Waight, P., Farrington, P., Crowcroft, N., Stowe, J., and Taylor, B. (2001). Does oral polio vaccine cause intussusception in infants? Evidence from a sequence of three self-controlled case series studies in the United Kingdom. *European Journal of Epidemiology*, 17(8):701–706.

Andrews, N. J. (2002). Statistical assessment of the association between vaccination and rare adverse events post-licensure. *Vaccine*, 30:S49–S53.

Armstrong, B. G., Gasparrini, A., and Tobias, A. (2014). Conditional Poisson models: a flexible alternative to conditional logistic cross-over analysis. *BMC Medical Research Methodology*, 14:122.

Baker, M. A., Lieu, T. A., Li, L., Hua, W., Qiang, Y., Kawai, A. T., Fireman, B. H., Martin, D. B., and Nguyen, M. D. (2015). A vaccine study design selection framework for the Postlicensure Rapid Immunization Safety Monitoring program. *American Journal of Epidemiology*, 181(8):608–618.

Barlow, W. E., Davis, R. L., Glasser, J. W., Rhodes, P. H., Thompson, R. S., Mulooly, J. P., Black, S. B., Shinefield, H. R., Ward, J. I., Marcy, S. M., DeStefano, F., and Chen, R. T. (2001). The risk of seizures after receipt of whole-cell pertussis or measles, mumps and rubella vaccine. *New England Journal of Medicine*, 345(9):656–661.

Becker, N. G., Li, Z., and Kelman, C. W. (2004). The effect of transient exposures on the risk of an acute illness with low hazard rate. *Biostatistics*, 5(2):239–248.

Becker, N. G., Salim, A., and Kelman, C. W. (2006). Analysis of a potential trigger of an acute illness. *Biostatistics*, 7(1):16–28.

Brauer, R., Smeeth, L., Anaya-Izquierdo, K., Timmis, A., Denaxas, S., Farrington, C. P., Whitaker, H., Hemingway, H., and Douglas, I. (2015). Antipsychotic drugs and risks of myocardial infarction: a self-controlled case series study. *European Heart Journal*, 36(16):984–992.

Breslow, N. E. and Day, N. E. (1980). *Statistical Methods in Cancer Research*, volume I: The analysis of case-control studies. IARC Publications No. 32.

Chernick, M. R. and Liu, C. Y. (2002). The saw-toothed behaviour of power versus sample size and software solutions: Single binomial proportion using exact methods. *The American Statistician*, 56:149–155.

Cook, R. J. and Lawless, J. F. (2007). *The Statistical Analysis of Recurrent Events*. New York: Springer.

Cox, D. R. (1972). The statistical analysis of dependencies in point processes. In Lewis, P. A. W., editor, *Stochastic Point Processes: Statistical Analysis, Theory and Applications*, pages 55–66. New York: Wiley.

Cox, D. R. and Oakes, D. (1984). *Analysis of Survival Data*. London: Chapman and Hall.

Davison, A. C. and Hinkley, D. V. (1997). *Bootstrap Methods and their Application*. Cambridge: Cambridge University Press.

Douglas, I. J., Evans, S. J., Pocock, S., and Smeeth, L. (2009). The risk of fractures associated with thiazolidinediones: A self-controlled case-series study. *PLoS Medicine*, 6(9):e1000154.

Douglas, I. J. and Smeeth, L. (2008). Exposure to antipsychotics and risk of stroke: self-controlled case series study. *British Medical Journal*, 337(7670):616–618.

Dunn, P. M. (1997). James Lind (1716-94) of Edinburgh and the treatment of scurvy. *Archives of Disease in Childhood*, 76:F64–F65.

Escolano, S., Farrington, C. P., Hill, C., and Tubert-Bitter, P. (2011). Intussusception after rotavirus vaccination – Spontaneous reports. *New England Journal of Medicine*, 365(22):2139.

Escolano, S., Hill, C., and Tubert-Bitter, P. (2013). A new self-controlled case series method for analyzing spontaneous reports of adverse events after vaccination. *American Journal of Epidemiology*, 178(9):1496–1504.

Farrington, C. P. (1995). Relative incidence estimation from case series for vaccine safety evaluation. *Biometrics*, 51(1):228–235.

Farrington, C. P. (2004). Control without separate controls: evaluation of vaccine safety using case-only methods. *Vaccine*, 22:2064–2070.

Farrington, C. P., Anaya-Izquierdo, K., Whitaker, H. J., Hocine, M. N., Douglas, I., and Smeeth, L. (2011). Self-controlled case series analysis with event-dependent observation periods. *Journal of the American Statistical Association*, 106(494):417–426.

Farrington, C. P. and Hocine, M. N. (2010). Within-individual dependence in self-controlled case series models for recurrent events. *Journal of the Royal Statistical Society, Series C*, 59(3):457–475.

Farrington, C. P., Miller, E., and Taylor, B. (2001). MMR and autism: further evidence against a causal association. *Vaccine*, 19:3632–3635.

Farrington, C. P., Nash, J., and Miller, E. (1996). Case series analysis of adverse reactions to vaccines: A comparative evaluation. *American Journal of Epidemiology*, 143(11):1165–1173. Erratum 1998; *147*, 93.

Farrington, C. P. and Whitaker, H. J. (2006). Semiparametric analysis of case series data (with discussion). *Journal of the Royal Statistical Society, Series C*, 55(5):553–594.

Farrington, C. P., Whitaker, H. J., and Hocine, M. N. (2009). Case series analysis for censored, perturbed, or curtailed post-event exposures. *Biostatistics*, 10(1):3–16.

Farrington, P., Pugh, S., Colville, A., Flower, A., Nash, J., Morgan-Capner, P., Rush, M., and Miller, E. (1995). A new method for active surveillance of adverse events from diphtheria/tetanus/pertussis and measles/mumps/rubella vaccines. *Lancet*, 345(8949):567–569.

Feldmann, U. (1993a). Design and analysis of drug safety studies, with special reference to sporadic drug use and acute adverse reactions. *Journal of Clinical Epidemiology*, 46(3):237–244.

Feldmann, U. (1993b). Epidemiologic assessment of risks of adverse reactions associated with intermittent exposure. *Biometrics*, 49:419–428.

Fujinaga, T., Motegi, Y., Tamura, H., and Kuroume, T. (1991). A prefecture-wide survey of mumps meningitis associated with measles, mumps and rubella vaccine. *Pediatric Infectious Disease Journal*, 10:204–209.

Galeotti, F., Massari, M., D'Alessandro, R., Beghi, E., Chió, A., Logroscino, G., Filippini, G., Benedetti, M. D., Pugliatti, M., Santiccio, C., and Raschetti, R. (2013). Risk of Guillain–Barré syndrome after 2010-2011 influenza vaccination. *European Journal of Epidemiology*, 28(5):433–444.

Galindo-Sardiñas, M. A., Zambrano-Cárdenas, A., Coutin-Marie, G., Santin-Peña, M., Aliño-Santiago, M., Valcárcel-Sanchez, M., and Farrington, C. P. (2001). Lack of association between intussusception and oral polio vaccine in Cuban children. *European Journal of Epidemiology*, 17(8):783–787.

Gault, N., Castañeda-Sanabria, J., Rycke, Y. D., Guillo, S., Foulon, S., and Tubacj, F. (2017). Self-controlled designs in pharmacoepidemiology involving electronic healthcare databases: a systematic review. *BMC Medical Research Methodology*, 17:25.

Ghebremichael-Weldeselassie, Y., Farrington, C. P., and Whitaker, H. J. (2018). Use of the self-controlled case series method beyond vaccine safety: a review and discussion. *Open University Statistics Group Technical Report*, 18/02. Available from www.mathematics.open.ac.uk/research/statistics/technical-reports/2018.

Ghebremichael-Weldeselassie, Y., Whitaker, H. J., Douglas, I. J., Smeeth, L., and Farrington, C. P. (2017a). Self-controlled case series model with multiple event types. *Computational Statistics and Data Analysis*, 113:64–72.

Ghebremichael-Weldeselassie, Y., Whitaker, H. J., and Farrington, C. P. (2014). Self-controlled case series method with smooth age effect. *Statistics in Medicine*, 33:639–649.

Ghebremichael-Weldeselassie, Y., Whitaker, H. J., and Farrington, C. P. (2016). Flexible modelling of vaccine effect in self-controlled case series models. *Biometrical Journal*, 58(3):607–622.

Ghebremichael-Weldeselassie, Y., Whitaker, H. J., and Farrington, C. P. (2017b). Spline-based self-controlled case series model. *Statistics in Medicine*, 36:3022–3038.

Greenland, S. (1999). A unified approach to the analysis of case-distribution (case-only) studies. *Statistics in Medicine*, 18:1–15.

Hagen, K., Stovner, L. J., Vatten, L., Holmen, J., Zwart, J.-A., and Bovim, G. (2002). Blood pressure and risk of headache: A prospective study of 22 685 adults in Norway. *Journal of Neurology, Neurosurgery and Psychiatry*, 72:463–466.

Hausman, J., Hall, B. H., and Griliches, Z. (1984). Econometric models for count data with an application to the patents-R & D relationship. *Econometrica*, 52(4):909–938.

Hocine, M., Guillemot, D., Tubert-Bitter, P., and Moreau, T. (2005). Testing independence between two Poisson-generated multinomial variables in case-series and cohort studies. *Statistics in Medicine*, 24:4035–4044.

Hocine, M. N. and Chavance, M. (2010). La méthode de la série de cas. *Revue d'Epidémiologie et de Santé Publique*, 58(6):435–440.

Hocine, M. N., Musonda, P., Andrews, N. J., and Farrington, C. P. (2009). Sequential case series analysis for pharmacovigilance. *Journal of the Royal Statistical Society Series A*, 172(1):213–236.

Höfler, M. (2005). Causal inference based on counterfactuals. *BMC Medical Research Methodology*, 5:28.

Hua, W., Sun, G., Dodd, C. N., Romio, S. A., Whitaker, H. J., Izurieta, H. S., Black, S., Sturkenboom, M. C. J. M., Davis, R. L., Deceuninck, G., and Andrews, N. J. (2013). Simulation study to compare three self-controlled case series approaches: correction for violation of assumption and evaluation of bias. *Pharmacoepidemiology and Drug Safety*, 22:819–825.

Hubbard, R., Farrington, P., Smith, C., Smeeth, L., and Tattersfield, A. (2003). Exposure to tricyclic and selective serotonin reuptake inhibitor antidepressants and the risk of hip fracture. *American Journal of Epidemiology*, 158(1):77–84.

Hubbard, R., Lewis, S., Smith, C., Godfrey, C., Smeeth, L., Farrington, P., and Britton, J. (2005a). Use of nicotine replacement therapy and the risk of acute myocardial infarction, stroke and death. *Tobacco Control*, 14:416–421.

Hubbard, R., Lewis, S., West, J., Smith, C., Godfrey, C., Smeeth, L., Farrington, P., and Britton, J. (2005b). Bupropion and the risk of sudden death: a self-controlled case series analysis using The Health Improvement Network. *Thorax*, 60:848–850.

Hunsberger, S. and Proschan, M. A. (2017). Simple approaches to analysing self-controlled case series (SCCS) data. *Statistics in Biopharmaceutical Research*, 9(1):65–72.

Jensen, A. K. G., Gerds, T. A., Weeke, P., Torp-Pedersen, C., and Andersen, P. K. (2014). On the validity of the case-time-control design for autocorrelated exposure histories. *Epidemiology*, 25(1):110–113.

Jesus, J. and Chandler, R. E. (2011). Estimating functions and the generalized method of moments. *Interface Focus*, 1:871–885.

Joly, P., Commenges, D., and Letenneur, L. (1998). A penalized likelihood approach for arbitrarily censored and truncated data: Application to age-specific incidence of dementia. *Biometrics*, 54:185–194.

Kalbfleisch, J. D. and Prentice, R. L. (2002). *The Statistical Analysis of Failure Time Data*. New Jersey: Wiley. Second edition.

King, M., Lodwick, R., Jones, R., Whitaker, H., and Petersen, I. (2017). Death following partner bereavement: A self-controlled case series analysis. *PLOS One*, 12(3):e0173870.

Kramarz, P., F., D., Gargiullo, P. M., Davis, R. L., Chen, R. T., Mullooly, J. P., Black, S. B., Shinefield, H. R., Bohlke, K., Ward, J. I., and Marcy, M. S. (2000). Does influenza vaccination exacerbate asthma? *Archives of Family Medicine*, 9:617–623.

Kuhnert, R., Hecker, H., Poethko-Müller, C., Schlaud, M., Vennemann, M., Whitaker, H. J., and Farrington, C. P. (2011). A modified self-controlled case series method to examine association between multidose vaccinations and death. *Statistics in Medicine*, 30:666–677.

Kuhnert, R., Schlaud, M., Poethko-Müller, C., Vennemann, M., Fleming, P., Blair, P. S., Mitchell, E., Thompson, J., and Hecker, H. (2012). Reanalyses of case-control studies examining the temporal association between sudden infant death syndrome and vaccination. *Vaccine*, 30:2349–2356.

Lancaster, T. (2000). The incidental parameter problem since 1948. *Journal of Econometrics*, 95:391–413.

Lee, K. J. and Carlin, J. B. (2014). Fractional polynomial adjustment for time-varying covariates in a self-controlled case series analysis. *Statistics in Medicine*, 33:105–116.

Li, L., Kulldorff, M., Russek-Cohen, E., Kawai, A. T., and Hua, W. (2015). Quantifying the impact of time-varying baseline risk adjustment in the self-controlled risk interval design. *Pharmacoepidemiology and Drug Safety*, 24:1304–1312.

Li, R., Stewart, B., and Weintraub, E. (2016). Evaluating efficiency and statistical power of self-controlled case series and self-controlled risk interval designs in vaccine safety. *Journal of Biopharmaceutical Statistics*, 26(4):686–693.

Liu, B., Anderson, G., Mittman, N., To, T., Axcell, T., and Shear, N. (1998). Use of selective serotonin-reuptake inhibitors or tricyclic antidepressants and risk of hip fracture in elderly people. *Lancet*, 351:1303–1307.

Lumley, T. and Levy, D. (2000). Bias in the case-crossover design: Implications for studies of air pollution. *Environmetrics*, 11:689–704.

Maclure, M. (1991). The case-crossover design: A method for studying transient effects on the risk of acute events. *American Journal of Epidemiology*, 133(2):144–153.

Madsen, K. M., Hviid, A., Vestergaard, M., Schendel, D., Wohlfahrt, J., Thorsen, P., Olsen, J., and Melbye, M. (2002). A population-based study of measles, mumps, and rubella vaccinations and autism. *New England Journal of Medicine*, 347(19):1477–1482.

Manly, B. F. J. (1997). *Randomization, Bootstrap and Monte Carlo Methods in Biology*. London: Chapman & Hall. Second edition.

Mardia, K. V., Kent, J. T., and Bibby, J. M. (1979). *Multivariate Analysis*. London: Academic Press. Sixth printing, 1988.

Marshall, R. J. and Jackson, R. T. (1993). Analysis of case-crossover designs. *Statistics in Medicine*, 12:2333–2341.

McCullagh, P. and Nelder, J. A. (1989). *Generalized Linear Models*. London: Chapman & Hall. Second edition.

Miller, E., Goldacre, M., Pugh, S., Colville, A., Farrington, P., Flower, A., Nash, J., MacFarlane, L., and Tettmar, R. (1993). Risk of aseptic meningitis after measles, mumps and rubella vaccine in UK children. *Lancet*, 341(8851):979–982.

Miller, E., Waight, P., Farrington, P., Andrews, N., Stowe, J., and Taylor, B. (2001). Idiopathic thrombocytopenic purpura and MMR vaccine. *Archives of Disease in Childhood*, 84:227–229.

Mittleman, M. A., Maclure, M., and Robins, J. M. (1995). Control sampling techniques for case-crossover studies: An assessment of relative efficiency. *American Journal of Epidemiology*, 142(1):91–98.

Moghaddass, R., Rudin, C., and Madigan, D. (2016). The factorized self-controlled case series method: An approach for estimating the effects of many drugs on many outcomes. *Journal of Machine Learning Research*, 17:1–24.

Mohammed, A. M., Şentürk, D., Dalrymple, L. S., and Nguyen, D. V. (2012). Measurement error case series models with application to infection-cardiovascular risk in older patients on dialysis. *Journal of the Americal Statistical Association*, 107(500):1310–1323.

Mohammed, S. M., Dalrymple, L. S., Şentürk, D., and Nguyen, D. V. (2013a). Design considerations for case series models with exposure onset measurement error. *Statistics in Medicine*, 32:772–786.

Mohammed, S. M., Dalrymple, L. S., Şentürk, D., and Nguyen, D. V. (2013b). Naive hypothesis testing for case series analysis with time-varying exposure onset measurement error: Inference for infection-cardiovascular risk in patients on dialysis. *Biometrics*, 69:520–529.

Murphy, T. V., Gargiullo, P. ., Massoudi, M. S., Nelson, D. B., Jumaan, A. O., Okoro, C. A., Zanardi, L. R., Setia, S., Fair, E., LeBaron, C. W., Wharton, M., and Livingood, J. R. (2001). Intussusception among infants given an oral rotavirus vaccine. *New England Journal of Medicine*, 344(8):564–572.

Musonda, P., Farrington, C. P., and Whitaker, H. J. (2006). Sample sizes for self-controlled case series. *Statistics in Medicine*, 25:2618–2631. Erratum 2008; *27*, 4854-4855.

Musonda, P., Hocine, M. N., Andrews, N. J., Tubert-Bitter, P., and Farrington, C. P. (2008a). Monitoring vaccine safety using case series cumulative
sum charts. *Vaccine*, 26:5358–5367.

Musonda, P., Hocine, M. N., Whitaker, H. J., and Farrington, C. P. (2008b).
Self-controlled case series analyses: Small sample performance. *Computational Statistics and Data Analysis*, 52(4):1942–1957.

Navidi, W. (1998). Bidirectional case-crossover designs for exposures with
time trends. *Biometrics*, 54:596–605.

Nordmann, S., Biard, L., Ravaud, P., Esposito-Farèse, M., and Tubach, F.
(2012). Case-only designs in pharmacoepidemiology: A systematic review.
PLoS One, 7(11):e49444.

O'Sullivan, F. (1988). Fast computation of fully automated log-density and
log-hazard estimators. *SIAM Journal on Scientific and Statistical Computing*, 9(2):363–379.

Pan, J.-R., He, H.-Q., Yan, R., and Fu, J. (2013). Self-controlled case series (SCCS) method as a tool for the evaluation on the safety of vaccine.
Zhonghua Liu Xing Bing Xue Za Zhi, 34(8):836–839.

Petersen, I., Gilbert, R., Evans, S., Ridolfi, A., and Nazareth, I. (2010). Oral
antibiotic prescribing during pregnancy in primary care: UK population-
based study. *Journal of Antimicrobial Chemotherapy*, 65:2238–2246.

Prentice, R. L., Vollmer, W. M., and Kalbfleisch, J. D. (1984). On the use of
case series to identify disease risk factors. *Biometrics*, 40:445–458.

Quantin, C., Benzenine, E., Velten, M., Huet, F., Farrington, C. P., and
Tubert-Bitter, P. (2013). Self-controlled case series and misclassification
bias induced by case selection from administrative databases: Application
to febrile convulsions in pediatric vaccine pharmacoepidemiology. *American
Journal of Epidemiology*, 178(12):1731–1739.

R Core Team (2015). *R: A Language and Environment for Statistical Computing*. R Foundation for Statistical Computing, Vienna, Austria.

Ramsay, J. O. (1988). Monotone regression splines in action. *Statistical Science*, 3(4):425–441.

Rathouz, P. J. (2004). Fixed-effects models for longitudinal binary data with
dropouts missing at random. *Statistica Sinica*, 14:969–988.

Ray, W. A. and Griffin, M. R. (1989). Use of Medicaid data for pharmacoepidemiology. *American Journal of Epidemiology*, 129(4):837–849.

Rondeau, V. and Gonzalez, J. R. (2005). Frailtypack: A computer program
for the analysis of correlated failure time data using penalized likelihood
estimation. *Computer Methods and Programs in Biomedicine*, 80:154–164.

Roy, J., Alderson, D., Hogan, J. W., and Tashima, K. T. (2006). Conditional inference methods for incomplete Poisson data with endogenous time-varying covariates: Emergency Department use among HIV-infected women. *Journal of the American Statistical Association*, 101(474):424–434.

Scarborough, P., Peto, V., Bhatnagar, P., Kaur, A., Leal, J., Luengo-Fernandez, R., Gray, A., Rayner, M., and Allender, S. (2009). *Stroke Statistics 2009*. London: The British Heart Foundation and The Stroke Association.

Schuemie, M. J., Trifirò, G., Coloma, P. M., Ryan, P. B., and Madigan, D. (2016). Detecting adverse drug reactions following long-term drug exposure in longitudinal observational data: The exposure-adjusted self-controlled case series. *Statistical Methods in Medical Research*, 25(6):2577–2592.

Shaddox, T. R., Ryan, P. B., Schuemie, M. J., Madigan, D., and Suchard, M. A. (2016). Hierarchical models for multiple, rare outcomes using massive observational healthcare databases. *Statistical Analysis and Data Mining: The ASA Data Science Journal*, 9(4):260–268.

Simpson, S. E. (2013). A positive event dependence model for self-controlled case series with applications in postmarketing surveillance. *Biometrics*, 69(1):128–136.

Simpson, S. E., Madigan, D., Zorych, I., Schuemie, M. J., Ryan, P. B., and Suchard, M. A. (2013). Multiple self-controlled case series for large-scale longitudinal observational databases. *Biometrics*, 69(4):893–902.

Smeeth, L., Cook, C., Fombonne, E., Heavey, L., Rodrigues, L. C., Smith, P. G., and Hall, A. J. (2004a). MMR vaccination and pervasive developmental disorders: a case-control study. *Lancet*, 364:963–969.

Smeeth, L., Thomas, S. L., Hall, A. J., Hubbard, R., Farrington, P., and Vallance, P. (2004b). Risk of myocardial infarction and stroke after acute infection or vaccination. *New England Journal of Medicine*, 351:2611–2618.

Stowe, J., Andrews, N., Ladhani, S., and Miller, E. (2016). The risk of intussusception following monovalent rotavirus vaccination in England: A self-controlled case-series evaluation. *Vaccine*, 34:3684–3689.

Suissa, S. (1995). The case-time-control design. *Epidemiology*, 6(3):248–253.

Tata, L. J., Fortun, P. J., Hubbard, R. B., Smeeth, L., Hawkey, C. J., Smith, C. J. P., Whitaker, H. J., Farrington, C. P., Card, T. R., and West, J. (2005). Does concurrent prescription of selective serotonin reuptake inhibitors and non-steroidal anti-inflammatory drugs substantially increase the risk of upper gastrointestinal bleeding? *Alimentary Pharmacology and Therapeutics*, 22:175–181.

Taylor, B., Miller, E., Farrington, C. P., Petropoulos, M.-C., Favot-Mayaud, I., Li, J., and Waight, P. A. (1999). Autism and measles, mumps and rubella vaccine: no epidemiological evidence for a causal association. *Lancet*, 353:2026–2029.

Therneau, T. M. (2015). *A Package for Survival Analysis in S*. Version 2.38.

Turner, H. and Firth, D. (2015). *Generalized nonlinear models in R: An overview of the gnm package*. R package version 1.0-8.

Van der Vaart, A. W. and Wellner, J. A. (1996). *Weak Convergence and Empirical Processes*. New York: Springer.

Vines, S. K. and Farrington, C. P. (2001). Within-subject exposure dependency in case-crossover designs. *Statistics in Medicine*, 20:3039–3049.

von Kries, R., Toschke, A. M., Strassburger, K., Kundi, M., Kalies, H., Nennstiel, U., Jorch, G., Rosenbauer, J., and Giani, G. (2005). Sudden and unexpected deaths after the administration of hexavalent vaccines (diphtheria, tetanus, pertussis, poliomyelitis, hepatitis B, *Haemophilus inluenzae* type b). *European Journal of Pediatrics*, 164:61–69.

Weldeselassie, Y. G., Whitaker, H. J., and Farrington, C. P. (2011). Use of the self-controlled case-series method in vaccine safety studies: review and recommendations for best practice. *Epidemiology and Infection*, 139(12):1805–1817.

Whitaker, H. J., Farrington, C. P., Spiessens, B., and Musonda, P. (2006). Tutorial in biostatistics: The self-controlled case series method. *Statistics in Medicine*, 25:1768–1797.

Whitaker, H. J., Ghebremichael-Weldeselassie, Y., Douglas, I. J., Smeeth, L., and Farrington, C. P. (2018a). Investigating the assumptions of the self-controlled case series method. *Statistics in Medicine*, 37(4):643–658.

Whitaker, H. J., Hocine, M. N., and Farrington, C. P. (2007). On case-crossover methods for environmental time series data. *Environmetrics*, 18(2):157–171.

Whitaker, H. J., Hocine, M. N., and Farrington, C. P. (2009). The methodology of self-controlled case series studies. *Statistical Methods for Medical Research*, 18(1):7–26.

Whitaker, H. J., Steer, C. D., and Farrington, C. P. (2018b). Self-controlled case series studies: just how rare does a rare non-recurrent outcome need to be? *Open University Statistics Group Technical Report*, 18/01. Available from www.mathematics.open.ac.uk/research/statistics/technical-reports/2018.

Xu, S., Hambidge, S. J., McClure, D., Daley, M. F., and Glanz, J. M. (2013). A scan statistic for identifying optimal risk windows in vaccine safety studies using self-controlled case series design. *Statistics in Medicine*, 32(19):3290–3299.

Xu, S., Newcomer, S., Nelson, J., Qian, L., McClure, D., Pan, Y., Zeng, C., and Glanz, J. (2014). Signal detection of adverse events with imperfect confirmation rates in vaccine safety studies using self-controlled case series design. *Biometrical Journal*, 56(3):513–525.

Xu, S., Zhang, L., Nelson, J. C., Zeng, C., Mullooly, J., McClure, D., and Glanz, J. (2011). Identifying optimal risk windows for self-controlled case series studies of vaccine efficacy. *Statistics in Medicine*, 30(7):742–752.

Zeng, C., Newcomer, S. R., Glanz, J. M., Stroup, J. A., Daley, M. F., Hambidge, S. J., and Xu, S. (2013). Bias correction or risk estimates in vaccine safety studies with rare adverse events using a self-controlled case series design. *American Journal of Epidemiology*, 178(12):1750 1759.

Index

adrug, 53
aedrug, 53
aend, 51
aevent, 51
agegrp, 53
alpha, 299
astart, 51
censor, 257
covariates, 264
dataformat, 59
data, 53
dob, 97
eage, 304
eexpo, 299
eventdepenexp, 231
eventdepenobs, 256
expogrp, 53
formatdata, 55, 329, 330
indiv, 51
lrtsccs, 75
multi, 59
nonparasccs, 184
power, 299
p, 299
quantsccs, 209
regress, 275
risk, 299
sameexpopar, 64
samplesize, 298
seasongrp, 97
semiscccs, 160
simulatesccsdata, 298
smoothagesccs, 169
smoothexposccs, 184
stack, 59
standardsccs, 51
verbose, 252

washout, 58

absolute risk, 335
absorption, 50, 215
administrative database, 3, 40
age group, 23, 50, 100, 143, 147, 157,
    181, 183, 285, 292
AIC, 274
air pollution, 215
antibiotic, 294
antibiotic resistance, 223
antidepressant, 57, 68, 81, 134, 173,
    293, 294, 331
antidiabetic, 84, 187, 201
antipsychotic, 105, 119, 262
aseptic meningitis, 7, 27, 33, 150, 292
asthma, 17, 215
asymptotic, 54, 149–154, 164, 166,
    201, 214, 298, 302, 309, 318,
    325, 327–329
asymptotic efficiency, 285, 314, 325,
    328
asymptotic theory, 159, 166
attributable fraction, 285, 335
attributable risk, 285, 336
autism, 5, 14, 87, 162, 176, 185, 323
autocorrelation, 214

Bartlett identity, 180
Bayes' Theorem, 40
Bayesian framework, 223
beta density, 306
bias
    asymptotic, 106, 318
    correction, 154, 284
    direction, 38, 39, 84, 115, 127,
        226, 318

non-ignorable, 115
of estimator, 107, 115, 117, 121,
    126, 127, 157, 226
relative, 104–107
small-sample, 154, 319
birth process, 284
blood pressure, 209
bootstrap, 337
Bupropion, 277

calendar time, 22, 51, 52, 92, 93, 101,
    116, 159, 286
car accident, 226
cardiovascular disease, 3, 322
case, 21, 24, 26, 34, 42
case series, 9, 20, 26, 104, 108
case-control, 2, 8, 19, 21, 40, 46, 50,
    51, 285, 316, 317
case-crossover
    bidirectional, 46, 212
    design, 223
    method, 2, 46
    time-stratified, 46, 212, 213
case-time-control, 46
causal pathway, 254
censoring, 108, 115, 116, 120, 125,
    126, 253–255, 270, 272, 273,
    275
centred plot
    event, 128–130, 134, 137,
        143–145, 197, 334
    observation, 128, 130, 137,
        143–145, 197, 334
chi-squared
    distribution, 75, 149, 150, 214,
        239
    test, 237, 239
chronic condition, 60
cohort, 3, 8, 19, 21, 24, 26, 33, 40,
    41, 44–46, 108, 285
conditional logistic regression, 50
confidence band, 110, 183–185, 193,
    194
confounding, 2, 9, 11, 16, 26, 84, 89,

115, 176, 177, 212, 214, 218,
    323, 328
constraint, 168, 181, 182, 194
continuity correction, 303
contra-indication, 127, 226, 227
controlled trial, 1, 298
convulsion, 13, 62, 66, 70, 73, 105,
    111, 144, 147, 197, 290
counterfactual, 226, 229, 230,
    244–248
covariate
    exogenous, 127
    external, 127
    multiplicative, 26, 36, 77
    time-invariant, 3, 10, 11, 22, 26,
        32, 36, 48, 49, 51, 77, 78,
        100, 101, 158, 167, 196, 256,
        270, 286
    time-varying, 142
coverage probability, 309, 310
cross-validation, 169, 170, 179, 183,
    184, 194
cumulative
    hazard, 106, 108–110, 112, 114
    incidence, 29, 34, 35
    intensity, 32
    relative age effect, 158, 159, 161,
        163, 164, 334

data-driven, 143, 146, 155
date of birth, 93, 97
death, 206, 225, 254, 275, 277, 280,
    282
degrees of freedom, 75, 149, 150, 166,
    181, 214, 239
dementia, 119
dependence, 154, 197, 205
design
    study, 285, 292, 301
    value, 298, 299
developmental disorder, 19
dose, 59, 60, 70, 73

effect
    additive, 148

age, 25, 47, 48, 78, 84, 100, 101,
   106, 115, 143, 157, 159, 166,
   167, 181, 184, 193, 194, 207,
   212, 222
dose, 60, 64, 65, 72
exposure, 25, 47, 49, 78, 84, 100,
   101, 143, 157, 163, 167, 179,
   181–184, 193, 194, 207, 208,
   212, 218, 223
homogeneous, 143, 147
main, 26, 48, 77
modifier, 77, 78, 161
multiplicative, 143, 148
relative age, 158, 181, 183
seasonal, 49, 92, 95, 97, 101,
   103, 218
temporal, 159, 208, 324
time-invariant, 48, 213
efficiency, 16, 20, 84, 166, 167, 223,
   275, 313, 318, 325
empirical process theory, 166
environmental epidemiology, 46, 212
epidemiology, 1, 5, 7, 9, 19, 40, 45, 47
episode, 107, 109, 114
estimability, 322
estimating equation, 225–229, 243,
   245, 249, 251
estimating function
   elementary, 227, 245, 247, 250,
      251
   unbiased, 227, 245–247, 249, 251
event
   clustered, 107, 109, 114
   competing, 206
   count, 108, 208, 285, 329
   first, 108, 115, 254
   incidental, 197, 206, 207
   multi-type, 195, 203
   non-recurrent, 21, 25, 39, 44,
      205, 225, 248, 254
   order, 108, 109
   rare, 25, 36, 45, 46, 104, 107,
      108, 142, 205, 206, 225, 271
   recurrent, 21, 26, 44, 107, 108,
      115, 140, 195, 197, 203, 205

event-dependence
   duration, 129
   long-term, 128, 137
   of exposure, 38, 104, 127–130,
      134, 137, 140, 225, 276
   of observation period, 38, 104,
      114–116, 120, 126, 225,
      253–255, 276
   short-term, 127, 129, 140
exchangeability, 46
exponential density, 274
exposure
   binary, 207, 212
   discrete, 48, 157
   environmental, 157, 323
   event-dependent, 38, 104,
      127–130, 134, 137, 140, 225,
      276
   exogenous, 38, 212
   external, 38
   history, 270
   homogeneity, 143
   individual, 214
   level, 23, 33, 101
   multi-type, 157
   multiple, 134
   population, 212, 214
   quantitative, 13, 48, 157, 207,
      212
   repeated, 59, 60, 65, 120
   terminal, 115
   time-invariant, 322
   timimg, 100
   transient, 20, 322
   type, 59, 65, 66, 68, 72, 101, 161

follow-up, 108
fractional polynomial, 223
fracture, 84, 187, 201
frailty, 205
full model, 75–77

gamma density, 274
gap time, 108, 109
gastro-intestinal bleed, 60, 68, 81,
   134, 294, 331

generalised linear model, 50, 212–214
goodness of fit, 214, 220
graphical display, 47, 333
Guillain–Barré syndrome, 93, 137,
      232, 290

hazard, 21, 36, 37, 39, 44, 46, 47,
      106, 125, 126, 205–207, 270
headache, 209
Hessian, 180, 181, 183, 194, 252, 280
high-dimensional, 50, 159
hip fracture, 16, 57, 173, 290, 293
history
    event, 39, 107, 125, 126, 140,
      141, 270, 284
    exposure, 20, 22, 23, 27, 38–41,
      48, 84, 100, 101, 125, 127,
      140, 141, 149, 152, 182, 183,
      206, 227–229, 254, 255, 270,
      284
    exposure and observation, 22,
      27, 32, 34, 35, 37, 38, 41,
      43, 203
    observation, 39, 255
hospital admission, 26, 37, 51, 107
hypothesis
    generating, 143, 155
    null, 74–76, 115, 126, 129, 166,
      214, 298
    test, 74, 115, 182, 284, 302

identifiability, 275, 285, 313,
      322–325, 328
incidence, 22, 45, 47–49, 103, 143,
      159, 203
independence, 27, 37, 40, 203, 205
infection, 240, 259
intensity, 21, 22, 26, 32, 36, 43, 44,
      47, 107, 115, 127, 140, 255
interaction, 26, 48, 49, 77, 78, 81,
      101, 103, 108, 116, 125, 126,
      143, 147, 161, 196, 199
intermittent treatment, 60
interval
    age, 23, 33, 100, 101
    notation, 32

risk, 48
intussusception, 38, 95, 224, 226,
      233, 236, 338
ITP, 51, 75, 78, 109, 130, 151, 160,
      170, 329, 337

Jacobian, 251
jitter, 5

kernel, 48, 50, 158, 159, 165, 167,
      182, 183, 196, 208, 212, 272
knot, 167, 168, 170, 179, 181

leave-one-out estimator, 180
likelihood
    asymptotic theory, 103, 149, 159
    binomial, 106
    cohort, 22, 34, 35, 42–44, 204,
      205, 271, 325, 327
    conditional, 10, 27, 38, 43–45,
      142, 204, 205, 271, 313
    contribution, 24, 193–195, 204,
      206, 208, 213
    log, 25, 31, 168, 180, 181
    marginal, 34, 35, 43, 44
    maximum, 22, 32, 46, 48, 75,
      106, 149, 158, 163, 164, 194,
      227, 266, 273, 275, 309, 314,
      318, 327
    multimodal, 266
    multinomial, 24, 33, 75, 77
    partial, 51
    penalised, 168, 179–181, 183,
      184, 194
    Poisson, 213
    profile, 133, 166
    pseudo-Poisson, 252
    ratio test, 74–77, 108, 115, 116,
      129, 143, 149–151, 153, 161,
      197, 200, 201
    SCCS, 21, 22, 29, 31, 34, 35,
      43–45, 48, 164, 168, 179,
      183, 184, 194, 207, 213, 314,
      325, 327
    SCCS, general, 32, 41, 45, 125,
      142, 157

SCCS, modified, 125, 254, 256, 269
SCCS, multi-type, 195, 196, 203–205, 207
SCCS, semiparametric, 159, 165
SCCS, standard, 25, 127, 208, 245, 247
SCCS, type-specific, 205
score, 227, 245–248
surface, 31

mean squared error, 318, 321
measurement error, 284
misclassification, 154
missing value, 65
mixture
    model, 266, 273–275
    probability, 274
model formula, 49, 53, 63, 67, 76–78, 93, 116, 160, 196
Monte Carlo standard error, 149, 151, 153, 302
mortality, 18, 115, 120, 253, 255
multinomial
    category, 47, 75, 76, 201
    distribution, 24, 50
    likelihood, 24
    probability, 24
    product, 25, 50, 159, 163, 165, 213
mumps meningitis, 7
myocardial infarction, 18, 19, 37, 90, 107, 117, 240, 257, 259, 323

negative binomial, 37
Nelson–Aalen estimator, 108, 110, 112
nested model, 75, 76, 146
Newton–Raphson, 180
nicotine replacement therapy, 90, 117, 257, 323
nonparametric, 158
notional cohort, 26
NSAID, 60, 68, 81, 134, 294, 331
null distribution, 149–151, 153

number needed to harm, 335, 336
number under observation, 129, 131, 137

observation period
    actual, 116, 117, 119, 254, 271, 276
    censoring, 115, 116, 119, 121, 125, 126, 253, 254, 275
    choice, 285, 289
    conditioning, 38, 115
    definition, 12, 22, 34, 39, 41, 116
    disjoint, 292
    event-dependent, 38, 114–117, 119, 120, 122, 124, 126, 225, 253, 255
    notation, 32
    planned, 117, 119
    plot, 57, 61, 333
    short, 90, 92
opioid analgesic, 226
outlier, 222
output, 53–55
overdispersion, 214, 217, 222
overlap, 73, 74, 135, 136

parameter
    common, 64, 72
    dispersion, 37, 214, 218, 220, 222
    dose-specific, 64, 72, 73
    estimate, 22, 32, 53, 115, 129, 159
    finite-dimensional, 166
    free, 93, 227
    high-dimensional, 166
    identifiability, 266, 275, 314
    incidental, 45, 50, 213, 214
    infinite-dimensional, 166
    initial value, 254, 256, 258, 266, 275
    not estimable, 248
    seasonal, 98
    smoothing, 169, 170, 179, 181, 183, 184, 193, 194
    space, 132, 201

parameterisation, 25, 30, 47, 49, 60, 73, 78, 79, 81, 82, 98, 100, 159, 208, 325
partner bereavement, 282
Pearson
    chi-square, 214
    residual, 214
penalty, 169, 180
permutation test, 149–152
person-time, 285, 329
pharmaceutical drug, 18, 48, 101
pharmacodynamics, 287
pharmacoepidemiology, 5, 23, 38, 207, 223, 226, 254, 286
point event, 140
point exposure, 48, 57, 128
Poisson
    assumption, 25, 36, 104, 107, 114, 151, 214, 218
    conditional, 45, 50, 212
    count, 45
    distribution, 214
    model, 157, 213–215, 313, 314
    probability, 35
    process, 22, 42, 44, 45, 103, 107, 108, 140, 195, 203, 205, 284
    pseudo, 251, 252
    trick, 50, 213
population attributable fraction, 285, 335
positive dependence, 154, 284
power, 119, 122, 285, 298, 301, 306, 308
precision, 176
pregnancy, 294
proportional hazards model, 51
proportional incidence model, 47, 143, 286

R package, 5, 51
random effect, 26
random sample, 336
rank, 165
reduced model, 75–77

reference level, 23, 49, 97, 98, 100, 101, 158, 168
relative incidence
    age-dependent, 92
    age-related, 92
    age-specific, 55, 86
    average, 55
    bias, 39, 84, 104–107, 115, 116, 126, 127, 154
    calendar time, 93
    confidence interval, 54
    estimator, 46, 107
    function, 93, 101, 182–184, 193, 194
    interpretation, 3, 21, 49, 322
    parameter, 10, 49, 73, 100, 101, 129
    time-dependent, 86, 88
residual, 214, 220, 222
respiratory syncytial virus, 218
respiratory tract infection, 240
risk
    absolute, 335
    communication, 334, 335
    competing, 195, 197, 205, 206
    gradient, 322, 323
    level, 23
risk period
    actual, 182
    choice, 143, 155, 285, 287
    combined, 55, 75, 149, 153, 154
    common, 106
    contiguous, 53, 169
    definition, 23, 27, 34, 57, 68, 106
    dose-related, 64
    extremal, 83, 84, 90
    indefinite, 83, 84, 87, 162, 182
    initial, 90
    long, 83, 87
    measurement error, 154
    multiple, 168
    nominal, 182
    overlap, 60, 73, 135, 136
    plot, 61
    pre-exposure, 129, 131–133, 135,

136, 138, 140, 142, 146, 147, 226
  short, 83, 87
  terminal, 115, 118, 124, 125
robustness, 114, 116, 129, 134, 137, 154

sample size, 285, 298, 299, 304
sampling, 19, 40, 103, 108
sampling distribution, 309, 310
sandwich estimator, 251
SCCS model
  assumption, 18, 19, 27, 33, 36, 43, 103, 127, 143, 225
  conditioning, 38
  extension, 4, 12, 104, 117, 128, 154, 225, 253, 254, 272
  factorised, 223
  for quantitative exposures, 207, 208
  fractional polynomial, 223
  framework, 214, 215
  genesis, 7
  likelihood, 29, 31, 33, 41, 43
  measurement error, 284
  multi-type, 157, 196, 197, 199
  multiple, 223
  nonparametric, 183, 184, 194, 223
  parameterisation, 25
  positive dependence, 284
  properties, 26
  R package, 51
  semiparametric, 157–160, 162, 163, 165–167, 222, 324
  sequential, 223
  spline-based, 157, 166, 167, 179, 181, 184, 193, 194, 222
  standard, 20–22, 37, 45, 47, 50, 51, 53, 93, 100, 103, 116, 140, 143, 157, 159, 160, 162, 163, 167, 168, 183, 196, 208, 223, 256, 325
season group, 93, 97, 99, 100
seasonality, 11, 96–98, 100, 286

self-control, 2, 26, 45, 46
self-controlled risk interval, 92, 295
sensitivity, 19, 104, 107–109, 115, 126, 140, 146, 154, 335
shrinkage, 223
significance level, 298
simulation, 285
smoothness, 166, 168, 183, 184
sparseness, 143, 149, 154, 214
spline
  basis, 167, 168, 179, 182, 184, 193
  cubic, 167
  function, 157, 167, 168, 181–183
  I-spline, 168, 179, 193
  integrated, 167
  M-spline, 167, 168, 179, 181–183, 193
spontaneous reporting, 40
standard error, 53, 159, 176, 217, 239
stratification, 10, 77, 78
stroke, 18, 38, 105, 119, 254, 255, 262
sudden death, 277
sudden infant death syndrome, 280
survivor function, 125

target population, 299
temperature, 218
thinning effect, 255
time
  line, 10, 11, 22, 94, 95, 157, 160, 285, 286
  series, 213, 215
  trend, 159, 286
  unit, 286
treatment duration, 57
turning point, 166
two-stage model, 254, 256

uncertainty, 104

vaccine
  DTP, 62, 70, 73
  hexavalent, 280
  Hib, 66, 70
  influenza, 93, 137, 232

MMR, 5, 7, 27, 33, 51, 66, 75,
        78, 87, 105, 109, 111, 130,
        144, 147, 150, 151, 160, 162,
        170, 176, 185, 197, 290, 292,
        299, 301, 323, 329, 337, 338
    oral polio, 95, 236
    rotavirus, 38, 226, 233
    routine childhood, 127
    safety, 39, 224
    with thiomersal, 19

washout period, 48, 57, 58, 169, 173
Weibull density, 274
weighting, 255, 256, 272, 274

Printed in the United States
by Baker & Taylor Publisher Services

Printed in the United States
by Baker & Taylor Publisher Services